上海市重点图书

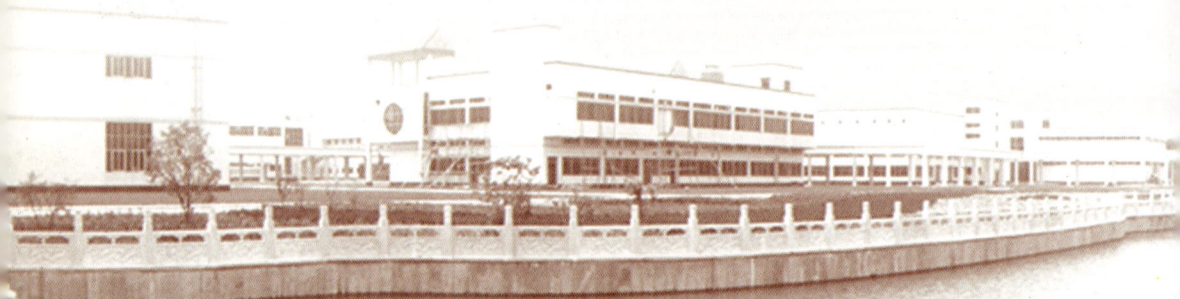

Full View of Yangtze River Pharmaceuticals Group（Taizhou,Jiangsu,China）
扬子江药业集团全景（中国·江苏·泰州）

Compilation Board of the Library

Translation Committee of the Library

Approval Committee of the Library

Foreword I

As we are walking into the 21st century, "health for all" is still an important task for the World Health Organization (WHO) to accomplish in the new century. The realization of "health for all" requires mutual cooperation and concerted efforts of various medical sciences, including traditional medicine. WHO has increasingly emphasized the development of traditional medicine and has made fruitful efforts to promote its development. Currently the spectrum of diseases is changing and an increasing number of diseases are difficult to cure. The side effects of chemical drugs have become more and more evident. Furthermore, both the governments and peoples in all countries are faced with the problem of high cost of medical treatment. Traditional Chinese medicine (TCM), the complete system of traditional medicine in the world with unique theory and excellent clinical curative effects, basically meets the need to solve such problems. Therefore, bringing TCM into full play in medical treatment and healthcare will certainly become one of the hot points in the world medical business in the 21st century.

Various aspects of work need to be done to promote the course of the internationalization of TCM, especially the compilation of works and textbooks suitable for international readers. The impending new century has witnessed the compilation of such a

序 一

人类即将迈入 21 世纪,"人人享有卫生保健"仍然是新世纪世界卫生工作面临的重要任务。实现"人人享有卫生保健"的宏伟目标,需要包括传统医药学在内的多种医学学科的相互协作与共同努力。世界卫生组织越来越重视传统医药学的发展,并为推动其发展做出了卓有成效的工作。目前,疾病谱正在发生变化,难治疾病不断增多,化学药品的毒副作用日益显现,日趋沉重的医疗费用困扰着各国政府和民众。中医药学是世界传统医学体系中最完整的传统医学,其独到的学科理论和突出的临床疗效,较符合当代社会和人们解决上述难题的需要。因此,科学有效地发挥中医药学的医疗保健作用,必将成为 21 世纪世界卫生工作的特点之一。

加快中医药走向世界的步伐,还有很多的工作要做,特别是适合国外读者学习的中医药著作、教材的编写是极其重要的方面。在新千年来临之际,由南京中医药大学

series of books known as *A Newly Compiled Practical English-Chinese Library of Traditional Chinese Medicine* published by the Publishing House of Shanghai University of TCM, compiled by Nanjing University of TCM and translated by Shanghai University of TCM. Professor Zuo Yanfu, the general compiler-in-chief of this Library, is a person who sets his mind on the international dissemination of TCM. He has compiled *General Survey on TCM Abroad*, a monograph on the development and state of TCM abroad. This Library is another important works written by the experts organized by him with the support of Nanjing University of TCM and Shanghai University of TCM. The compilation of this Library is done with consummate ingenuity and according to the development of TCM abroad. The compilers, based on the premise of preserving the genuineness and gist of TCM, have tried to make the contents concise, practical and easy to understand, making great efforts to introduce the abstruse ideas of TCM in a scientific and simple way as well as expounding the prevention and treatment of diseases which are commonly encountered abroad and can be effectively treated by TCM.

This Library encompasses a systematic summarization of the teaching experience accumulated in Nanjing University of TCM and Shanghai University of TCM that run the collaborating centers of traditional medicine and the international training centers on acupuncture and moxibustion set by WHO. I am sure that the publication of this Library will further promote the development of traditional Chinese med-

主编、上海中医药大学主译、上海中医药大学出版社出版的《〈英汉对照〉新编实用中医文库》的即将问世,正是新世纪中医药国际传播更快发展的预示。本套文库总主编左言富教授是中医药学国际传播事业的有心人,曾主编研究国外中医药发展状况的专著《国外中医药概览》。本套文库的编撰,是他在南京中医药大学和上海中医药大学支持下,组织许多著名专家共同完成的又一重要专著。本套文库的作者们深谙国外的中医药发展现状,编写颇具匠心,在注重真实、不失精华的前提下,突出内容的简明、实用,易于掌握,力求科学而又通俗地介绍中医药学的深奥内容,重点阐述国外常见而中医药颇具疗效的疾病的防治。

本套文库蕴含了南京中医药大学和上海中医药大学作为 WHO 传统医学合作中心、国际针灸培训中心多年留学生教学的实践经验和系统总结,更为全面、系统、准确地向世界传播中医药学。相信本书的出版将对中医更好地走向世界,让世界更好地了解中医产生更

icine abroad and enable the whole world to have a better understanding of traditional Chinese medicine.

为积极的影响。

Professor Zhu Qingsheng

Vice-Minister of Health Ministry of the People's Republic of China

Director of the State Administrative Bureau of TCM

December 14, 2000 Beijing

朱庆生教授

中华人民共和国卫生部副部长

国家中医药管理局局长

2000年12月14日于北京

Foreword II

Before the existence of the modern medicine, human beings depended solely on herbal medicines and other therapeutic methods to treat diseases and preserve health. Such a practice gave rise to the establishment of various kinds of traditional medicine with unique theory and practice, such as traditional Chinese medicine, Indian medicine and Arabian medicine, etc. Among these traditional systems of medicine, traditional Chinese medicine is a most extraordinary one based on which traditional Korean medicine and Japanese medicine have evolved.

Even in the 21st century, traditional medicine is still of great vitality. In spite of the fast development of modern medicine, traditional medicine is still disseminated far and wide. In many developing countries, most of the people in the rural areas still depend on traditional medicine and traditional medical practitioners to meet the need for primary healthcare. Even in the countries with advanced modern medicine, more and more people have begun to accept traditional medicine and other therapeutic methods, such as homeopathy, osteopathy and naturopathy, etc.

With the change of the economy, culture and living style in various regions as well as the aging in the world population, the disease spectrum has changed. And such a change has paved the way for the new application of traditional medicine. Besides,

序　二

在现代医学形成之前,人类一直依赖草药和其他一些疗法治病强身,从而发展出许多有理论、有实践的传统医学,例如中医学、印度医学、阿拉伯医学等。中医学是世界林林总总的传统医学中的一支奇葩,在它的基础上还衍生出朝鲜传统医学和日本汉方医学。在跨入 21 世纪的今天,古老的传统医学依然焕发着活力,非但没有因现代医学的发展而式微,其影响还有增无减,人们对传统医学的价值也有了更深刻的体会和认识。在许多贫穷国家,大多数农村人口仍然依赖传统医学疗法和传统医务工作者来满足他们对初级卫生保健的需求。在现代医学占主导地位的许多国家,传统医学及其他一些"另类疗法",诸如顺势疗法、整骨疗法、自然疗法等,也越来越被人们所接受。

伴随着世界各地经济、文化和生活的变革以及世界人口的老龄化,世界疾病谱也发生了变化。传统医学有了新的应用,而新疾病所引起的新需求以及现代医学的成

the new requirements initiated by the new diseases and the achievements and limitations of modern medicine have also created challenges for traditional medicine.

WHO sensed the importance of traditional medicine to human health early in the 1970s and have made great efforts to develop traditional medicine. At the 29th world health congress held in 1976, the item of traditional medicine was adopted in the working plan of WHO. In the following world health congresses, a series of resolutions were passed to demand the member countries to develop, utilize and study traditional medicine according to their specific conditions so as to reduce medical expenses for the realization of "health for all".

WHO has laid great stress on the scientific content, safe and effective application of traditional medicine. It has published and distributed a series of booklets on the scientific, safe and effective use of herbs and acupuncture and moxibustion. It has also made great contributions to the international standardization of traditional medical terms. The safe and effective application of traditional medicine has much to do with the skills of traditional medical practitioners. That is why WHO has made great efforts to train them. WHO has run 27 collaborating centers in the world which have made great contributions to the training of acupuncturists and traditional medical practitioners. Nanjing University of TCM and Shanghai University of TCM run the collaborating centers with WHO. In recent years it has, with the cooperation of WHO and other countries, trained about ten thousand international students from over

就与局限又向传统医学提出了挑战,推动它进一步发展。世界卫生组织早在20世纪70年代就意识到传统医学对人类健康的重要性,并为推动传统医学的发展做了努力。1976年举行的第二十九届世界卫生大会将传统医学项目纳入世界卫生组织的工作计划。其后的各届世界卫生大会又通过了一系列决议,要求各成员国根据本国的条件发展、使用和研究传统医学,以降低医疗费用,促进"人人享有初级卫生保健"这一目标的实现。

世界卫生组织历来重视传统医学的科学、安全和有效使用。它出版和发行了一系列有关科学、安全、有效使用草药和针灸的技术指南,并在专用术语的标准化方面做了许多工作。传统医学的使用是否做到安全和有效,是与使用传统疗法的医务工作者的水平密不可分的。因此,世界卫生组织也十分重视传统医学培训工作。它在全世界有27个传统医学合作中心,这些中心对培训合格的针灸师及使用传统疗法的其他医务工作者做出了积极的贡献。南京中医药大学、上海中医药大学是世界卫生组织传统医学合作中心之一,近年来与世界卫生组织和其他国家合作,培训了近万名来自90多个国

90 countries.

In order to further promote the dissemination of traditional Chinese medicine in the world, *A Newly Compiled Practical English-Chinese Library of Traditional Chinese Medicine*, compiled by Nanjing University of TCM with Professor Zuo Yanfu as the general compiler-in-chief and published by the Publishing House of Shanghai University of TCM, aims at systematic, accurate and concise expounding of traditional Chinese medical theory and introducing clinical therapeutic methods of traditional medicine according to modern medical nomenclature of diseases. Undoubtedly, this series of books will be the practical textbooks for the beginners with certain English level and the international enthusiasts with certain level of Chinese to study traditional Chinese medicine. Besides, this series of books can also serve as reference books for WHO to internationally standardize the nomenclature of acupuncture and moxibustion.

The scientific, safe and effective use of traditional medicine will certainly further promote the development of traditional medicine and traditional medicine will undoubtedly make more and more contributions to human health in the 21st century.

Zhang Xiaorui

WHO Coordination Officer

December, 2000

家和地区的留学生。

在南京中医药大学左言富教授主持下编纂的、由上海中医药大学出版社出版的《(英汉对照)新编实用中医文库》,旨在全面、系统、准确、简要地阐述中医基础理论,并结合西医病名介绍中医临床治疗方法。因此,这套文库可望成为具有一定英语水平的初学中医者和具有一定中文水平的外国中医爱好者学习基础中医学的系列教材。这套文库也可供世界卫生组织在编写国际针灸标准术语时参考。

传统医学的科学、安全、有效使用必将进一步推动传统医学的发展。传统医学一定会在 21 世纪为人类健康做出更大的贡献。

张小瑞

世界卫生组织传统医学协调官员

2000 年 12 月

Preface

The Publishing House of Shanghai University of TCM published *A Practical English-Chinese Library of Traditional Chinese Medicine* in 1990. The Library has been well-known in the world ever since and has made great contributions to the dissemination of traditional Chinese medicine in the world. In view of the fact that 10 years has passed since its publication and that there are certain errors in the explanation of traditional Chinese medicine in the Library, the Publishing House has invited Nanjing University of TCM and Shanghai University of TCM to organize experts to recompile and translate the Library.

Nanjing University of TCM and Shanghai University of TCM are well-known for their advantages in higher education of traditional Chinese medicine and compilation of traditional Chinese medical textbooks. The compilation of *A Newly Compiled Practical English-Chinese Library of Traditional Chinese Medicine* has absorbed the rich experience accumulated by Nanjing University of Traditional Chinese Medicine in training international students of traditional Chinese medicine. Compared with the previous Library, the Newly Compiled Library has made great improvements in many aspects, fully demonstrating the academic system of traditional Chinese medicine. The whole series of books has systematically introduced the basic theory and thera-

前 言

上海中医药大学出版社于 1990 年出版了一套《(英汉对照)实用中医文库》,发行 10 年来,在海内外产生了较大影响,对推动中医学走向世界起了积极作用。考虑到该套丛书发行已久,对中医学术体系的介绍还有一些欠妥之处,因此,上海中医药大学出版社特邀南京中医药大学主编、上海中医药大学主译,组织全国有关专家编译出版《(英汉对照)新编实用中医文库》。

《(英汉对照)新编实用中医文库》的编纂,充分发挥了南京中医药大学和上海中医药大学在高等中医药教育教学和教材编写方面的优势,吸收了作为 WHO 传统医学合作中心之一的两校,多年来从事中医药学国际培训和留学生学历教育的经验,对原《(英汉对照)实用中医文库》整体结构作了大幅度调整,以突出中医学术主体内容。全套丛书系统介绍了中医基础理论和中医辨证论治方法,讲解了中药学和方剂学的基本理论,详细介绍了 236 味中药、152 首常用方剂和 100 种常用中成药;详述

peutic methods based on syndrome differentiation,
expounding traditional Chinese pharmacy and prescriptions; explaining 236 herbs, 152 prescriptions
and 100 commonly-used patent drugs; elucidating
264 methods for differentiating syndromes and treating commonly-encountered and frequently-encoun-
tered diseases in internal medicine, surgery, gynecology, pediatrics, traumatology and orthopedics,
ophthalmology and otorhinolaryngology; introducing
the basic methods and theory of acupuncture and
moxibustion, massage (tuina), life cultivation and
rehabilitation, including 70 kinds of diseases suitable
for acupuncture and moxibustion, 38 kinds of diseases for massage, examples of life cultivation and
over 20 kinds of commonly encountered diseases
treated by rehabilitation therapies in traditional Chinese medicine. For better understanding of traditional Chinese medicine, the books are neatly illustrated. There are 296 line graphs and 30 colored pic-
tures in the Library with necessary indexes, making
it more comprehensive, accurate and systematic in
disseminating traditional Chinese medicine in the
countries and regions where English is the official
language.

This Library is characterized by following features:

1. Scientific　Based on the development of
TCM in education and research in the past 10 years,
efforts have been made in the compilation to high-
light the gist of TCM through accurate theoretical
exposition and clinical practice, aiming at introducing authentic theory and practice to the world.

2. Systematic　This Library contains 14 sepa-

264 种临床内、外、妇、儿、骨伤、眼、
耳鼻喉各科常见病与多发病的中
医辨证论治方法；系统论述针灸、
推拿、中医养生康复的基本理论和
基本技能，介绍针灸治疗病种 70
种、推拿治疗病种 38 种、各类养生
实例及 20 余种常见病证的中医康
复实例。为了更加直观地介绍中
医药学术，全书选用线图 296 幅、
彩图 30 幅，并附有必要的索引，从
而更加全面、系统、准确地向使用
英语的国家和地区传播中医学术，
推进中医学走向世界，造福全
人类。

本丛书主要具有以下特色：
(1) 科学性：在充分吸收近 10 余年
来中医教学和科学研究最新进展
的基础上，坚持突出中医学术精
华，理论阐述准确，临床切合实用，
向世界各国介绍"原汁原味"的中
医药学术；(2) 系统性：本套丛书包
括《中医基础理论》、《中医诊断
学》、《中药学》、《方剂学》、《中医内

rate fascicles, i. e. *Basic Theory of Traditional Chinese Medicine*, *Diagnostics of Traditional Chinese Medicine*, *Science of Chinese Materia Medica*, *Science of Prescriptions*, *Internal Medicine of Traditional Chinese Medicine*, *Surgery of Traditional Chinese Medicine*, *Gynecology of Traditional Chinese Medicine*, *Pediatrics of Traditional Chinese Medicine*, *Traumatology and Orthopedics of Traditional Chinese Medicine*, *Ophthalmology of Traditional Chinese Medicine*, *Otorhinolaryngology of Traditional Chinese Medicine*, *Chinese Acupuncture and Moxibustion*, *Chinese Tuina (Massage)*, and *Life Cultivation and Rehabilitation of Traditional Chinese Medicine*.

3. Practical   Compared with the previous Library, the Newly Compiled Library has made great improvements and supplements, systematically introducing therapeutic methods for treating over 200 kinds of commonly and frequently encountered diseases, focusing on training basic clinical skills in acupuncture and moxibustion, tuina therapy, life cultivation and rehabilitation with clinical case reports.

4. Standard   This Library is reasonable in structure, distinct in categorization, standard in terminology and accurate in translation with full consideration of habitual expressions used in countries and regions with English language as the mother tongue.

This series of books is not only practical for the beginners with certain competence of English to study TCM, but also can serve as authentic textbooks for international students in universities and colleges of TCM in China to study and practice TCM. For those from TCM field who are going to go

科学》、《中医外科学》、《中医妇科学》、《中医儿科学》、《中医骨伤科学》、《中医眼科学》、《中医耳鼻喉科学》、《中国针灸》、《中国推拿》、《中医养生康复学》14 个分册,系统反映了中医各学科建设与发展的最新成果;(3)实用性:临床各科由原来的上下两册,根据学科的发展进行大幅度的调整和增补,比较详细地介绍了 200 多种各科常见病、多发病的中医治疗方法,重点突出了针灸、推拿、养生康复等临床基本技能训练,并附有部分临证实例;(4)规范性:全书结构合理,层次清晰,对中医各学科名词术语表述规范,对中医英语翻译执行了更为严格的标准化方案,同时又充分考虑到使用英语国家和地区人们的语言习惯和表达方式。

本丛书不仅能满足具有一定英语水平的初学中医者系统学习中医之用,而且也为中医院校外国留学生教育及国内外开展中医双语教学提供了目前最具权威的系列教材,同时也是中医出国人员进

abroad to do academic exchange, this series of books will provide them with unexpected convenience.

Professor Xiang Ping, President of Nanjing University of TCM, is the director of the Compilation Board. Professor Zuo Yanfu from Nanjing University of TCM, General Compiler-in-Chief, is in charge of the compilation. Zhang Wenkang, Minister of Health Ministry, is invited to be the honorary director of the Editorial Board. Li Zhenji, Vice-Director of the State Administrative Bureau of TCM, is invited to be the director of the Approval Committee. Chen Keji, academician of China Academy, is invited to be the General Advisor. International advisors invited are Mr. M. S. Khan, Chairman of Ireland Acupuncture and Moxibustion Fund; Miss Alessandra Gulí, Chairman of "Nanjing Association" in Rome, Italy; Doctor Secondo Scarsella, Chief Editor of YI DAO ZA ZHI; President Raymond K. Carroll from Australian Oriental Touching Therapy College; Ms. Shulan Tang, Academic Executive of ATCM in Britain; Mr. Giovanni Maciocia from Britain; Mr. David, Chairman of American Association of TCM; Mr. Tzu Kuo Shih, director of Chinese Medical Technique Center in Connecticut, America; Mr. Helmut Ziegler, director of TCM Center in Germany; and Mr. Isigami Hiroshi from Japan. Chen Ken, official of WHO responsible for the Western Pacific Region, has greatly encouraged the compilers in compiling this series of books. After the accomplishment of the compilation, Professor Zhu Qingsheng, Vice-Minister of Health Ministry and Director of the State Administrative Bureau of TCM, has set a high value on the books in his fore-

行中医药国际交流的重要工具书。

全书由南京中医药大学校长项平教授担任编委会主任、左言富教授任总主编,主持全书的编写。中华人民共和国卫生部张文康部长担任本丛书编委会名誉主任,国家中医药管理局李振吉副局长担任审定委员会主任,陈可冀院士欣然担任本丛书总顾问指导全书的编纂。爱尔兰针灸基金会主席萨利姆先生、意大利罗马"南京协会"主席亚历山大·古丽女士、意大利《医道》杂志主编卡塞拉·塞肯多博士、澳大利亚东方触觉疗法学院雷蒙特·凯·卡罗院长、英国中医药学会学术部长汤淑兰女士、英国马万里先生、美国中医师公会主席大卫先生、美国康州中华医疗技术中心主任施祖谷先生、德国中医中心主任赫尔木特先生、日本石上博先生担任本丛书特邀外籍顾问。世界卫生组织西太平洋地区官员陈恩先生对本丛书的编写给予了热情鼓励。全书完成后,卫生部副部长兼国家中医药管理局局长朱庆生教授给予了高度评价,并欣然为本书作序;WHO 传统医学协调官员张小瑞对于本丛书的编写给予高度关注,百忙中也专为本书作序。我国驻外教育机构,特别是中国驻英国曼彻斯特领事张益群先生、中国驻美国休斯敦领事严美华

word for the Library. Zhang Xiaorui, an official
from WHO's Traditional Medicine Program, has
paid great attention to the compilation and written a
foreword for the Library. The officials from the educational organizations of China in other countries
have provided us with some useful materials in our
compilation. They are Mr. Zhang Yiqun, China
Consul to Manchester in Britain; Miss Yan Meihua,
Consul to Houston in America; Mr. Wang Jiping,
First Secretary in the Educational Department in the
Embassy of China to France; and Mr. Gu Sheng-
ing, the Second Secretary in the Educational Department in the Embassy of China to Germany. We are
grateful to them all.

The Compilers
December, 2000

女士、中国驻法国使馆教育处一秘
王季平先生、中国驻德国使馆教育
处二秘郭胜英先生在与我们工作
联系中,间接提供了不少有益资
料。在此一并致以衷心感谢!

编 者
2000 年 12 月

Note for compilation

This book mainly deals with the basic theory of traditional Chinese medicine (TCM). It covers a wide range of content, including the theories of yin and yang, five elements, zangxiang (viscera and their manifestations), qi and blood, body fluid, meridians and collaterals, etiology, pathogenesis, prevention of disease and therapeutic principles. In the compilation, traditional terms and expressions are adopted in order to maintain the classical style of TCM while modern Chinese is used to expound the abstruse theory and methods of TCM so as to make it easy to read and understand.

In order to make the content concise, great efforts have been made to polish the contents and avoid repetition. For example, the running areas of the meridians, syndrome differentiation of the viscera, cultivation of health and prevention of disease are not discussed in detail in this book because they are thoroughly described in the other fascicles.

One point should be made clear here is that TCM is a unique medical system different from modern medicine. So the terms used in this book, such as the heart, the liver, the spleen, the lung and the kidney, are quite different from those used in modern medicine.

编写说明

本分册主要讲述中医学的基础理论，内容非常丰富，涉及阴阳五行、藏象、气血津液、经络、病因、病机、预防及治疗原则等。在编写方式上，尽量保留中医固有的术语，以保持中医传统特色不变。并采用全白话文形式，以使行文流畅易读。

为了防止篇幅冗长，编写中除了在文字上反复修饰，使其更加精炼外，还在内容详略上进行了恰当的处理，以防止与其他分册内容重复。如经络的循行部位、脏腑辨证、养生防病等内容，可参阅《中国针灸》、《中医诊断学》、《中医养生康复学》等分册，本书不作详细介绍。

中医学是不同于现代医学的一个独特的医学体系，所以本书中所涉及的一些名词术语，如心、肝、脾、肺、肾等，与现代医学的同名词语在概念上有很大差别，希望读者在学习时加以注意。

Contents

Introduction ·· (1)

1　Yin-yang and the five elements ·· (11)

　1. 1　Yin-yang ··· (11)

　　1. 1. 1　The implication of yin-yang and the categorization of things according to
　　　　　the nature of yin-yang ··· (11)

　　　1. 1. 1. 1　The implication of yin-yang ······························· (12)

　　　1. 1. 1. 2　The categorization of things according to yin and yang ·············· (12)

　　1. 1. 2　Interaction between yin and yang ······························· (13)

　　　1. 1. 2. 1　Opposition of yin and yang ······························· (14)

　　　1. 1. 2. 2　Interdependence between yin and yang ··················· (14)

　　　1. 1. 2. 3　Wane and wax between yin and yang ····················· (15)

　　　1. 1. 2. 4　Mutual transformation between yin and yang ············· (16)

　　1. 1. 3　Application of the theory of yin and yang in TCM ··········· (17)

　　　1. 1. 3. 1　Explanation of the histological structure of the human body ········ (17)

　　　1. 1. 3. 2　Explanation of the relationship between structure and function ········· (17)

　　　1. 1. 3. 3　Explanation of pathogenesis ····························· (18)

　　　1. 1. 3. 4　Diagnosis and syndrome differentiation ················· (21)

　　　1. 1. 3. 5　Guiding clinical treatment ····························· (22)

　1. 2　Wuxing (the five elements) ··· (24)

　　1. 2. 1　The implication of the five elements and the categorization of things
　　　　　according to the theory of the five elements ················· (25)

　　　1. 2. 1. 1　Implication of the five elements ······················· (25)

　　　1. 2. 1. 2　Categorization of things according to the properties of the five
　　　　　　　elements ··· (26)

　　1. 2. 2　Interactions among the five elements ························· (29)

　　　1. 2. 2. 1　Inter-promotion and inter-restraint among the five elements ········ (29)

　　　1. 2. 2. 2　Over restraint and reverse restraint ····················· (31)

　　1. 2. 3　Application of the theory of the five elements in TCM ····················· (33)

目 录

绪论 ……………………………………………………………（ 1 ）

第一章　阴阳五行 ……………………………………………（11）

　第一节　阴阳 ………………………………………………（11）

　　一、阴阳的含义与事物阴阳属性的划分 ………………（11）

　　　（一）阴阳的含义 …………………………………………（12）

　　　（二）事物阴阳属性的划分 ……………………………（12）

　　二、阴阳之间的相互作用 ………………………………（13）

　　　（一）阴阳对立 …………………………………………（14）

　　　（二）阴阳互根 …………………………………………（14）

　　　（三）阴阳消长 …………………………………………（15）

　　　（四）阴阳转化 …………………………………………（16）

　　三、阴阳学说在中医学中的应用 ………………………（17）

　　　（一）用于说明人体组织结构的属性 …………………（17）

　　　（二）用于说明人体结构与功能的关系 ………………（17）

　　　（三）用于说明基本病机变化 …………………………（18）

　　　（四）用于诊断与辨证 …………………………………（21）

　　　（五）用于指导临床治疗 ………………………………（22）

　第二节　五行 ………………………………………………（24）

　　一、五行的含义与事物五行属性的划分 ………………（25）

　　　（一）五行的含义 ………………………………………（25）

　　　（二）事物五行属性的划分 ……………………………（26）

　　二、五行之间的相互作用 ………………………………（29）

　　　（一）五行的相生与相克 ………………………………（29）

　　　（二）五行的相乘与相侮 ………………………………（31）

　　三、五行学说在中医学中的应用 ………………………（33）

1. 2. 3. 1　Explaining the physiological functions of the five zang-organs and the relationships among them ………………………………………… (33)

1. 2. 3. 2　Explaining interactions among the five zang-organs ……………… (34)

1. 2. 3. 3　Guiding clinical diagnosis ………………………………………… (36)

1. 2. 3. 4　Guiding the treatment of disease ………………………………… (37)

2　Zangxiang (viscera and their manifestations) ………………………… (41)

2. 1　The five zang-organs ………………………………………………… (44)

2. 1. 1　The heart …………………………………………………………… (45)

2. 1. 1. 1　The physiological functions of the heart ………………………… (45)

2. 1. 1. 2　The relationships between the heart and the body, the sensory organs and the orifices ……………………………………………… (47)

Appendix: The pericardium ………………………………………………… (49)

2. 1. 2　The lung …………………………………………………………… (49)

2. 1. 2. 1　The physiological functions of the lung ………………………… (50)

2. 1. 2. 2　The relationships between the lung and the body, the sensory organs and the orifices ……………………………………………… (54)

2. 1. 3　The liver …………………………………………………………… (55)

2. 1. 3. 1　The physiological functions of the liver ………………………… (56)

2. 1. 3. 2　The relationships between the liver and the body, the sensory organs and the orifices ……………………………………………… (60)

2. 1. 4　The spleen ………………………………………………………… (61)

2. 1. 4. 1　The physiological functions of the spleen ……………………… (62)

2. 1. 4. 2　The relationships between the spleen and the body, the sensory organs and the orifices ……………………………………………… (64)

2. 1. 5　The kidney ………………………………………………………… (65)

2. 1. 5. 1　The physiological functions of the kidney ……………………… (65)

2. 1. 5. 2　The relationships between the kidney and the body, the sensory organs and the orifices ……………………………………………… (71)

Appendix: Mingmen (life-gate) …………………………………………… (73)

2. 2　The six fu-organs …………………………………………………… (73)

2. 2. 1　The gallbladder …………………………………………………… (74)

2. 2. 2　The stomach ……………………………………………………… (75)

2. 2. 3　The small intestine ………………………………………………… (76)

2. 2. 4　The large intestine ………………………………………………… (77)

2. 2. 5　The bladder ………………………………………………………… (78)

（一）用于说明五脏的生理特性及其相互关系 ······················（33）
（二）用于说明五脏病变的相互影响 ·································（34）
（三）用于疾病的诊断 ···（36）
（四）用于疾病的治疗 ···（37）

第二章　藏象 ···（41）
　第一节　五脏 ···（44）
　　一、心 ···（45）
　　（一）心的生理功能 ···（45）
　　（二）心与形体官窍的关系 ·····································（47）
　　　附：心包 ···（49）
　　二、肺 ···（49）
　　（一）肺的生理功能 ···（50）
　　（二）肺与形体官窍的关系 ·····································（54）
　　三、肝 ···（55）
　　（一）肝的生理功能 ···（56）
　　（二）肝与形体官窍的关系 ·····································（60）
　　四、脾 ···（61）
　　（一）脾的生理功能 ···（62）
　　（二）脾与形体官窍的关系 ·····································（64）
　　五、肾 ···（65）
　　（一）肾的生理功能 ···（65）
　　（二）肾与形体官窍的关系 ·····································（71）
　　　附：命门 ···（73）
　第二节　六腑 ···（73）
　　一、胆 ···（74）
　　二、胃 ···（75）
　　三、小肠 ···（76）
　　四、大肠 ···（77）
　　五、膀胱 ···（78）

2. 2. 6   Sanjiao (the triple energizer) ……………………………………… (79)
2. 2. 6. 1   The conception of the triple energizer ……………………… (79)
2. 2. 6. 2   The physiological function of the triple energizer ………… (79)
2. 3   The extraordinary fu-organs ……………………………………………… (82)
2. 3. 1   The characteristics of the extraordinary fu-organs …………… (82)
2. 3. 2   The physiological functions of the extraordinary fu-organs ……… (82)
2. 3. 2. 1   The brain …………………………………………………… (83)
2. 3. 2. 2   The uterus ………………………………………………… (84)
2. 4   The relationships among the zang-organs and the fu-organs ……… (87)
2. 4. 1   The relationships among the five zang-organs ………………… (87)
2. 4. 1. 1   The relationship between the heart and the lung ………… (87)
2. 4. 1. 2   The relationship between the heart and the spleen ……… (88)
2. 4. 1. 3   The relationship between the heart and the liver ………… (88)
2. 4. 1. 4   The relationship between the heart and the kidney ……… (89)
2. 4. 1. 5   The relationship between the lung and the liver ………… (90)
2. 4. 1. 6   The relationship between the lung and the spleen ……… (91)
2. 4. 1. 7   The relationship between the lung and the kidney ……… (91)
2. 4. 1. 8   The relationship between the liver and the spleen ……… (92)
2. 4. 1. 9   The relationship between the liver and the kidney ……… (92)
2. 4. 1. 10   The relationship between the spleen and kidney ……… (93)
2. 4. 2   The relationships among the six fu-organs …………………… (94)
2. 4. 3   The relationship between the five zang-organs and the six fu-organs ……… (95)
2. 4. 3. 1   The internal and external relationship between the heart and the
small intestine ………………………………………………… (96)
2. 4. 3. 2   The internal and external relationship between the lung and the large
intestine ………………………………………………………… (97)
2. 4. 3. 3   The internal and external relationship between the spleen and the
stomach ………………………………………………………… (97)
2. 4. 3. 4   The internal and external relationship between the liver and the
gallbladder ……………………………………………………… (99)
2. 4. 3. 5   The internal and external relationship between the kidney and the
bladder ………………………………………………………… (100)
3   Qi, blood and body fluid ……………………………………………… (102)
3. 1   Qi …………………………………………………………………… (102)
3. 1. 1   The basic concept of qi …………………………………… (102)

六、三焦 ……………………………………………………………（79）

　　（一）三焦的概念 ………………………………………………（79）

　　（二）三焦的生理功能 …………………………………………（79）

第三节　奇恒之腑 …………………………………………………（82）

一、奇恒之腑的特点 ………………………………………………（82）

二、奇恒之腑的功能 ………………………………………………（82）

　　（一）脑 …………………………………………………………（83）

　　（二）女子胞 ……………………………………………………（84）

第四节　脏腑之间的关系 …………………………………………（87）

一、五脏之间的关系 ………………………………………………（87）

　　（一）心与肺 ……………………………………………………（87）

　　（二）心与脾 ……………………………………………………（88）

　　（三）心与肝 ……………………………………………………（88）

　　（四）心与肾 ……………………………………………………（89）

　　（五）肺与肝 ……………………………………………………（90）

　　（六）肺与脾 ……………………………………………………（91）

　　（七）肺与肾 ……………………………………………………（91）

　　（八）肝与脾 ……………………………………………………（92）

　　（九）肝与肾 ……………………………………………………（92）

　　（十）脾与肾 ……………………………………………………（93）

二、六腑之间的关系 ………………………………………………（94）

三、五脏与六腑之间的关系 ………………………………………（95）

　　（一）心合小肠 …………………………………………………（96）

　　（二）肺合大肠 …………………………………………………（97）

　　（三）脾合胃 ……………………………………………………（97）

　　（四）肝合胆 ……………………………………………………（99）

　　（五）肾合膀胱 …………………………………………………（100）

第三章　气血津液 …………………………………………………（102）

第一节　气 …………………………………………………………（102）

一、气的基本概念 …………………………………………………（102）

3. 1. 2   The production of qi ················ (103)

3. 1. 3   The physiological functions of qi ·············· (103)

   3. 1. 3. 1   Propelling function ················ (104)

   3. 1. 3. 2   Warming function ················ (104)

   3. 1. 3. 3   Protecting function ················ (105)

   3. 1. 3. 4   Fixating function ················ (105)

   3. 1. 3. 5   Qi-transforming function ·············· (106)

3. 1. 4   The moving styles of qi ················ (106)

3. 1. 5   The classification of qi and its production, distribution and functional
characteristics ················ (109)

   3. 1. 5. 1   Yuan-qi (primordial qi) ·············· (109)

   3. 1. 5. 2   Zong-qi (the pectoral qi) ·············· (110)

   3. 1. 5. 3   Ying-qi (nutrient qi) and wei-qi (defensive qi) ·············· (111)

3. 2   Blood ················ (113)

3. 2. 1   The basic concept of blood ·············· (113)

3. 2. 2   The production of blood ················ (114)

3. 2. 3   The physiological functions of blood ·············· (115)

3. 2. 4   The circulation of blood ················ (115)

3. 3   Body fluid ················ (117)

3. 3. 1   The basic concept of body fluid ·············· (117)

3. 3. 2   The production of body fluid ·············· (118)

3. 3. 3   The physiological functions of body fluid ·············· (119)

   3. 3. 3. 1   Moistening and nourishing ·············· (119)

   3. 3. 3. 2   The transformation of blood ·············· (119)

   3. 3. 3. 3   The transportation of the turbid qi ·············· (119)

3. 3. 4   The transportation and metabolism of body fluid ·············· (120)

   Appendix: The five zang-organs transforming five kinds of liquids ·············· (121)

3. 4   The relationships among qi, blood and body fluid ·············· (123)

3. 4. 1   The relationship between qi and blood ·············· (123)

   3. 4. 1. 1   The effect of qi on blood ·············· (124)

   3. 4. 1. 2   The effect of blood on qi ·············· (125)

3. 4. 2   The relationship between qi and body fluid ·············· (126)

   3. 4. 2. 1   The effect of qi on body fluid ·············· (126)

   3. 4. 2. 2   The effect of body fluid on qi ·············· (128)

3. 4. 3   The relationship between blood and body fluid ·············· (129)

二、气的生成 ……………………………………………… (103)

三、气的生理作用 ………………………………………… (103)

（一）推动作用 ………………………………………… (104)

（二）温煦作用 ………………………………………… (104)

（三）防御作用 ………………………………………… (105)

（四）固摄作用 ………………………………………… (105)

（五）气化作用 ………………………………………… (106)

四、气的运动形式 ………………………………………… (106)

五、气的分类及其生成、分布与功能特点 ……………… (109)

（一）元气 ……………………………………………… (109)

（二）宗气 ……………………………………………… (110)

（三）营气与卫气 ……………………………………… (111)

第二节　血 ………………………………………………… (113)

一、血的基本概念 ………………………………………… (113)

二、血的生成 ……………………………………………… (114)

三、血的生理作用 ………………………………………… (115)

四、血的运行 ……………………………………………… (115)

第三节　津液 ……………………………………………… (117)

一、津液的基本概念 ……………………………………… (117)

二、津液的生成 …………………………………………… (118)

三、津液的生理作用 ……………………………………… (119)

（一）滋润与营养 ……………………………………… (119)

（二）化生血液 ………………………………………… (119)

（三）运输浊气 ………………………………………… (119)

四、津液的运行代谢 ……………………………………… (120)

附：五脏化五液 ……………………………………… (121)

第四节　气血津液之间的关系 …………………………… (123)

一、气与血的关系 ………………………………………… (123)

（一）气对血的作用 …………………………………… (124)

（二）血对气的作用 …………………………………… (125)

二、气与津液的关系 ……………………………………… (126)

（一）气对津液的作用 ………………………………… (126)

（二）津液对气的作用 ………………………………… (128)

三、血与津液的关系 ……………………………………… (129)

4 The meridians and collaterals ·········· (131)
  4.1 The content of the theory of meridians and collaterals ·········· (131)
    4.1.1 The twelve meridians ·········· (133)
      4.1.1.1 The names of the twelve meridians ·········· (133)
      4.1.1.2 The flowing and infusing order of the twelve meridians ·········· (134)
      4.1.1.3 The distribution of the twelve meridians ·········· (135)
      4.1.1.4 The external and internal relationships ·········· (136)
    4.1.2 The eight extraordinary vessels ·········· (137)
      4.1.2.1 The nomenclature ·········· (137)
      4.1.2.2 The running features of the eight extraordinary vessels ·········· (138)
    Appendix: The twelve branches of the meridians, the twelve tendons, the twelve skin divisions, the fifteen divergent collaterals, the floating collaterals and the minute collaterals ·········· (140)
  4.2 The basic functions of the meridians and collaterals ·········· (141)
    4.2.1 To connect the external with the internal as well as to connect the viscera with other organs ·········· (141)
      4.2.1.1 The relationships between the viscera, the body, the sensory organs and the orifices ·········· (142)
      4.2.1.2 The relationships between the zang-organs and fu-organs ·········· (142)
      4.2.1.3 The relationships among the meridians ·········· (142)
    4.2.2 To transport qi, blood, yin and yang to nourish the viscera and the body ·········· (143)
    Appendix: The functional characteristics of the eight extraordinary vessels ·········· (143)
  4.3 The clinical application of the theory of meridians and collaterals ·········· (144)
    4.3.1 To explain pathogenesis and pathological transmission ·········· (144)
      4.3.1.1 To explain the pathogenesis ·········· (144)
      4.3.1.2 To explain pathological transmission ·········· (144)
    4.3.2 To guide the diagnosis and treatment of disease ·········· (145)
      4.3.2.1 To guide the diagnosis of disease ·········· (145)
      4.3.2.2 To guide the treatment of disease ·········· (146)
5 Causes of disease ·········· (148)
  5.1 The six climatic factors ·········· (148)
    5.1.1 Wind ·········· (151)

第四章　经络 …………………………………………………………… (131)

第一节　经络学说的内容 ………………………………………………… (131)

一、十二经脉 …………………………………………………………… (133)

（一）名称 …………………………………………………………… (133)

（二）流注次序 ……………………………………………………… (134)

（三）分布规律 ……………………………………………………… (135)

（四）表里关系 ……………………………………………………… (136)

二、奇经八脉 …………………………………………………………… (137)

（一）名称 …………………………………………………………… (137)

（二）循行特点 ……………………………………………………… (138)

附：十二经别、十二经筋、十二皮部、十五别络、浮络、孙络 ……… (140)

第二节　经络的基本功能 ………………………………………………… (141)

一、沟通表里上下，联络脏腑器官 …………………………………… (141)

（一）脏腑与形体官窍之间的联系 ………………………………… (142)

（二）脏腑之间的联系 ……………………………………………… (142)

（三）经络之间的联系 ……………………………………………… (142)

二、通行气血阴阳，濡养脏腑形体 …………………………………… (143)

附：奇经八脉的功能特点 …………………………………………… (143)

第三节　经络学说的临床应用 …………………………………………… (144)

一、说明疾病发生与传变的机理 ……………………………………… (144)

（一）说明疾病发生的机理 ………………………………………… (144)

（二）说明疾病传变的机理 ………………………………………… (144)

二、指导疾病的诊断和治疗 …………………………………………… (145)

（一）指导疾病的诊断 ……………………………………………… (145)

（二）指导疾病的治疗 ……………………………………………… (146)

第五章　病因 …………………………………………………………… (148)

第一节　外感六淫 ………………………………………………………… (148)

一、风 ………………………………………………………………… (151)

5. 1. 2　Cold ……………………………………………………… (152)

5. 1. 3　Summer-heat ……………………………………………… (154)

5. 1. 4　Dampness ………………………………………………… (155)

5. 1. 5　Dryness …………………………………………………… (157)

5. 1. 6　Heat (fire) ………………………………………………… (158)

　　　Appendix: Pestilence and five endogenous pathogenic factors …………… (160)

5. 2　Internal impairment due to seven emotions ……………………… (163)

5. 2. 1　Directly impairing the internal organs ……………………… (164)

5. 2. 2　Disordering the activity of qi ………………………………… (164)

　5. 2. 2. 1　Excessive joy relaxing the activity of qi ………………… (165)

　5. 2. 2. 2　Excessive anger driving qi to move upwards …………… (165)

　5. 2. 2. 3　Excessive anxiety inhibiting qi …………………………… (165)

　5. 2. 2. 4　Excessive contemplation stagnating qi ………………… (166)

　5. 2. 2. 5　Excessive grief exhausting qi …………………………… (166)

　5. 2. 2. 6　Excessive terror driving qi to move downwards ………… (166)

　5. 2. 2. 7　Excessive fear disturbing qi …………………………… (166)

5. 2. 3　Causing or aggravating certain diseases ………………… (167)

5. 3　Improper diet ……………………………………………………… (167)

5. 3. 1　Starvation and overeating …………………………………… (167)

5. 3. 2　Unhygienic food ………………………………………………… (168)

5. 3. 3　Food partiality ………………………………………………… (169)

5. 4　Overwork and over-rest ………………………………………… (170)

5. 4. 1　Overwork ……………………………………………………… (171)

5. 4. 2　Over-rest ……………………………………………………… (171)

5. 5　Diseases caused by phlegm, rheum and blood stasis ………… (172)

5. 5. 1　Phlegm and rheum …………………………………………… (172)

　5. 5. 1. 1　The basic concept of phlegm and rheum ……………… (172)

　5. 5. 1. 2　The formation of phlegm and rheum ………………… (173)

　5. 5. 1. 3　The characteristics of phlegm and rheum in causing diseases …… (174)

5. 5. 2　Blood stasis …………………………………………………… (176)

　5. 5. 2. 1　The basic concept of blood stasis ……………………… (176)

　5. 5. 2. 2　The formation of blood stasis …………………………… (176)

　5. 5. 2. 3　The characteristics of blood stasis in causing diseases ………… (179)

6　Pathogenesis ………………………………………………………… (181)

6. 1　Causes of disease ………………………………………………… (181)

二、寒 ……………………………………………………………… (152)

三、暑 ……………………………………………………………… (154)

四、湿 ……………………………………………………………… (155)

五、燥 ……………………………………………………………… (157)

六、热(火) ………………………………………………………… (158)

　　附：疫疠、内生五邪 ………………………………………… (160)

第二节　内伤七情 ………………………………………………… (163)

一、直接伤及内脏 ………………………………………………… (164)

二、导致气机紊乱 ………………………………………………… (164)

　(一) 喜则气缓 …………………………………………………… (165)

　(二) 怒则气上 …………………………………………………… (165)

　(三) 忧则气郁 …………………………………………………… (165)

　(四) 思则气结 …………………………………………………… (166)

　(五) 悲则气消 …………………………………………………… (166)

　(六) 恐则气下 …………………………………………………… (166)

　(七) 惊则气乱 …………………………………………………… (166)

三、引发或加重某些疾病 ………………………………………… (167)

第三节　饮食失宜 ………………………………………………… (167)

一、饥饱失度 ……………………………………………………… (167)

二、饮食不洁 ……………………………………………………… (168)

三、饮食偏嗜 ……………………………………………………… (169)

第四节　劳逸过度 ………………………………………………… (170)

一、过劳 …………………………………………………………… (171)

二、过逸 …………………………………………………………… (171)

第五节　痰饮、瘀血致病 ………………………………………… (172)

一、痰饮 …………………………………………………………… (172)

　(一) 痰饮的基本概念 …………………………………………… (172)

　(二) 痰饮的形成 ………………………………………………… (173)

　(三) 痰饮致病的特点 …………………………………………… (174)

二、瘀血 …………………………………………………………… (176)

　(一) 瘀血的基本概念 …………………………………………… (176)

　(二) 瘀血的形成 ………………………………………………… (176)

　(三) 瘀血致病的特点 …………………………………………… (179)

第六章　病机 ……………………………………………………… (181)

第一节　发病机理 ………………………………………………… (181)

6.1.1   Occurrence of disease and the relationship between pathogenic factors and
        the healthy qi ·· (182)
  6.1.1.1   Deficiency of healthy qi and invasion of pathogenic factors: two
            important aspects of the occurrence of disease ·························· (182)
  6.1.1.2   The effect of healthy qi and pathogenic factors on the occurrence of
            disease ·· (183)
6.1.2   Constitution and disease ··· (187)
  6.1.2.1   The definition of constitution ··· (187)
  6.1.2.2   The formation of constitution ··· (187)
  6.1.2.3   The classification of constitution ······································ (188)
  6.1.2.4   The influence of constitution on disease ······························ (192)
6.2   Mechanism of pathological changes ·· (194)
6.2.1   Predomination and decline of pathogenic factors and healthy qi ········ (195)
  6.2.1.1   Predomination and decline of pathogenic factors and healthy qi and
            the changes of deficiency and excess ···································· (195)
  6.2.1.2   The relationship between the prognosis of disease and the state
            of pathogenic factors and healthy qi ···································· (198)
6.2.2   Imbalance between yin and yang ··· (200)
  6.2.2.1   Relative predomination and decline of yin and yang ················· (201)
  6.2.2.2   Inter-consumption of yin and yang ····································· (204)
  6.2.2.3   Inter-rejection of yin and yang ··· (205)
  6.2.2.4   Inter-transformation of yin and yang ·································· (206)
  6.2.2.5   Loss of yin and yang ··· (207)
6.2.3   Disorder of qi, blood and body fluid ······································· (208)
  6.2.3.1   Disorder of qi ··· (209)
  6.2.3.2   Disorder of blood ··· (210)
  6.2.3.3   Disorder of body fluid ·· (211)
7   Prevention and therapeutic principles ··· (212)
7.1   Principles of prevention ·· (212)
7.1.1   Theory of prevention ··· (213)
  7.1.1.1   Importance of prevention ·· (213)
  7.1.1.2   The theoretical basis of the principles of prevention ················ (213)
  7.1.1.3   The guiding ideology of the principles of prevention ················ (214)
7.1.2   The preventive methods ·· (215)
  7.1.2.1   Giving prevention the priority ··· (215)

一、邪正与发病 ·· (182)

　（一）正虚、邪侵是发病的两个重要因素 ························· (182)

　（二）正气与邪气在发病过程中的不同作用 ····················· (183)

二、体质与发病 ·· (187)

　（一）体质的定义 ·· (187)

　（二）体质的形成 ·· (187)

　（三）体质的分类 ·· (188)

　（四）体质对发病的影响 ·· (192)

第二节　病变机理 ·· (194)

一、邪正盛衰 ·· (195)

　（一）邪正盛衰与虚实变化 ·· (195)

　（二）邪正盛衰与疾病转归 ·· (198)

二、阴阳失调 ·· (200)

　（一）阴阳盛衰 ··· (201)

　（二）阴阳互损 ··· (204)

　（三）阴阳格拒 ··· (205)

　（四）阴阳互转 ··· (206)

　（五）阴阳亡失 ··· (207)

三、气血津液失常 ·· (208)

　（一）气失常 ·· (209)

　（二）血失常 ·· (210)

　（三）津液失常 ··· (211)

第七章　预防与治则 ··· (212)

第一节　预防原则 ·· (212)

一、中医预防思想 ·· (213)

　（一）预防的重要性 ·· (213)

　（二）预防原则的理论基础 ·· (213)

　（三）预防原则的指导思想 ·· (214)

二、中医预防方法 ·· (215)

　（一）未病先防 ··· (215)

7. 1. 2. 2 Preventing transmission and change ……………………… (217)

7. 2 Therapeutic principles ……………………………………………… (218)

7. 2. 1 Concentrating treatment on the root cause ……………………… (219)

7. 2. 1. 1 Significance ……………………………………………………… (219)

7. 2. 1. 2 Application …………………………………………………… (220)

7. 2. 2 Strengthening healthy qi and eliminating pathogenic factors …………… (225)

7. 2. 2. 1 Significance ……………………………………………………… (225)

7. 2. 2. 2 Application of strengthening healthy qi and eliminating pathogenic
          factors …………………………………………………………… (226)

7. 2. 3 Regulation of yin and yang ………………………………………… (228)

7. 2. 3. 1 Reducing excess ……………………………………………… (229)

7. 2. 3. 2 Supplementing insufficiency …………………………………… (229)

7. 2. 4 Abidance by individuality, locality and seasons ………………… (231)

7. 2. 4. 1 Abidance by individuality …………………………………… (232)

7. 2. 4. 2 Abidance by locality ………………………………………… (234)

7. 2. 4. 3 Abidance by seasonal variation ……………………………… (235)

Postscript ……………………………………………………………………… (237)

（二）既病防变 ……………………………………………（217）

第二节　治疗原则 ………………………………………………（218）

一、治病求本 ……………………………………………………（219）

（一）治病求本的意义 ……………………………………（219）

（二）治病求本的运用 ……………………………………（220）

二、扶正祛邪 ……………………………………………………（225）

（一）扶正祛邪的意义 ……………………………………（225）

（二）扶正祛邪的运用 ……………………………………（226）

三、调整阴阳 ……………………………………………………（228）

（一）损其有余 ……………………………………………（229）

（二）补其不足 ……………………………………………（229）

四、因人、因地、因时制宜 ……………………………………（231）

（一）因人制宜 ……………………………………………（232）

（二）因地制宜 ……………………………………………（234）

（三）因时制宜 ……………………………………………（235）

后记 ……………………………………………………………（237）

Introduction

绪　论

TCM, a great treasure-house of culture, is an indispensable part of the splendid classic Chinese culture. In its long course of development, it has absorbed the quintessence of classical Chinese philosophy, culture and science, and summarized the experience of the Chinese people in fighting against disease. It is rich in theory and practical in treatment. Today modern medicine is quite advanced, but TCM is still widely used because of its significant clinical curative effect. In recent decades, TCM is understood and adopted in more and more countries and regions in the world.

中医学是一个博大精深的文化宝库,是灿烂的中国古代文化的一部分。由于中医学一方面汲取了中国古代深邃的哲学、文化和科学思想,另一方面又是对中华民族数千年来与疾病作斗争的经验总结,所以她不但具有极其丰富的理论思辨性和创造性,而且临床实用性极强。即使在现代医学十分发达的今天,中医学依然具有很强的生命力,其重要原因之一,就在于其卓越的临床疗效。近几十年来,中医学的独特优势逐渐被国际医学界所认识,这一古老的传统医学正一步步走向世界。

1. The origination, formation and development of the theoretical system of TCM

TCM originated in antiquity. Early in the primitive society, human beings began to accumulate medical knowledge. In Chinese classics there are many records concerning medicine or drugs, such as "Fuxi made nine needles" and "Shennong tasted hundreds of herbs and was poisoned seventy times in a single day". These records indicate that the Chinese ancestors made great efforts to explore medicine in their life and work. In the Spring and Autumn Period and the Warring States, China was greatly advanced in politics, economy, science and culture. In

1. 中医学理论体系的起源、形成和发展

中医学起源于中国远古时代。早在原始部落时代,人类就开始了医药知识的初步积累。如中国古典文献有"伏羲制九针"、"神农尝百草,一日而遇七十毒"等记载,就是对上古时期中华民族的祖先在生活和生产实践中努力探索医药知识的真实写照。到了春秋战国时期,人们对疾病

medicine, disease was well understood and medical experience was further enriched. Such a rapid development in
medicine made it possible to develop a new theoretical
system of medicine by combining the medical knowledge
passed on from the previous generations with latest theoretical ideas. The publication of *Huangdi Neijing*
(*Huangdi's Canon of Medicine*), the earliest extant
medical canon in China, symbolized the formation of such
a new theoretical system of medicine. *Huangdi Neijing*
appeared around the time from the Warring States to the
Qin and the Han Dynasties. It collected a great quantity of
materials concerning medical practice done by the previous generations, summarized and synthesized knowledge
of astronomy, geography, biology and meterology in the
light of the theories of yin-yang and five elements popular
then. It systematicaliy expounded the physiology and the
pathology of human body as well as the diagnosis, treatment and prevention of disease, consequently establishing
a unique theoretical system for TCM and laying a solid
foundation for the theoretical and clinical development of
TCM.

Since the publication of *Huangdi Neijing*, doctors of
all generations have made great efforts to further enrich
and improve the theory of TCM, thus promoting the development of this medical system.

Nanjing (*Canon of Difficult Issues*), another important medical classic after *Huangdi Neijing*, expounded
the main contents of *Huangdi Neijing* in a style of question and answer and supplemented what *Huangdi Neijing*
lacked. As an indispensable classic in the theoretical

的认识已经相当深刻,医疗实
践经验也已经非常丰富,再加
上此时的社会快速进入了一
个文明昌盛的时代,政治、经
济、科学、文化都有显著的发
展,学术思想也空前活跃。因
此,把代代相传的医药知识和
最新的理论思想结合起来,创
造一个崭新的医学理论体系,
就成了自然而然的事情。中
国现存最早的医学经典《黄帝
内经》的出现,就是这种崭新
的医学理论体系形成的重要
标志。《黄帝内经》成书于战
国至秦汉时代,它收集了前人
大量的医疗实践资料,运用当
时盛行的阴阳、五行等学说,
以及天文、地理、生物、气象等
各种自然科学知识进行归纳、
综合,系统地阐述了人体生
理、病理和关于疾病的诊断、
治疗、预防等内容,形成了中
医学独特的理论体系,为中医
学理论和临床的发展奠定了
坚实的基础。

自《黄帝内经》以后,历代
医家对中医学理论不断进行
充实和提高,推动了中医学理
论体系的进一步发展和完善。

《难经》是稍晚于《黄帝内
经》问世的另一部重要的古典
医籍,它以问答的行文方式,
针对《黄帝内经》的某些重要
内容进一步进行阐发、论述,

works of TCM, *Nanjing* put forward a number of important ideas, such as "taking pulse only at the area of cunkou" and "the left is the kidney and the right is mingmen (life gate)" which exerted great impact on the theoretical development of TCM.

In the last years of the East Han Dynasty, Zhang Zhongjing, based on *Huangdi Neijing* and *Nanjing* as well as his own clinical practice, wrote *Shanghan Zabing Lun* (*Treatise on Exogenous Febrile Disease and Miscellaneous Diseases*), the first monograph on clinical medicine. This book contributed much to the formation and development of syndrome differentiation and treatment in clinical medicine. Taking syndrome differentiation of the six meridians (taiyang, shaoyang, yangming, taiyin, shaoyin and jueyin) and syndrome differentiation of the viscera as the principles for the differentiation of syndrome, Zhang formulated effective therapeutic methods and prescriptions for the diagnosis and treatment of exogenous and endogenous diseases. These methods and prescriptions are still widely used in and out of China now. Zhang himself was worshiped as the "sage of medicine" by the later generations.

The Jin, Sui and Tang Dynasties witnessed extensive summarization, enrichment and completion of the theory and clinical practice of TCM. In the Jin Dynasty, Wang Shuhe wrote *Maijing* (*Canon of Pulse*), the first monograph on diagnostics of TCM in China; in the Sui Dynasty, Chao Yuanfang compiled the first monograph on pathogenesis and symptomology; in the Tang Dynasty, Wang Tao wrote *Waitai Miyao* (*Medical Secrets of An Official*) and Sun Simiao wrote *Beiji Qianjin Yaofang* (*Valuable*

对《黄帝内经》的某些不足进行了重要补充,是研究中医学经典理论必不可少的一部医学典籍。如《难经》提出的诊脉"独取寸口"及"左为肾、右为命门"等理论,对后世医学理论的发展产生了巨大的影响。

东汉末年,张仲景在继承《黄帝内经》、《难经》等理论的基础上,结合临床实际,撰写了中国第一部临床医学专著《伤寒杂病论》,为中医临床医学辨证论治体系的形成和发展作出了杰出的贡献。张仲景以六经(太阳、少阳、阳明、太阴、少阴、厥阴)辨证和脏腑辨证等方法为辨证纲领,对外感疾病和内伤杂病的诊治制订了许多卓有疗效的治法和方剂,至今仍为国内外医学界所推崇,因此后人尊称张仲景为"医圣"。

晋、隋、唐时期,是对中医学理论和临床进行大规模总结、充实,并形成完整理论体系的重要时期。晋代王叔和所著《脉经》,是第一部关于中医诊断学的专门著作;隋代巢元方等人编撰了中国医学史上第一部病机证候学专著;唐代王焘著《外台秘要》、孙思邈

Prescriptions for Emergency) which thoroughly summarized the theoretical study and clinical practice made before the Tang Dynasty.

　　From the Song Dynasty to the Jin and Yuan Dynasties, various schools of medicine appeared, promoting the
development of TCM from different angles. Liu Wansu,
Zhang Congzheng, Li Gao and Zhu Zhenheng were the
representatives of these medical schools. Liu Wansu believed that "fire and heat" were the main causes of diseases and that diseases should be treated with drugs cold and
cool in nature. So his theory was known as "the school of
cold and cool" by the later generations; Zhang Congzheng
believed that all diseases were caused by exogenous pathogenic factors and advocated that pathogenic factors should
be eliminated by means of diaphoresis, emesis and purgation. Elimination of pathogenic factors ensures the resto-
ration of the healthy qi and cure of disease, so his theory
was known as the "school of purgation". Li Gao held that
internal impairment of the spleen and the stomach would
bring about various diseases and therefore emphasize that
the most important thing in clinical treatment should be to
warm and invigorate the spleen and the stomach. So he
was regarded as the founder of the "school for reinforcing
the earth". Zhu Zhenheng believed that "yang is usually
redundant while yin is frequently deficient" and that yin-
deficiency and fire-exuberance were the commonly encountered syndromes. Clinically he usually used the prescriptions for nourishing yin and reducing fire to treat diseases. So his theory was known as the "school for nourishing yin". Though different from each other, these theories enriched TCM and promoted its development because
they were all developed from clinical practice. That is why
they were called "four great doctors in the Jin and the Yuan
Dynasties" by the later generations.

著《备急千金要方》等书,是对
唐以前医学理论和实践经验
进行全面总结的集大成之作。

　　宋代以后至金元时期,涌
现了很多各具特色的医学流
派,从不同的角度发展了中医
学理论,其中具有典型代表性
的医家当推刘完素、张从正、
李杲、朱震亨四人。刘完素提
出疾病的性质多为火热之证,
用药以寒凉为主,后人称为
"寒凉派";张从正认为疾病的
发生主要是由邪气侵袭人体
所致,若邪气去则正气复而疾
病痊愈,主张用发汗、涌吐、泻
下三法治疗,后人称为"攻下
派";李杲指出脾胃是元气之
本,脾胃一伤,元气即虚,抗邪
无力,各种疾病就会随之而
生,故治疗重在调补脾胃,后
人称为"补土派";朱震亨则认
为人体常处于阴气不足、阳气
有余的状态(即所谓"阳常有
余,阴常不足"),阴虚火旺是
疾病的常见证候,所以临床治
疗善用滋阴降火的方法,后人
称为"滋阴派"。 由于他们的
理论都是从临床实践中来,各
有不同的创见,对丰富中医学
理论都起了重要的促进作用,
所以受到后人的重视和推崇,
把他们尊称为"金元四大家"。

In the Ming and Qing Dynasties, wenbing (seasonal febrile disease), a new branch in TCM, appeared. Wu Youke in the Ming Dynasty first put forward the idea that the cause of pestilence was different from liuyin (six abnormal climatic factors). He believed it is "a special pathogenic factor in the natural world". This was a new explanation of pestilence. In the Qing Dynasty, Ye Tianshi, Xue Shengbai, Wu Jutong and Wang Mengying made extensive study on the route of infection, pathogenesis and pathological changes of seasonal febrile disease through clinical practice, gradually establishing a theoretical system of seasonal febrile disease with syndrome differentiation of wei (defensive qi), qi, ying (nutrient qi), xue (blood) and sanjiao (triple energizer) as its core. This theoretical system is now a specialty of TCM.

With the rapid development of modern medicine, TCM now encounters another chance to develop. On the basis of the theoretical study and clinical practice made by the previous generations and with the adoption of modern scientific theory and technology, TCM will certainly develop into a new era.

2. The basic characteristics of TCM

Concept of holism and syndrome differentiation and treatment are the two basic characteristics of TCM in understanding human physiology and pathology as well as diagnosis, treatment and prevention of disease.

(1) Concept of holism: The concept of holism means that the human body is an organic whole and that human beings are interrelated with nature.

到了明清时代,中医温病学说异军突起。明代吴又可首先提出,温疫病的病因不同于一般的六淫,是"天地间别有一种异气"感染人体所致,对温疫病的病因提出了新的见解。之后,清代的叶天士、薛生白、吴鞠通、王孟英等医家,通过大量的临床实践,对温病的传染途径、发病机制、病理变化等,都获得了更深刻的认识,于是创立了以卫气营血辨证和三焦辨证为核心的温病学理论体系,在中医学理论体系中逐步形成了一个新的专门学科。

由于现代医学科学的出现,今天的中医学正面临着一次新的发展机遇。我们在整理继承前人理论和实践经验的基础上,可以结合现代科学理论、运用现代技术手段来研究中医,中医学理论的发展将会进入一个新的历史阶段。

2. 中医学的基本特点

中医学有两个基本特点,一是整体观念,二是辨证论治,它体现在对人体生理功能和病理变化的认识以及对疾病的诊断和治疗等各个方面。

(1) 整体观念:整体观念,即指人体是一个统一的整体以及人与自然是一个相互关联的整体的思想。

1) Organic wholeness of the body　TCM believes that the human body is composed of various tissues and organs, including the viscera, the meridians, the five sensory organs, the nine orifices, the four limbs and all the skeletal parts. These different tissues and organs are united into an organic whole because they are closely related to each other in structure, physiology and pathology. In structure, the body centers around the five zang-organs, namely the heart, the liver, the spleen, the lung and the kidney. Through the system of the meridians and the functional activities of the corresponding six fu-organs, the five constituents, the five sensory organs and the nine orifices, the body becomes a unified whole that is connected with the upper and lower as well as the internal and external. In physiology, the viscera, though different in functional activities, cooperate with each other in functions. Take food for example. When it enters the mouth, the stomach digests it first and then transmits it to the small intestine where it is further digested with the functions of the spleen to transform and the small intestine to separate the clear from the turbid. Then the nutrients are absorbed and transformed into qi and blood to be transported to all parts of the body. The waste part is transmitted to the large intestine where it is transformed into feces and then discharged through the anus. Actually the liver, the gallbladder and the triple energizer are also involved in this digestion process. It is obvious that the digestion of food, the absorption of nutrients and the discharge of waste are accomplished by concerted action of a number of organs. In pathology, morbid change in any part of the body will affect the other viscera and tissues or even the whole body. Similarly, general pathological change of the body will affect the functions of the local viscera. Take the liver for example. If it fails to dredge and disperse, it

1) 人体是一个统一的整体　中医学认为，人体由许多组织器官所构成，包括脏腑经络、五官九窍、四肢百骸等，但彼此之间在结构上、生理上、病理上却有着密切的联系，是一个统一的整体。如在结构上，以心、肝、脾、肺、肾五脏为中心，通过经络系统联系到相应的六腑、五体、五官九窍等各组织器官，形成一个上下沟通、表里相连的统一整体。在生理方面，虽然脏腑各有不同的功能活动，但相互之间也是密切配合协作的。如饮食入口，首先通过胃的受纳腐熟功能，进行初步的消化而输送到小肠，然后依靠脾的运化和小肠受盛化物、分别清浊的功能，在进一步充分消化的基础上，吸收其中的精微物质而化生气血营养周身，剩余的食物糟粕又继续输送至大肠，再通过大肠的传导功能形成粪便而排出体外。在这一过程中，还有肝、胆、三焦等内脏功能的帮助。由此可见，食物的消化吸收及其糟粕的排泄过程，是由多个脏腑的生理功能互相配合而完成的。在病理方面，人体任何部位发生病变，都可影响到其他的脏腑组织甚至整个机体，而整体的病变也可影响到局部脏腑器官

may lead to dysfunction of the spleen, affecting the digestion and absorption of food. Take the heart for another example. Stagnation of heart-blood will inhibit the flow of lung-qi, leading to disorder of respiration. So in clinical diagnosis and treatment of disease, thorough examination of the five sensory organs, physical condition, complexion and pulse must be made to analyze the pathological changes of the viscera so as to decide correct therapeutic principles and methods.

2) Correlation between man and nature   Human beings live in nature and nature provides them with various necessities, such as sunlight, air and water. On the other hand, various changes taking place in nature may directly or indirectly affect the human body and bring on corresponding physiological or pathological responses. For example, warmth in spring, heat in summer, coolness in autumn and cold in winter may affect the human body in different ways. In spring and summer it is warm and hot, and yang-qi is in predominance. In these two seasons, the skin is loose and the sweat pores are open. That is why there is profuse sweating and infrequent urination in spring and summer. In autumn and winter it is cool and cold, and yang-qi gradually declines. In these two seasons the skin is tense and sweat pores are closed. That is why there is frequent urination and scanty sweating in autumn and winter. This shows that the metabolism of water in the body is regulated automatically with the variations of the four seasons. If the variations of the seasons are too violent and beyond the automatic adjustment of the body, or if the body resistance declines and the self-regulation function becomes abnormal, frequently encountered seasonal disease and epidemic disease will be caused. Usually

的功能。如肝的疏泄功能失常，可引起脾失健运，从而影响食物的消化吸收；心血瘀阻，使肺气运行不畅，可导致呼吸失调等。因此，在临床上诊治疾病时，必须从整体出发，通过五官、形体、色脉等外在的变化，来分析和判断内脏的病变，从而在整体观的指导下制定正确的治疗原则和方法。

2）人与自然是一个相互关联的整体　人类生活在自然界之中，自然界存在着各种人类赖以生存的必要条件，如阳光、空气、水源等。同时自然界的各种变化又可以直接或间接地影响着人体，使人体产生生理或病理上的相应反应。例如，一年四季有春温、夏热、秋凉、冬寒等不同的气候变化，会对人体产生不同的影响。春夏季节，天气比较温热，阳气旺盛，人体皮肤松弛，毛窍开张，汗出较多而排尿减少；秋冬季节，天气比较寒凉，阳气渐衰，人体皮肤收缩，毛窍固密，排尿增多而出汗减少，这说明人体的水液代谢是随着四时气候的变化而自动进行调节的。如果气候变化过于剧烈，超过了人体的调节能力，或人体本身抵抗力下降，调节功能失常时，就可引

wind disease tends to occur in spring, summer-heat disease in summer, dry disease in autumn and cold disease in winter. Take some old people or patients with chronic disease for example. They tend to have ailments when the season changes. Such ailments may further lead to the onset or aggravation of diseases.

Geographical conditions, similar to the seasonal variations, also affect the physiological activity and pathological state of the body. In the warm areas with sufficient rain, for example, people are easily to be affected by exogenous pathogenic factors because their skin is loose and their constitution is comparatively weak. But in the dry areas, people are prone to endogenous impairment because their skin is tense and their constitution is comparatively strong, making it difficult for exogenous pathogenic factors to invade them. It is obvious that different geographical conditions are responsible for different constitutions of the human beings. That is why it is difficult for people to be quickly accustomed to new geographical conditions when they have moved to a new place.

(2) Bianzheng lunzhi (Syndrome differentiation and treatment):

1) Implication of syndrome differentiation and treatment   Syndrome differentiation and treatment means to analyze, induce, synthesize, judge and summarize the clinical data of symptoms and signs collected with the four diagnostic methods (namely inspection, listening and smelling, inquiry, taking pulse and palpation) into certain syndrome. Then the therapeutic methods are decided according to the result of syndrome differentiation. Syndrome differentiation and treatment is a basic principle in TCM to understand and treat disease.

起季节性的多发病、流行病，如春多风病，夏多暑病，秋多燥病，冬多寒病等。又如某些老年人或慢性病患者，由于适应能力比较差，往往在季节转换之际感到身体不舒服，导致疾病发作或加重。

不仅季节气候变化对人体有影响，地理环境的不同也影响着人体的生理活动和病理状态。如气候温热多雨的地区，人体的肌肤疏松，体质较弱，容易感受外邪；而气候寒冷干燥的地区，人体肌肤致密，体质较强，一般外邪不易侵犯，其病多为内伤。正因为不同的地理条件造成了人的体质上的差异，故一旦易地而居，原来的体质状况不能适应新的地理环境，短期内就会出现相应的病变和不适反应，称为"水土不服"。

(2) 辨证论治：

1) 辨证论治的含义   辨证论治，就是将通过四诊(望、闻、问、切)所收集的症状、体征等临床资料，进行分析、归纳和综合，判断、概括为某种性质的证，然后再根据辨证的结果，确定相应的治疗方法。辨证论治是中医学认识疾病和治疗疾病的基本原则。

"Zheng" (syndrome) is a summarization of the pathological changes of a disease at a certain stage in its course of development, including the location, cause and nature of the disease as well as the state of xie (pathogenic factors) and zheng (the healthy qi). Compared with single symptom, syndrome can more extensively, completely and correctly demonstrate the nature of a disease. For example, if a patient has clinical manifestations of serious aversion to cold, light fever, headache, body pain, anhidrosis and floating-tense pulse, it can be analyzed that the disease is caused by wind-cold, the location is superficial, the nature of the disease is cold, and the relationship between the pathogenic factors and healthy qi is excess. According to such a differentiation it can be induced that the patient is suffering from external excess syndrome due to wind-cold which can be treated by dispersing wind and dissipating cold with drugs acrid in flavor and warm in property for relieving superficial pathogenic factors. It is obvious that syndrome differentiation is prerequisite to treatment, while treatment is the aim of syndrome differentiation and the method to test whether syndrome differentiation is correct. In fact, syndrome differentiation and treatment are two interrelated and indispensable aspects in the diagnosis and treatment of disease.

2) Differentiation of syndrome and differentiation of disease   Clinically differentiation of syndrome and differentiation of disease are intrinsically interrelated on the one hand, and different on the other. It is generally thought that disease includes the whole pathological course while syndrome is just the summarization of disease at a certain stage of its development. For this reason one disease may display different syndromes while different diseases may demonstrate the same syndrome in their course of development. Therefore in TCM, the understanding

所谓"证",即"证候",是对疾病发生、发展过程中某一阶段的病理变化的概括,包括了疾病的部位、原因、性质以及邪正关系等内容,它比单一的症状能更全面、更深刻、更正确地反映出疾病的本质。例如,患者表现出恶寒重、发热轻、头身疼痛、无汗、脉浮紧等临床症状,通过分析归纳,辨清病因为风寒之邪,病位在表,疾病性质为寒,邪正关系是实,于是就概括判断为风寒表实证,治以疏风散寒,辛温解表。可见,辨证是决定治疗的前提和依据,论治是辨证的目的,也是检验辨证是否正确的方法和手段,辨证与论治是诊治疾病过程中相互联系而不可分割的两个方面。

2) 辨证与辨病的关系
在临床上,疾病与证候之间既有内在的联系,又有一定的区别。通常认为,疾病是包括其整个病理过程在内的,而证候则是疾病过程中某一阶段的病理概括,因此同一种疾病可表现出不同的证,而不同的疾病在发展过程中又可出现相同的证,所以中医认识疾病和

and treatment of disease mainly focuses on differentiating syndrome and analyzing the common nature or difference of syndrome in the course of differentiating disease. For example, one disease may demonstrate different syndromes which should be treated with different therapies due to difference in constitution, onset of disease, geographic conditions, or stage of development. Take common cold for example. Clinically it is divided into wind-cold syndrome and wind-heat syndrome due to difference in pathogenic factors. The former is treated by relieving superficial pathogenic factors with drugs acrid in taste and warm in property while the latter with drugs acrid in taste and cool in property, which is known as "treating the same disease with different methods" in TCM. However, same therapeutic method can be used to treat different diseases with the emergence of the same syndrome in their course of development. Take dysentery and jaundice for example. They are two different diseases. But if they all demonstrate damp-heat syndrome, both of them can be treated by the therapeutic method for clearing away damp-heat, which is known as "treating different diseases with the same method" in TCM. It is clear that syndrome differentiation and treatment can truly reveal the relationship between disease and syndrome. It emphasizes the role of syndrome in treatment and advocates the idea of "treating the same syndrome with the same method" and "treating different syndromes with different methods."

治疗疾病,主要是着眼于辨证,着眼于在辨病的过程中找出证的共性或差异性。如同一种疾病,由于患者的体质不同,或发病的时间、地区不同,或处于不同的发展阶段等,可以表现出不同的证候,因而治法也不一样。以感冒为例,由于患者感受的邪气不同,临床上有风寒证与风热证的区别,前者治以辛温解表,后者治以辛凉解表,中医学把这种情形叫做"同病异治"。又如不同的疾病,在其发展过程中,只要出现相同的证候,便可采用相同的治疗方法,如痢疾与黄疸,是两种不同的疾病,但如果都表现为湿热证,就都可用清利湿热的方法来进行治疗,中医学把这种情形叫做"异病同治"。由此可见,辨证论治能够从本质上理解病和证的关系,强调"证"在治疗中的首要作用,认为"证同治亦同,证异治亦异"。

1 Yin-yang and the five elements

1.1 Yin-yang

The theory of yin-yang originated in antiquity in China. It is a theory dealing with the origination of the universe as well as the motion and variation of all things in the natural world. It holds that the natural world is made up of materials and that the material world conceives, develops and constantly varies under the interaction of yin and yang. The philosophers and doctors in ancient China explained all the phenomena and the nature of the universe and life with the theory of yin-yang. They regarded the opposition, the wane and wax as well as the variation of yin-yang as "the law of the universe".

1.1.1 The implication of yin-yang and the categorization of things according to the nature of yin-yang

People in ancient China held that the original state of the universe was "qi" and that the motion and variation of "qi" produced two poles known as "yin" and "yang". Such a process of transformation was called "to divide one into two". Since all the things in the universe are produced through the motion and variation of qi, everything can be divided into the aspects of yin and yang, such as the heaven and the earth, the day and the night, the water and fire, upper and lower, cold and heat as well as man and

第一章 阴阳 五行

第一节 阴阳

阴阳学说产生于中国远古时代,是一种关于宇宙起源及万物运动变化的最高法则的理论,认为世界是由物质构成的,物质世界是在阴阳二气的相互作用下孳生、发展和不断运动变化着的,古代哲学家和医学家们用阴阳学说来解释整个宇宙和生命的一切现象和本质,并把阴阳对立和消长运动变化的规律称之为"天地之道"。

一、阴阳的含义与事物阴阳属性的划分

古代中国人认为,宇宙的原初状态是"气",由"气"的运动变化而产生了相反的两极,即"阴"和"阳"。这一过程叫做"一分为二"。宇宙间万事万物都由气的运动变化而生成,所以一切事物都可以分为阴和阳两个方面,如天地、昼夜、水火、上下、寒热、男女等。

woman, etc.

1.1.1.1　The implication of yin-yang

The original meaning of yin and yang is simple and specific, mainly referring to the sides facing and opposite to the sun. That is to say that the things facing the sun pertain to yang while the things opposite to the sun pertain to yin. In Chinese "yang" means "sunshine" while "yin" means "shadow". Later on specific things related to yin and yang were abstracted to induce a series of properties in the light of yin and yang. In this way yin and yang, two special signifiers, gradually evolved into a theory of extensive application. Consequently the implication of yin and yang was extended.

The properties of things signified by yin and yang are quite abstract. In order to make the meaning of yin and yang explicit, people in ancient China used specific things, namely water and fire, as metaphors to analogize. Since water and fire are opposite to each other in nature and reflect the basic characteristics of yin and yang, they are used as the signifiers of yin and yang in *Huangdi Neijing*. Comparatively speaking, fire is warm, bright, active and up-flaming; while water is cold, dim, static and downward-moving. That is why it is stipulated in *Huangdi Neijing* that "water is yin and fire is yang".

1.1.1.2　The categorization of things according to yin and yang

Fire and water are the evidences used to categorize things because they are the signifiers of yin and yang. Generally speaking, the things and the phenomena that bear the properties of being warm, bright, active, rising and dispersing pertain to yang; while the things and the

（一）阴阳的含义

阴阳的最初含义是比较直观、具体的，主要指阳光的向背。即事物向阳的一面属阳，背阴的一面属阴，这就是"阴阳"二字的来历。后来，人们把与阴阳相关的具体事物抽象化，归纳出一系列能够表明其阴阳归属的事物属性，从而使"阴阳"由特定的指代概念上升为能够普遍运用的理论，这样，阴阳的含义就变得更加宽广了。

由于阴阳所表达的事物属性是很抽象的，所以古人为了清晰明了地表达阴阳的概念，就借具体事物——水火来比喻。由于水火性质相反，并且集中地体现了阴阳的一些特征，所以《黄帝内经》称水火为"阴阳之征兆"。"征兆"，就是象征的意思。相对于"火"温热、明亮、运动、向上的特性而言，"水"的特性则是寒凉、晦暗、静止、向下，等等，所以《内经》规定："水为阴"，"火为阳"。

（二）事物阴阳属性的划分

由于有了水火的象征性比喻，因而就有了划分事物阴阳属性的依据。一般地说，凡是具有温热、明亮、运动、上升、发散等特征的事物和现象

phenomena that bear the properties of being cold, dim, static, descending and astringing pertain to yin.

According to such criteria, all things and phenomena can be categorized into either yin or yang group. However, the yin and yang properties of things are relative, not absolute. In the categorization of things according to the nature of yin and yang, two points have to be taken into consideration.

（1）The yin or yang properties of things may vary with the change of time and application. Take spring and summer for example. It is comparatively hot in summer and cold in spring, so summer pertains to yang and spring to yin. Take spring and winter for another example. It is comparatively cold in winter and warm in spring, so winter pertains to yin while spring to yang.

（2）Any aspect of yin and yang in an object can be further and infinitely divided. In this case there exists yin within yang and yang within yin. Take daytime and night for example. Daytime pertains to yang while night to yin. However, daytime can be further divided into two phases: morning and afternoon. Since yang-qi ascends in the morning and descends in the afternoon, morning pertains to yang（yang within yang）and afternoon to yin（yin within yang）. Similarly, night can be divided into anterior night and posterior night. Since yin-qi increases in the anterior night and decreases in the posterior night, anterior night pertains to yin（yin within yin）while posterior night to yang（yang within yin）.

1.1.2 Interaction between yin and yang

The yin and yang aspects within an object or phenom-

都属于阳,凡是具有寒凉、晦暗、静止、下降、收敛等特征的事物和现象都属于阴。

根据上述划分事物阴阳属性的依据,就可以对任何事物和现象进行阴阳属性的划分了。但是,事物的阴阳属性是相对的,而不是绝对的,所以在划分事物阴阳属性时,必须注意到以下两点。

（1）事物的阴阳属性,随着时间的推移和适用范围的不同,可以发生相应的变化。如春与夏相对,夏热而春冷,故夏属阳而春属阴;若春与冬相对,冬寒而春温,则冬属阴而春属阳。

（2）事物的阴阳属性的每一方面还可以再分阴阳,并且可以无限地分下去,这就形成了阴中有阳、阳中有阴的现象。如以昼夜分阴阳,则昼为阳而夜为阴。但昼还可以分为上午和下午,则上午阳气上升故属阳（阳中之阳）,下午阳气下降故属阴（阳中之阴）。同理,夜可分为前半夜和后半夜,则前半夜阴气增长故属阴（阴中之阴）,后半夜阴气消退故属阳（阴中之阳）。

二、阴阳之间的相互作用

事物或现象之间的阴阳

enon are not simply arbitrary divisions. In fact they are in constant and complicated interaction. Such interactions between yin and yang give rise to the origination, development and change of things. The interactions between yin and yang are various in manifestations. The following is a brief description of the major ones.

1.1.2.1　Opposition of yin and yang

Since yin and yang are opposite to each other in nature, they constantly repel and restrain each other. If both yin and yang are quite powerful, such a mutual repelling and restraining activity will maintain general equilibrium of things. If one side is weak and the other side is strong, the strong side will restrain the weak side, consequently damaging the general balance of things. The so-called "contrary treatment", one of the basic therapeutic principles in TCM, is developed in the light of the opposition between yin and yang. For example, the treatment of cold disease with drugs hot in nature means to use heat (yang) to control cold (yin) while the treatment of febrile disease with drugs cold in nature means to use cold drugs (yin) to restrict heat (yang). Since the drugs used and the disease treated are different in nature, such a treatment is termed "contrary treatment". "Contrary" means "opposite".

1.1.2.2　Interdependence between yin and yang

Interdependence between yin and yang, literarily yin and yang rooting in each other, indicates that yin and yang depend on each other for existence in an object. In conception, yin and yang must exist in pair and no side can exist solitarily. In nature, yin and yang within an object can transform into each other under certain condition,

两个方面,不是一种简单的划分,而是处于十分复杂的相互作用中。正是阴阳之间的这种相互作用,导致了事物的发生、发展和变化。阴阳之间相互作用的形式多种多样,可以表现在以下几个主要方面。

(一)阴阳对立

阴阳对立,是说阴阳双方由于其性质相反,总是处于相互排斥、相互制约之中。如果阴阳双方力量相当,那么这种相互排斥和相互制约就会导致事物整体的平衡。若阴阳双方力量有强弱盛衰的变化,那么弱者将受强者制约,事物整体的平衡就会被破坏。根据阴阳对立的作用原理,中医治疗疾病的基本原则之一是"逆治"。如寒性疾病用热药治疗,即用热(阳)制约寒(阴);热性疾病用寒药治疗,即用寒(阴)制约热(阳)。由于药性与病性相反,所以称为"逆治"。逆,就是"反向"的意思。

(二)阴阳互根

阴阳互根,是说阴阳双方存在于一个统一体中,二者相互依赖,互为根基。从概念上说,阴阳双方必须成对存在,任何一方都不能孤立地存在。从实质上讲,事物内部的阴阳

implying that no one can exist without the existence of the other. That is why it is said in the theory of TCM that "solitary yang cannot exist" and "solitary yin cannot grow". In the light of interdependence between yin and yang, TCM pays much attention to mutual transformation between qi and blood as well as yin and yang in the treatment of diseases due to deficiency of qi and blood as well as of yin and yang. For example, the patients with blood deficiency can be treated by supplementing qi to produce blood, the patients with qi deficiency can be treated by supplementing blood to promote qi, the patients with yin deficiency can be treated by supplementing yang to generate yin (also called "drawing yin from yang") and the patients with yang deficiency can be treated by supplementing yin to promote yang (also called "drawing yang from yin").

1.1.2.3 Wane and wax between yin and yang

Wane and wax between yin and yang implies that, in the interaction between yin and yang, one side is developing while the other side is declining and vice versa. Such a state manifests in different ways, such as yin waning while yang waxing, yin waxing while yang waning, yang waning leading to yin waxing, and yang waxing leading to yin waning.

Under normal condition, wane and wax between yin and yang are maintained to a certain range. Waning to a certain degree will turn to waxing and waxing to a certain level will change into waning. In this way wane and wax will never be excessive. Alternation and repetition of wane and wax maintain a dynamic balance between yin and yang.

If wane and wax between yin and yang exceeds the

之间可以相互化生,体现了一种共存共亡的关系,任何一方都不能脱离另一方而单独存在。因此,中医理论中有"独阳不生"、"孤阴不长"的说法。根据阴阳互根的原理,中医在治疗气血阴阳不足的病证时,特别重视气血的相互化生和阴阳的互根互化。如血虚者可以补气以生血,气虚者可以补血以助气;阴虚者可以补阳以生阴(称为"阳中求阴"),阳虚者可以补阴以助阳(称为"阴中求阳")。

(三) 阴阳消长

阴阳消长,是说在阴阳的相互作用过程中,双方总是表现出此消则彼长,此长则彼消的运动变化形式。其具体表现形式如:阴消则阳长,阴长则阳消,阳消则阴长,阳长则阴消。

在正常情况下,阴阳双方的互为消长总是保持在一定的范围之内。"消"至一定程度会转为"长","长"至一定程度则转为"消",因此"消"与"长"都不会过度。"消"与"长"相互交替,周而复始,形成一种动态的阴阳平衡。

如果阴阳消长超出了正

normal level, relative predominance or relative decline of either yin or yang will arise, consequently damaging the dynamic balance between yin and yang and leading to imbalance of yin and yang.

1.1.2.4 Mutual transformation between yin and yang

If yin or yang wanes or waxes to the extreme point, it will turn to the opposite. That means yin will change into yang and yang into yin. The key element involved in such a mutual transformation is the degree of wane and wax. The degree that leads to transformation is termed "extreme point" or "excess" in TCM. In *Huangdi Neijing*, it suggests that "extreme cold generates heat", "extreme heat generates cold", "excessive yin turns into yang" and "excessive yang changes into yin", all reflecting mutual transformation relationship between yin and yang.

The typical mutual transformation process of yin and yang is well signified by the variations of yin and yang in the four seasons of a year. From spring to summer, yang waxes while yin wanes. However when such a transformation reaches the peak — the Summer Solstice, yin begins to wax while yang starts to wane. From autumn to winter, yin waxes while yang wanes. But when such a transformation reaches the peak — the Winter Solstice, yang begins to wax while yin starts to wane. Such a change exactly explains the idea that "excessive yin turns into yang" and "excessive yang changes into yin". With the wane and wax of yin and yang, cold and heat in the climate also alternate. Such an alternation vividly demonstrates the theory that "extreme cold generates heat" and "extreme heat generates cold".

常范围,就出现阴阳偏盛或偏衰的变化,于是动态的阴阳平衡就会被打破,从而导致阴阳失调。

(四)阴阳转化

阴阳转化,是说在阴阳消长的前提下,如果"消"或"长"至极点,可以向相反的方面转化,即阴可以转变为阳,阳可以转变为阴。值得注意的是,引起阴阳转化的关键因素是消长的量度,必须到达特定的转折点。这一转折点,中医学用"极"、"重"等字来形容。《黄帝内经》提出"寒极生热"、"热极生寒"、"重阴必阳"、"重阳必阴"等理论,都属于阴阳转化的范畴。

从一年四季的阴阳变化中,可以看到一个阴阳转化的典型过程。从春至夏,属于阳长而阴消,但到达特定的时间转折点——夏至,阴阳消长出现逆转,转变为阴长而阳消;秋冬阴长而阳消,到达另一个特定的时间转折点——冬至,又逆转为阳长而阴消,这就体现了"重阴必阳、重阳必阴"的过程。随着阴阳消长的变化,气候也出现寒热的交替,从而表现为"寒极生热、热极生寒"。

1.1.3　Application of the theory of yin and yang in TCM

1.1.3.1　Explanation of the histological structure of the human body

TCM believes that the human body is an organic whole and that all the tissues and organs in the body depend on each other in function. Such an interdependence between these tissues and organs can also be explained according to the theory of yin and yang. That is why it is said in *Huangdi Neijing* that "man has a physical shape which is inseparable from yin and yang". Generally speaking, the upper part of the body pertains to yang while the lower part to yin; the exterior pertains to yang while the interior to yin; the back pertains to yang while the chest and the abdomen to yin; the chest pertains to yang because it is located in the upper part of the body while the abdomen to yin because it is located in the lower part of the body; the lateral sides of the four limbs pertain to yang while the medial sides to yin. As to the zang-organs and the fu-organs, the five zang-organs pertain to yin because they store essence, but never discharge it; the six fu-organs pertain to yang because they transport and transform food, but never store it. Among the five zang-organs, the heart and the lung are located in the chest, so they pertain to yang; but the liver, the spleen and the kidney are located in the abdomen, so they pertain to yin. Each organ itself can be further divided into yin and yang aspects, such as heart-yin and heart-yang, kidney-yin and kidney-yang, etc.

1.1.3.2　Explanation of the relationship between structure and function

The theory of yin and yang holds that the normal activities of life result from the balance between yin and

三、阴阳学说在中医学中的应用

(一) 用于说明人体组织结构的属性

中医学认为,人体是一个有机的整体,其体内一切相关组织结构之间,都存在着阴阳对立依存的关系,因此也都可用阴阳来说明这些组织结构的属性,故《黄帝内经》有"人生有形,不离阴阳"的说法。从大体部位来说,人体上部属阳,下部属阴;体表属阳,体内属阴;背部属阳,胸腹部属阴;胸在上属阳,腹在下属阴;四肢外侧属阳,四肢内侧属阴。若以脏腑来分,五脏藏精气而不泻,属阴;六腑传化物而不藏,属阳。五脏之中,心肺居胸中,属阳;肝脾肾居腹中,属阴。而每一脏腑又各有阴阳之分,如心阴、心阳、肾阴、肾阳等。

(二) 用于说明人体结构与功能的关系

阴阳学说认为,人体的正常生命活动,是阴阳两个方面

yang and that the close relationship between histological structure and physiological functions signifies the opposition and the unity between yin and yang. The histological structure of the body, including the viscera, the meridians, qi, blood and body fluid, all pertains to yin because they are all substantial. However, their functions all pertain to yang. Thus there is an intrinsical relationship between substances that pertain to yin and functions that pertain to yang, i.e. the mutual opposition, interdependence, wane and wax as well as transformation of yin and yang. In terms of the interdependence between yin and yang, the human body relies on the viscera, the meridians, qi, blood and body fluid to perform and maintain its physiological functions. On the other hand, the metabolism of qi, blood and body fluid depends on the functional activities of the related viscera. Similarly, the performance of various functional activities will inevitably consume qi, blood and body fluid. This process is marked by wax of yang and wane of yin. Besides, constant transformation and generation of nutrients must rely on the functional activities of the viscera and consume certain amount of energy. This process is characterized by wax of yin and wane of yang. This process of metabolism is also accompanied by mutual transformation of yin and yang between substances and functions. Only when the balance between yin and yang is ensured in this series of physiological process can normal state of life be maintained.

1.1.3.3　Explanation of pathogenesis

When the balance between yin and yang in the body is damaged, it leads to various diseases known as "imbalance between yin and yang". Though complicated, pathological

保持着协调平衡的结果，而组织结构与生理功能之间的密切联系，正是阴阳对立统一的一种体现形式。人体的组织结构，包括脏腑经络和气血津液等物质基础均属于阴，其功能活动则属于阳。属阴的物质与属阳的功能之间，存在着阴阳的对立、依存、消长以及转化的关系。若从阴阳依存方面来说，人体生理功能的产生和维持，要以脏腑经络、气血津液等作为物质基础，而气血津液的新陈代谢过程，也要依赖有关脏腑的功能活动。同时，人体各种功能活动的产生，必然要消耗气血津液等营养物质，这属于阳长阴消的运动变化过程；而营养物质的不断化生，又必须依赖于脏腑的功能活动并消耗一定的能量，这又属于阴长阳消的运动变化过程。在此新陈代谢的运动变化过程中，还存在着物质与功能之间阴阳转化的关系。只有这一系列的生理过程保持阴阳相对平衡的状态，人体才能维持"阴平阳秘"的正常生命状态。

（三）用于说明基本病机变化

当人体阴阳之间的平衡协调关系遭到破坏时，便会出现一系列病理变化而产生各

changes generally fall into two categories: relative predominance of yin or yang and relative decline of yin or yang, according to the analysis of pathogenesis with the theory of yin and yang.

1. Relative predominance of yin or yang

Relative predominance of yin and yang, a pathological change due to excessive increase of yin and yang, includes two aspects: relative predominance of yin and relative predominance of yang. Yin or yang that becomes predominant inevitably turns into a pathogenic factor. So predominant yin becomes a pathogenic factor of yin nature and predominant yang a pathogenic factor of yang nature.

Relative predominance of yang, usually caused by invasion of pathogenic factors of yang nature or exuberant heat transforming from the pathogenic factors of yin nature activated by yang, is a manifestation of excess-heat syndrome known as "predominance of yang leading to heat" in *Huangdi Neijing*. Pathogenic factors of different nature impair the corresponding healthy qi in the body. So pathogenic factors of yang nature tends to consumption of yin-fluid in the course of pathological changes. That is why it is said in *Huangdi Neijing* that "predominance of yang leading to disease of yin." "Disease" here means impairment. For example, invasion of pathogenic heat into the body will make yang-qi in the body hyperactive, leading to high fever, sweating, reddish complexion and rapid pulse. With the progress of the morbid condition, pathogenic factors of yang nature consume yin-fluid in the body, bringing on thirst, scanty urine and constipation.

Relative predominance of yin is usually caused by invasion of pathogenic factors of yin nature into the body, leading to exuberance of yin-cold and bringing on excess-cold syndrome known as "predominance of yin leading to

种疾病,这叫做"阴阳失调"。人体的病理变化虽然复杂,但用阴阳学说来分析其基本的病机,不外乎阴阳偏盛和阴阳偏衰两个方面。

1.阴阳偏盛

阴阳偏盛,也可称阴阳偏胜,是由于阴阳增长超过了正常的范围而出现的一种病理变化,包括阳偏盛和阴偏盛两个方面。偏盛的阴或阳就成了致病的邪气,阴偏盛则属于阴邪,阳偏盛则属于阳邪。

阳偏盛,多由阳邪侵犯人体,或感受阴邪从阳化热,造成体内阳热之气亢盛,而表现出实热证的病证性质,此即《黄帝内经》所说的"阳胜则热"。由于不同性质的邪气能够损伤人体与之相对的正气,所以在病变过程中,阳邪还容易损伤人体的阴液,故《黄帝内经》指出:"阳胜则阴病"。这里的"病",是损伤的意思。例如热邪侵入人体,使体内阳气偏盛,出现高热、汗出、面红、脉数等实热证候,随着病情进一步发展,阳邪耗伤了机体的阴液,又可出现口渴、尿少、便秘等阴液受损的症状。

阴偏盛,多由阴邪侵犯人体,导致体内阴寒之气亢盛,从而引起实寒证的病证性质,此即《黄帝内经》所说的"阴胜

cold" in *Huangdi Neijing*. If pathogenic factors of yin nature further impair yang-qi in the body, a pathogenesis of "predominance of yin leading to disease of yang" will arise, as is recorded in *Huangdi Neijing*. Take pathogenic cold for example. When it invades the body, it leads to cold symptoms like aversion to cold, cold limbs and cold abdominal pain on the one hand, and symptoms due to yang-deficiency like floating whitish complexion, lassitude, frequent lying on bed, slow and weak pulse on the other hand.

Besides, when relative predominance of yin or yang develops to the extreme point, mutual transformation will occur under certain condition according to the principle of inter-transformation between yin and yang. That is to say that yin-cold syndrome will turn into yang-heat syndrome and vice versa.

2. Relative decline of yin or yang

Relative decline of yin or yang refers to pathological changes of yin or yang that declines below the normal level, including relative decline of yin and relative decline of yang. This morbid state mainly results from insufficiency of healthy qi in the body. To be specific, relative decline of yin refers to insufficiency of yin-fluid and relative decline of yang to insufficiency of yang-qi in the body. Usually relative decline of yin or yang leads to the imbalance between yin and yang which brings on hypofunction of the viscera.

Relative decline of yang refers to deficiency-cold syndrome due to insufficiency of yang-qi that fails to restrain yin-cold and warm the viscera. The usual clinical symptoms are whitish complexion, aversion to cold, spontaneous sweating, slow and weak pulse. This morbid state was described as "deficiency of yang leading to cold" in *Huangdi Neijing*.

则寒"。如果阴邪进一步损伤了人体的阳气，又可出现《黄帝内经》所说"阴胜则阳病"的病机变化。例如寒邪侵入人体，患者一方面可出现恶寒肢冷、腹部冷痛等实寒症状，另一方面也可表现出面色㿠白、倦怠喜卧、脉迟无力等阳虚之象。

此外，根据阴阳转化的原理，阴阳偏盛的病变发展到极点，还可在一定的条件下发生相互转化，如阴寒证可转化为阳热证，阳热证可转化为阴寒证。

2. 阴阳偏衰

阴阳偏衰，是由于阴阳消减超过了正常范围而出现的病理变化，包括阴偏衰和阳偏衰两个方面。阴阳偏衰属于人体正气不足的范畴，其中阴偏衰指人体的阴液不足，阳偏衰指人体的阳气不足。阴阳偏衰既引起阴阳失调，又导致脏腑功能减退。

阳偏衰，指人体阳气不足，不能制约阴寒之气，脏腑失于温养，出现虚寒证的病证性质，临床可见面白、畏寒、自汗、脉迟弱等症状，即《黄帝内经》所谓"阳虚则寒"。

Relative decline of yin refers to deficiency-heat syndrome due to insufficiency of yin-fluid that fails to restrain yang-heat and nourish the viscera. The usual clinical symptoms are reddish complexion, tidal fever, night sweating, thin and rapid pulse. This morbid state was described as "deficiency of yin leading to heat" in *Huangdi Neijing*.

Since yin and yang depend on each other and no one can exist without the other, relative decline of yin or yang may affect each other with the development of pathological changes. That is to say that prolonged deficiency of yin will lead to deficiency of yang and protracted deficiency of yang will bring on insufficiency of yin-fluid, eventually resulting in deficiency of both yin and yang.

When relative predominance of yin or yang and relative decline of yin or yang become extremely serious, it will lead to declination of healthy qi and bring on special changes of pathogenesis known as "loss of yin" and "loss of yang" which consequently cause death due to separation of yin and yang.

1.1.3.4 Diagnosis and syndrome differentiation

The occurrence, development and changes of disease, according to the theory of yin and yang, lie in the imbalance between yin and yang. Clinically all kinds of diseases, including pathological changes of complexion, voice and pulse condition as well as the nature of diseases, can be generalized and analyzed with the theory of yin and yang.

Diagnostically, the theory of yin and yang can be used to analyze the data collected with the four diagnostic methods and differentiate the nature of disease, which is an important method for making correct diagnosis. That is

阴偏衰,指人体阴液不足,不能制约阳热之气,脏腑失于滋养,出现虚热证的病证性质,临床可见面红、潮热、盗汗、脉细数等症状,即《黄帝内经》所谓"阴虚则热"。

由于阴阳双方互相依赖,互相化生,任何一方都不能脱离对方而单独存在,因此阴阳偏衰的病变进一步发展,还可以互相影响,即阴虚日久会引起阳气虚损,阳虚日久也会引起阴液不足,从而出现阴阳两虚证。

阴阳偏盛和阴阳偏衰发展到极其严重的程度,还可能导致人体正气衰竭,出现所谓"亡阴"和"亡阳"的特殊病机变化。亡阴、亡阳的最终结果是导致阴阳离决而死亡。

(四) 用于诊断与辨证

阴阳学说认为,由于疾病的发生、发展和变化的根本原因均在于阴阳失调,所以临床上各种疾病,包括其色泽、声音、脉象等症状表现,以及病证的性质,都可以用阴阳来加以概括和说明。

首先在诊断方面,可运用阴阳学说对四诊所收集的资料来进行具体地分析,首先判明疾病的阴阳性质,这是作出

why it is said in *Huangdi Neijing* that one should "observe complexion and take pulse, differentiating yin and yang first." Take complexion, voice, disposition, nature of disease and pulse for example. Bright complexion pertains to yang while grayish complexion to yin; sonorous voice pertains to yang while low and weak voice to yin; preference for cold and aversion to heat pertain to yang while preference for heat and aversion to cold to yin; floating, slippery, rapid and full pulse states pertain to yang while deep, unsmooth, slow and thin pulse conditions to yin.

In syndrome differentiation, syndromes are usually differentiated from the aspects of yin and yang, external and internal, deficiency and excess, cold and heat which are the general principles for differentiating disease and syndrome, known as "syndrome differentiation with eight principles". Among these eight principles, yin and yang are regarded as the general ones. According to such a gradation, external syndrome, excess syndrome and heat syndrome are yang syndromes while internal syndrome, deficiency syndrome and cold syndrome are yin syndromes. The theory of yin and yang are also used to differentiate visceral syndromes. Take visceral deficiency syndrome for example. It can be divided into heart-yin deficiency, heart-yang deficiency, kidney-yin deficiency, kidney-yang deficiency, spleen-yang deficiency and liver-yin deficiency. Clinically the basic principle for differentiating syndrome is to differentiate yin syndrome and yang syndrome.

1.1.3.5 Guiding clinical treatment

1. Deciding the therapeutic principles

(1) Therapeutic principles for relative predominance of yin and yang: Since the basic pathogenesis of relative predominance of yin and yang is the exuberance of patho-

正确诊断的重要方法。所以《黄帝内经》指出："察色按脉，先别阴阳。"如从色泽的明暗来看，色泽鲜明者为阳，色泽晦暗者为阴；从语声的高低来看，声音高亢洪亮者为阳，声音低微无力者为阴；从患者性情的喜恶来看，喜寒恶热者为阳，喜热恶寒者为阴；从脉象形态来看，凡浮、滑、数、洪等脉象皆属阳，凡沉、涩、迟、细等脉象皆属阴。

其次在辨证方面，临床上往往首先从疾病性质的阴阳、表里、虚实、寒热等方面来进行辨证，认为这是辨别一切病证的纲领，所以称之为"八纲辨证"。但其中的"阴阳"两纲，又可看作是八纲辨证的总纲。也就是说，表证、实证、热证皆属阳证，里证、虚证、寒证皆属阴证。又如在脏腑辨证中，也常结合阴阳来进行分析，如脏腑虚证分类中有心阴虚、心阳虚、肾阴虚、肾阳虚、脾阳虚、肝阴虚等证候。所以辨别疾病的阴证、阳证，是辨证的基本原则，在临床上具有重要的指导意义。

（五）用于指导临床治疗

1. 确定治疗原则

（1）阴阳偏盛的治疗原则

由于阴阳偏盛的基本病机均表现为邪气盛的实证，故治

genic factors, the treatment must follow the therapeutic principle that "excess should be reduced". To be specific, excess-heat syndrome due to the exuberance of pathogenic factors of yang nature should be treated by clearing away heat while excess-cold syndrome due to the exuberance of pathogenic factors of yin nature should be treated by eliminating cold. Further development of relative predominance of yin and yang may lead to consumption of yin-fluid by yang-heat or impairment of yang-qi by yin-cold, which should be treated by elimination of pathogenic factors in combination with deficiency-supplementing therapy, i. e. combination of the therapy for clearing away heat with the therapy for nourishing yin or combination of the therapy for eliminating cold with the therapy for tonifying yang.

(2) Therapeutic principle for relative decline of yin and yang: Since the basic pathogenesis of relative decline of yin and yang is insufficiency of the healthy qi, the treatment must follow the principle that "deficiency should be supplemented". To be specific, deficiency-cold syndrome due to insufficiency of yang-qi should be treated by nourishing yang while deficiency-heat syndrome due to deficiency of yin-fluid should be treated by nourishing yin. Further development of relative decline of yin and yang may lead to deficiency of yin due to prolonged deficiency of yang or deficiency of yang due to protracted deficiency of yin, bringing on deficiency of both yin and yang which should be treated by nourishing both yin and yang or mainly nourishing yang with the consideration of yin or mainly nourishing yin with the consideration of yang.

2. Generalization of the properties of drugs

TCM believes that all drugs possess four properties, five flavors and four acting tendencies (namely ascending, descending, sinking and floating) which are generalized according to the theory of yin and yang.

疗时须遵循"实者泻之"即祛除邪气的原则。具体来说,凡是阳邪偏盛所出现的实热证,可采用清热的治法;凡是阴邪偏盛所出现的实寒证,可采用祛寒的治法。如果阴阳偏盛的病变进一步发展,阳热之邪损伤了人体的阴液,或阴寒之邪损伤了人体的阳气,则应当在祛邪的同时兼顾补虚的方法,即用清热法配合补阴,或用祛寒法配合补阳。

（2）阴阳偏衰的治疗原则

阴阳偏衰的基本病机均表现为正气不足的虚证,故治疗时须遵循"虚者补之"即扶助正气的原则。具体来说,凡是阳气不足而出现的虚寒证,采用补阳的治法;凡是阴液亏虚而出现的虚热证,采用补阴的治法。如果阴阳偏衰的病变进一步发展,阳虚日久引起阴虚,或阴虚日久引起阳虚,从而出现阴阳两虚证,则又当阴阳双补,或补阳为主兼顾补阴,或补阴为主兼顾补阳。

2. 归纳药物性能

中医学认为,各种药物都具有四气、五味以及升降浮沉等性能,并用阴阳理论来归纳这些性能。

The four properties refer to cold, hot, warm and cool nature of drugs. Drugs of hot and warm nature pertain to yang while drugs of cold and cool nature belong to yin. The former are usually used to treat cold syndrome while the latter to treat heat syndrome.

The five flavors refer to acrid, sweet, sour, bitter and salty tastes of drugs. There is another flavor known as bland which is not as distinct as any of the five flavors. Drugs of different flavors bear different effects and are categorized differently in terms of yin and yang. For example, acrid flavor disperses, sweet flavor nourishes and bland flavor oozes. So the acrid, sweet and bland flavors pertain to yang. Sour flavor astringes, bitter flavor purges and salty flavor moistens. So the sour, bitter and salty flavors pertain to yin.

The concept of ascending, descending, sinking and floating is a generalization of the acting tendencies of drugs. Drugs tending to ascend and disperse pertain to yang while drugs tending to descend and tranquilize pertain to yin.

To generalize the properties and acting tendencies of drugs with the theory of yin and yang is to guide clinic differentiation of syndrome. Clinically only when relative predominance or decline of yin and yang is clearly differentiated, correct therapeutic principles are decided and proper drugs are selected according to their properties, flavors and effects can satisfactory curative effect be obtained and therapeutic aim be realized.

1.2　Wuxing（the five elements）

The theory of the five elements, just as the theory of yin and yang, originated in antiquity in China. It is the

四气也称四性,有寒、热、温、凉之别。其中热药、温药属阳,寒药、凉药属阴。温热性质的药物一般用来治疗寒证,寒凉性质的药物一般用来治疗热证。

五味指药味,包括辛、甘、酸、苦、咸五种。另有一种五味皆轻薄的称为淡味。不同的药味具有不同的作用,阴阳属性也不相同。如辛味能发散,甘味能补益,淡味能渗泄,故辛、甘、淡属阳;而酸味可收敛,苦味可泻降,咸味可润下,故酸、苦、咸属阴。

升降浮沉,是对药物作用趋向的一种概括。凡是具有升浮即上升、发散作用的药物均属阳,凡是具有降沉即下降、重镇作用的药物均属阴。

用阴阳理论归纳药物性能,是为临床辨证论治服务的。临床治疗疾病,只有在辨清阴阳偏盛或偏衰并制定正确治疗原则的基础上,再结合药物的性味功能,选用适宜的药物,才能收到良好的疗效,达到治愈疾病的目的。

第二节　五行

五行学说与阴阳学说一样,也产生于中国的远古时

cognition of the material world made by people in ancient China. This theory was used to explain and analyze things and their changes in the natural world in ancient times. The theory of the five elements, together with the theory of yin and yang, formed a special world outlook in ancient China. Later on the theory of the five elements was applied to TCM and became one of the important components in the theoretical system of TCM.

期,是古人在长期的生活和生产实践中所形成的对物质世界的一种认识,并成为古代用来解释和分析自然界中的所有事物及其变化的思维方法,它和阴阳学说一起构成了中国古代一种独特的宇宙观。五行学说后来被运用于中医学的领域,就成了中医学理论体系的组成部分之一。

1.2.1 The implication of the five elements and the categorization of things according to the theory of the five elements

一、五行的含义与事物五行属性的划分

People in ancient China believed that wood, fire, earth, metal and water are indispensable to daily life and productive labor and that these five elements were key to the normal variations in the natural world. For example, people drink water and use fire to cook food; metal and wood can be made into various tools; earth ensures the growth of all things. Besides, these elements are interrelated and influence each other. Such a cognition and understanding eventually evolved into the theory of the five elements.

远古时期的人们认为,木、火、土、金、水这五种物质是日常生活及生产劳动中不可缺少的东西,也是构成自然界正常变化的五种重要的基本元素,如水、火是人们饮食所需要的,金、木可制成各种用具,土则能化生万物,并且这些物质之间又是相互联系、相互作用的,这样就逐渐形成了五行理论。

1.2.1.1 Implication of the five elements

In Chinese, "wu" refers to five categories of things in the natural world, namely wood, fire, earth, metal and water; "xing" means movement and transformation. So "wuxing" (the five elements) actually refers to the movement and transformation of these five elements as well as their interrelationships.

The theory of the five elements holds that all things in the natural world are derived from wood, fire, earth,

(一) 五行的含义

"五",是指自然界中的木、火、土、金、水五类物质;"行",是指运动和变化。五行,就是指木、火、土、金、水这五类物质的运动变化及其相互之间的关系。

五行学说认为,世界上一切事物都是由木、火、土、金、

metal and water. So they all bear the basic properties of these five elements and maintain a harmonious balance through the activities of constant inter-promotion and inter-restraint among the five elements.

1.2.1.2　Categorization of things according to the properties of the five elements

Since wood, fire, earth, metal and water are five categories of the main objects in the natural world, possess specific properties and depend on each other to exist, people in ancient China divided and explained the properties of things according to the characteristics of the five elements.

As to the characteristics of the five elements, the early understanding concentrated on the primary properties of wood, fire, earth, metal and water in the natural world, such as "water moistens and flows downward", "fire flames up", "wood can be flexed and extended", "metal can be changed in form" and "earth can grow crops", etc. In order to explain the properties of more things, people abstracted the properties of the five elements for extensive application and extended their implications. For example, the properties of flexing and extending, growth and development as well as free activity all pertain to the category of wood; warmth, heat, ascending and brightness all pertain to the category of fire; reception, cultivation and transformation all pertain to the category of earth; change, depuration and astringency all pertain to the category of metal; and moistening, downward movement, cold and coolness as well as closure and storage all pertain to the category of water.

In the light of the basic properties of the five elements, analogy and induction can be used to categorize things in order to decide the properties of different things. The first step is to compare the image, properties

水这五类基本物质所衍化生成,都具有五行的基本特性,并且在不断的相互资生、相互制约的运动变化之中维持着整体的协调与平衡。

(二) 事物五行属性的划分

由于木、火、土、金、水是自然界中主要的五类物质,彼此之间各有特性,同时又相互依存,因此人们就利用五行的特性来划分和说明一切事物的属性。

关于五行特性,人们最早认识到的是自然界木、火、土、金、水五种物质的原始属性,如水性滋润、向下,火性炎热、向上,木可弯曲、伸直,金可进行变革,土可播种、收获等。为了说明和解释更多的事物属性,人们又将五行特性进一步抽象地加以引申运用,使其具有了更广泛的涵义,如曲直、生长、升发、舒畅等,均属于木的特性;温热、上升、明亮等,均属于火的特性;受纳、承载、生化等,均属于土的特性;变革、肃杀、收敛等,均属于金的特性;滋润、向下、寒凉、闭藏等,均属于水的特性。

在掌握了五行基本特性的基础上,就可以运用归类法和推演法,对所有的事物进行分类,以确定不同事物的五行

and functions of things with the abstracted properties of the five elements respectively. If it is similar to the properties of one element, then it pertains to the category of that element. For example, the sun rises in the east according to the geographical location of China. In this case the east is similar to wood in properties, so it pertains to wood. The south is hot and similar to fire in properties. So the south pertains to fire. The west is mountainous with high terrain and cold climate, similar to the properties of metal. That is why the west pertains to metal. The north is cold and snowy with deeply latent terrestrial qi, similar to the properties of water. Thus the north pertains to water. The central region of China is mild in climate and rich in crops, similar to the properties of earth. Therefore the central region pertains to earth. Take the four seasons for another example. Spring, characterized by gradual ascendance of yang-qi, warm weather and resuscitation of all things, is similar to the properties of wood. So spring pertains to wood. Summer, characterized by hot weather and luxuriant growth of all things, is similar to the properties of fire. That is why summer pertains to fire. Autumn, characterized by decrease of yang-qi and decline of all things in the natural world, is similar to the properties of metal. Thus autumn pertains to metal. Winter, characterized by cold weather and storage of all things, is similar to the properties of water. For this reason winter pertains to water.

For dealing with things difficult to compare directly with the abstract properties of the five elements, inference and deduction can be used to decide the properties of these things in the light of the properties of other related things induced according to the defined properties of the known things. Take the liver for example. The physiological characteristic of the liver is to function freely, quite similar

属性。首先将事物的形象、性质、作用等分别与五行的抽象特性进行比较,如果与某一行的特性相类似,就归属于某一行中。如就中国的地理环境而言,太阳从东方升起,与木的升发特性相类似,故东方属木;南方气候炎热,与火的温热特性相类似,故南方属火;西方多崇山峻岭,地势高而寒,与金的肃杀特性相类似,故西方属金;北方气候寒冷,多冰雪,地气潜藏,与水的寒凉、闭藏特性相类似,故北方属水;中国中原地区气候温适宜,物产丰富,与土的生化特性相类似,故中央之地属土。又如春天阳气渐升,天气温和,万物萌生,与木的舒展生发特性相类似,故春季属木;夏天气候炎热,万物盛长,与火的炎热升腾特性相类似,故夏季属火;秋天阳气下降,万物凋落,与金的收敛肃杀特性相类似,故秋季属金;冬天气候寒冷,万物潜藏,与水的寒凉闭藏特性相类似,故冬季属水,等等。

其次,对于一些与五行的抽象特性无法进行直接比较的事物,可以采用推演的方法,即根据已知的某些事物的五行属性,再推演至与其相关的其他事物,从而得知这些事物的五行属性。如人体肝的生理特性

to the properties of wood. So the liver pertains to wood in the five elements. However, the gallbladder, tendon and eyes are difficult to compare with the properties of the five elements directly. Because these organs and tissues are intrinsically related to the liver, they also pertain to wood.

In this way TCM classifies, with the methods of categorization, inference and deduction, various things in the natural world as well as the viscera, organs and tissues in the human body respectively into the categories of wood, fire, earth, metal and water according to their properties, thus formulating a structural system of the five elements with close interrelationship between the internal and external environments of the body. This structural system of the five elements mainly includes the five flavors, the five colors, the five transformations, the five kinds of qi, the five directions and the five seasons as well as the five zang-organs, the five fu-organs, the five sensory organs, five constituents (tendon, vessel muscle, skin and bone), the five emotions, the five kinds of liquids and the five states of pulse in the human body as illustrated in the following table.

是喜条达,这与木的舒畅特性相类似,故肝的五行属性为木,而胆、筋、目等却无法与五行的特性直接类比,但这些器官组织又与肝有着内在的密切联系,于是就随肝而归属于木。

因此,中医学理论用归类和推演的方法,将自然界的各种事物和人体的脏腑、器官、组织,按其不同的属性分别归类于木、火、土、金、水五行之中,从而形成人体内外环境相互联系的五行结构系统。五行结构系统的主要内容包括自然界中五味、五色、五化、五气、五方、五季及人体中五脏、五腑、五官、五体、五志、五液、五脉等。我们把上述内容与五行的对应关系归纳成"五行结构系统表"如下。

Table 1 - 1　The structural system of the five elements

Nature							Five Elements	Human body						
Five Notes	Five Flavors	Five Colours	Five Transformations	Five Kinds of Qi	Five Directions	Five Seasons		Five Zang-Organs	Five Fu-Organs	Five Sensory Organs	Five Constituents	Five Emotions	Five Kinds of Liquids	Five States of Pulse
Jue	Sour	Green	Germination	Wind	East	Spring	Wood	Liver	Gallbladder	Eye	Tendon	Anger	Tear	Taut
Zhi	Bitter	Red	Growth	Heat	South	Summer	Fire	Heart	Small Intestine	Tongue	Vessel	Joy	Sweating	Bounding
Gong	Sweet	Yellow	Transformation	Dampness	Center	Late Summer	Earth	Spleen	Stomach	Mouth	Muscle	Contemplation	Saliva	Moderate
Shang	Pungent	White	Reaping	Dryness	West	Autumn	Metal	Lung	Large Intestine	Nose	Skin & Hair	Grief	Snivel	Superficial
Yu	Salty	Black	Storing	Cold	North	Winter	Water	Kidney	Urinary Bladder	Ear	Bone	Fear	Spittle	Deep

五行结构系统表

自　　然　　界							五	人　　　　体						
五音	五味	五色	五化	五气	五方	五季	行	五脏	五腑	五官	五体	五志	五液	五脉
角	酸	青	生	风	东	春	木	肝	胆	目	筋	怒	泪	弦
徵	苦	赤	长	暑	南	夏	火	心	小肠	舌	脉	喜	汗	洪
宫	甘	黄	化	湿	中	长夏	土	脾	胃	口	肉	思	涎	缓
商	辛	白	收	燥	西	秋	金	肺	大肠	鼻	皮	悲	涕	浮
羽	咸	黑	藏	寒	北	冬	水	肾	膀胱	耳	骨	恐	唾	沉

1.2.2　Interactions among the five elements

The five elements possess specific properties respectively. They are related to each other and act on other. Though the five categories of things classified according to the properties of the five elements are complicated and changeable, they still can be expounded with the theory of the five elements. The interactions among the five elements are either normal or abnormal. The former includes inter-promotion and inter-restraint and the latter includes over restraint (or subjugation) and reverse restraint which are actually the abnormal manifestations of inter-restraint.

1.2.2.1　Inter-promotion and inter-restraint among the five elements

1. Inter-promotion

Inter-promotion means that one thing bears the effect of promoting or generating another in the five elements. The order of inter-promotion among the five elements follows certain rules and forms a circle, i. e. wood promoting fire, fire promoting earth, earth promoting metal, metal promoting water and water promoting wood. The

二、五行之间的相互作用

五行之间各有特性，又相互作用，相互联系，故根据五行特性而划分的五类事物，虽然彼此之间关系复杂而多变，但仍可用五行理论来进行说明。五行之间相互作用有正常和异常两种情形，五行的相生与相克属于正常的相互作用，五行的相乘与相侮属于异常的相互作用。相乘与相侮，实质上是相克作用的反常表现。

（一）五行的相生与相克

1. 相生

相生，是指五行之间一种事物对另一种事物具有促进和资生的作用。五行相生的次序是按一定的规律排列的，并构成一个循环相生环，即木生火，火生土，土生金，金生

one that generates is called "mother" while the one that is generated is termed "child". So the inter-promotion relationship among the five elements is also called mother-child relationship. Take fire for example. The one that generates fire is wood and the one that is generated by fire is earth. So wood is the mother of fire and earth is the child of fire.

2. Inter-restraint

Inter-restraint means that one thing controls and restrains another thing in the five elements. The order of inter-restraint also follows certain rules and forms a circle, i. e. wood restraining earth, earth restraining water, water restraining fire, fire restraining metal and metal restraining wood. Since the thing being restrained "cannot dominate the one that controls it" and the thing restraining another "dominates the one that it controls", the inter-restraint relationship among the five elements is also known as the relationship of domination and submission. Take water for example. The one that restrains water is earth and the one that is restrained by water is fire. For this reason, earth is called the dominator of water and fire is called the submitter of water.

3. The relationship between inter-promotion and inter-restraint

Inter-promotion and inter-restraint among the five elements are in fact inseparable. Without promotion, nothing can grow and develop; without restraint, there will be no way to prevent harm caused by excessive development of things. Only when restraint exists in promotion and promotion in restraint can the normal development and harmonious balance of things be maintained.

Besides, inter-promotion and inter-restraint among the five elements restrict each other to avoid harm resulting from

水,水生木。由于"生我"者为我之"母","我生"者为我之"子",所以五行相生关系又叫做母子关系。如以火行为例,生我者为木,我生者为土,故称木为火之母,土为火之子。

2. 相克

相克,是指五行之间一种事物对另一种事物具有制约的作用。其次序也有一定的规律,并构成一个循环相克环,即木克土,土克水,水克火,火克金,金克木。由于"克我"者制约我,为我之"所不胜","我克"者受我制约,为我之"所胜",因此五行相克关系又叫做所胜、所不胜关系。如以水行为例,克我者为土,我克者为火,故称土为水之所不胜,火为水之所胜。

3. 相生与相克的关系

五行的相生与相克,是不可分割的两个方面。没有生,就没有事物的发生和成长;没有克,就不能防止事物因过于发展而造成的危害,所以只有生中有克,克中有生,才能维持事物的正常发展变化及其平衡协调状态。

五行相生与相克之间还存在着相互制约关系,即相生

excessive promotion and over restraint. For example, wood restrains earth, earth generates metal and metal, in turn, restrains wood. If wood is too powerful, it will over restrain earth and bring on harm. However, metal generated by earth can protect earth by restricting wood. Again take wood for example. Only under the normal restraint of metal can wood generate fire. If wood excessively generates fire, fire will become superabundant and turn to restrain metal. Consequently metal will be weakened in restraining wood and wood will become feeble in generating fire. In such a way automatic regulation within the five elements is realized through mutual restriction between inter-promotion and inter-restraint.

1.2.2.2 Over restraint and reverse restraint

1. Over restraint

Over restraint refers to an abnormal state in which one element among the five elements excessively restrains another element. The order of over restraint is the same as that of inter-restraint, i. e. wood over restraining earth, earth over restraining water, water over restraining fire, fire over restraining metal and metal over restraining wood. There are two causes responsible for over restraint:

One is that one element among the five elements becomes too powerful and, in turn, excessively restrains the element that it normally restrains, damaging the normal restraint relationship between them. For example, if wood is too powerful, it will excessively restrain earth; if water is too strong, it will excessively restrain fire.

The other is that one element among the five elements becomes weak and therefore provides the element normally restraining it a chance to excessively restrain it, damaging the normal restraint relationship between them. For example, if earth becomes weak, it will be excessive-

作用能防止克制过度带来的不利影响,相克作用也能制约相生太过造成的危害。如木能克土,土能生金,金又克木;如果木太强,则克土太过,土即受害,但土所生之金制约了木,也就保护了土。又如木在金的正常克制下才能生火,如果木生火太过,火气旺而金受制,金克木的作用减弱,木生火的作用也就减弱。这样通过生与克的相互制约而实现了五行系统内部的自动调节。

（二）五行的相乘与相侮

1. 相乘

相乘,是指五行之间一种事物对另一种事物制约过度的异常状态。相乘的次序与相克的次序是一致的,即木乘土,土乘水,水乘火,火乘金,金乘木。引起相乘的原因有两方面:

一是五行中的某一行出现太过,导致对"所胜"的一行制约太过,从而破坏了两者之间正常的相克关系。如木旺则乘土,水盛则乘火等。

二是五行中的某一行出现不及,引起"所不胜"一行对它的制约过度,从而破坏了两者之间正常的相克关系。如土虚则木乘,水虚则土乘等。

ly restrained by wood; if water is weak, it will be excessively restrained by earth.

2. Reverse restraint

Reverse restraint refers to an abnormal state in
which one element among the five elements reversely restrains and bullies another element. That is why this
phenomenon is called reverse restraint. The order of reverse restraint is just opposite to that of inter-restraint,
i.e. wood reversely restraining metal, metal reversely
restraining fire, fire reversely restraining water, water
reversely restraining earth and earth reversely restraining
wood. There are two causes responsible for reverse restraint:

One is that one element among the five elements becomes very powerful and turns to restraint the element
that it is normally inferior to, damaging the normal inter-
restraint relationship between them. For example, if
wood becomes too powerful, it will reversely restrain
metal; if fire becomes too strong, it will reversely restrain water.

The other is that one element among the five elements becomes weak and is restrained by the one that it is
normally superior to, damaging the normal inter-restraint
relationship between them. For example, if metal becomes weak, it will be reversely restrained by wood; if
earth is weak, it will be reversely restrained by water.

Besides, the abnormal change of inter-promotion relationship is called mutual involvement of the mother and
the child. The mother involving or affecting the child
means that the disorder of the mother-element involving
or affecting the child-element. The order of such an involvement or affection is the same as that of inter-promotion. The child involving or affecting the mother means
that the disorder of the child-element involving or affect-

2. 相侮

相侮,是指五行之间一种事物对另一种事物反向制约欺侮的异常状态,故又叫"反侮"。相侮的次序与相克的次序是相反的,即木侮金,金侮火,火侮水,水侮土,土侮木。引起相侮的原因也有两方面:

一是五行中的某一行出现太过,便反向制约其"所不胜"一行,导致两者之间的相克关系出现异常。如木旺则侮金,火盛则侮水等。

二是五行中的某一行出现不及,反而受到其"所胜"一行的反向制约,导致两者之间的相克关系出现异常。如金虚而受木侮,土虚则受水侮等。

另外,相生关系的异常叫做子母相及。其中母及子,是指母行异常可影响及子行,其次序与相生次序是一致的;而子及母,是指子行异常可影响及母行,其次序与相生次序是相反的。

ing the mother-element. The order of such an involvement or affection is just opposite to that of inter-promotion.

1.2.3   Application of the theory of the five elements in TCM

1.2.3.1   Explaining the physiological functions of the five zang-organs and the relationships among them

The theory of the five elements explains the physiological characteristics and functions of the five zang-organs according to the attributes of the five elements, pairing each of the five zang-organs with the corresponding one of the five elements. For example, wood is characterized by free development while the liver prefers freedom to stagnation, so the liver pertains to wood; fire is hot and tends to flame up while heart-yang warms the whole body, so the heart pertains to fire; earth receives and generates while the spleen transforms food nutrients and is the source of qi and blood, so the spleen pertains to earth; metal depurates and astringes while lung-qi maintains inside and normally descends, so the lung pertains to metal; water moistens and closes while the kidney stores essence and manages water metabolism, so the kidney pertains to water.

Some of the intrinsic relationships among the functional activities of the five zang-organs also reflect the relationships of inter-promotion and inter-restraint. So they can be explained with the theory of inter-promotion and inter-restraint among the five elements. In terms of inter-promotion, the state of wood promoting fire corresponds to the state of the liver promoting the heart because liver-blood can nourish heart-spirit; the state of fire promoting earth corresponds to the state of the heart promoting the

三、五行学说在中医学中的应用

（一）用于说明五脏的生理特性及其相互关系

五行学说运用五行的特性来说明五脏的生理特性及功能特点,而将五脏分别归属于五行。如木性舒展升发,肝喜调畅而恶抑郁,故肝属木;火性温热炎上,心阳可温煦周身,故心属火;土性受纳生化,脾主运化饮食精微,为气血生化之源,故脾属土;金性肃杀收敛,肺气内守,以肃降为顺,故肺属金;水性滋润闭藏,肾藏精,主管水液代谢,故肾属水。

由于五脏功能活动之间的某些内在联系,也体现着相互资生与相互制约的关系,因此也可用五行相生相克的理论来加以说明。在相生方面:木生火,对应于肝生心,表现为肝血可营养心神;火生土,对应于心生脾,表现为心神可调节脾的运化功能;土生金,

spleen because heart-spirit can regulate the transporting and transforming functions of the spleen; the state of earth promoting metal corresponds to the state of the spleen promoting the lung because the spleen can transports and transforms food nutrients to nourish the lung; the state of metal promoting water corresponds to the state of the lung promoting the kidney because the lung depurates and descends qi to help the kidney receive qi; the state of water promoting wood corresponds to the state of the kidney promoting the liver because kidney-yin can nourish liver-yin. In terms of inter-restraint, the state of wood restraining earth corresponds to the state of the liver restraining the spleen because liver-qi relieves stagnation of spleen-earth to bring the transporting and transforming functions of the spleen into full play; the state of wood restraining water corresponds to the state of the spleen restraining the kidney because the spleen governs metabolism of water to prevent edema due to abnormal flow of kidney-water; the state of water restraining fire corresponds to the state of the kidney restraining the heart because sufficient kidney-yin can assist the heart to control hyperactivity of heart-fire; the state of fire restraining metal corresponds to the state of the heart restraining the lung because the warmth of heart-yang can prevent lung-qi from excessively depurating and descending; the state of metal restraining wood corresponds to the state of the lung restraining the liver because lung-qi depurates and descends to prevent liver-qi from excessively ascending.

1.2.3.2　Explaining interactions among the five zang-organs

　　The human body is an organic whole. The five zang-organs coordinate with each other physiologically and affect each other pathologically. Under pathological condition, disorder of one organ may be transmitted to another. According to the theory of the five elements, there

对应于脾生肺,表现为脾运化水谷精微可濡养于肺;金生水,对应于肺生肾,表现为肺主肃降有利于肾主纳气;水生木,对应于肾生肝,表现为肾阴可滋养肝阴。在相克方面:木克土,对应于肝克脾,表现为肝气调畅能疏泄脾土的壅滞,使脾主运化的功能得以正常发挥;土克水,对应于脾克肾,表现为脾主运化水液可防止肾水泛滥而生水肿等症;水克火,对应于肾克心,表现为肾阴充足而上济于心,可制约心火亢盛;火克金,对应于心克肺,表现为心阳温煦能抑制肺气肃降太过;金克木,对应于肺克肝,表现为肺气肃降下行能制约肝气,防止肝气过于升发而出现逆乱。

(二) 用于说明五脏病变的相互影响

　　人体是一个有机的整体,五脏之间不仅在生理功能上互相协调,互相配合,在病理上也会相互影响,相互传变,即一脏有病可以传及其他内

are two aspects of pathological transmission among the five zang-organs: one includes over restraint and reverse restraint, the other includes disorder of the mother-organ involving the child-organ and disorder of the child-organ involving the mother-organ.

Over restraint and reverse restraint are pathological transmissions due to abnormal change of inter-restraint relationship. Over restraint refers to transmission of disease due to excessive restraint, the order of which is the same as that of inter-restraint. For example, if liver-qi attacks the spleen, spleen-qi will be weakened, leading to dysfunction of the spleen. Reverse restraint refers to transmission of disease due to opposite restraint, the order of which is just contrary to inter-restraint. For example, the lung normally restrains the liver. But if liver-fire becomes hyperactive and invades the lung, it may lead to failure of the lung to depurate.

Mutual involvement or affection of the mother-organ and the child-organ reflects pathological transmission due to abnormal change of inter-promotion relationship. Disorder of the mother-organ involving or affecting the child-organ means that the disease is transmitted from the mother-organ into the child-organ, the order of which is the same as that of inter-promotion. For example, hyperactivity of liver-fire may affect the heart and bring on hyperactivity of heart-fire, leading to superabundance of both heart-fire and liver-fire. Such a transmission is called disorder of the mother-organ involving the child-organ. Disorder of the child-organ involving or affecting the mother-organ indicates that the disease is transmitted form the child-organ into the mother-organ, the order of which is just opposite to that of inter-promotion. For example, prolonged deficiency of liver-yin affects the kidney and causes deficiency of kidney-yin. Such a transmission is

脏。运用五行学说来说明五脏病变的相互影响,包括相乘相侮和子母相及两个方面。

相乘相侮是相克关系异常所导致的病理传变。相乘是相克太过而发生的疾病传变,其次序与相克一致,如肝气横逆犯脾,脾气受制而功能减退,可导致脾失健运。相侮是反向克制而引起的疾病传变,其次序与相克相反,如肺本克肝,若肝火太亢而反犯肺,可导致肺失清肃等。

子母相及是相生关系异常所导致的病理传变。母病及子是指疾病从母脏传变及子脏,次序与相生一致,如肝火亢盛,可影响及心,导致心火也亢盛,从而形成心肝火旺的证候,就属于母病及子的传变。子病及母是指疾病从子脏传变及母脏,次序与相生相反,如肝阴亏虚,日久及肾,引起肾阴也虚,则属于子病及母的传变,也叫"子盗母气"。

called disorder of the child-organ involving the mother-organ, also known as "the child-organ consuming qi of the mother-organ".

1.2.3.3 Guiding clinical diagnosis

Since the five zang-organs pair with the five elements, the five colors, the five flavors and the five pulses respectively, and because the disorders of the internal organs can manifest on the surface of the body, clinically the theory of the five elements can be used to analyze the changes of complexion, taste and pulse in order to decide which viscus and meridian are involved.

1. Diagnosis according to complexion, taste and pulse

The five colors, the five flavors and the five pulses correspond to the liver, the heart, the spleen, the lung and the kidney respectively. So they can be directly used to diagnose disease. For example, bluish complexion, preference for sour flavor or sour taste in the mouth and taut pulse indicate liver disease; reddish complexion, bitter taste in the mouth and full pulse indicate heart disease; yellowish complexion, sweet taste in the mouth and slow pulse indicate spleen disease; whitish complexion, acrid taste in the mouth and floating pulse indicate lung disease; and blackish complexion, salty taste in the mouth and deep pulse indicate kidney disease.

2. Deciding the transmission of disease according to complexion, taste and pulse

If the complexion, taste and pulse of the patient do not agree with the nature of visceral disorder, it shows that the disorder is already changed among the five zang-organs. Then the theory of the five elements must be used to analyze the transmission. Take spleen deficiency for example. Instead of displaying the manifestations of

（三）用于疾病的诊断

由于五脏分属于五行,五色、五味、五脉等与五脏都有着内在的联系,而内脏有病又可反映到体表,因此在临床上,可以应用五行学说来分析面部色泽、口味、脉象等变化,以推断病变的脏腑经络属性,从而诊断疾病。

1. 根据色、味、脉诊断疾病

五色、五味、五脉,分别对应肝、心、脾、肺、肾五脏,可直接用于五脏疾病的诊断。如面色青,喜食酸味,或口味酸,脉象弦,可诊断为肝病;面色赤,口味苦,脉象洪,可诊断为心病;面色黄,口味甘,脉象缓,可诊断为脾病;面色白,口味辛,脉象浮,可诊断为肺病;面色黑,口味咸,脉象沉,可诊断为肾病等。

2. 根据色、味、脉与五脏的关系判断疾病传变

如果病人色、味、脉的反应与病变内脏属性不一致,说明疾病在五脏之间发生了传变,可运用五行理论对这种传变进行分析。如脾虚病人,不见脾所主的面色黄、口味甘及

yellowish complexion, sweet taste in the mouth and slow pulse, there are signs of bluish complexion, sour taste in the mouth and taut pulse which are normally the manifestations of liver disorder. It shows that liver disease has been transmitted to the spleen, i. e. wood over restraining earth. Take lung disease for another example. Instead of displaying the manifestations of whitish complexion, acrid taste in the mouth and floating pulse, there are signs of reddish complexion, bitter taste in the mouth and full pulse which are normally the manifestations of heart disease. It shows that heart disease has been transmitted to the lung, i. e. fire over restraining metal.

Of course, using the theory of the five elements to diagnose disease is only one of the methods used in clinical diagnosis. In order to reveal the nature of disease and make correct diagnosis, this method should be used together with other methods for differentiation of syndrome, such as yin and yang, zangxiang (visceral and their manifestations), qi, blood and body fluid.

1.2.3.4 Guiding the treatment of disease

In the treatment of disease, the theory of the five elements is mainly used to control the transmission of disease and decide therapeutic principles.

1. Controlling the transmission of disease

The pathological changes of the five zang-organs, according to the phenomena of over restraint, reverse restraint and mutual involvement of the mother-element and the child-element among the five elements, can affect and transmit to each other. Thus in clinical treatment of the affected viscus, other viscera to be possibly involved must be taken into consideration by taking preventive measures in advance to control the transmission of disease. However, the following two points have to be borne in mind. One is to

缓脉,而出现肝所主的面色青、口味酸及脉象弦,则可知其脾病原因在于肝病传脾,即木乘土;又如肺病之人,不见肺所主的面色白、口味辛及浮脉,而出现心所主的面色赤、口味苦及脉象洪,则可知其肺病的原因在于心病传肺,即火乘金。

当然,运用五行理论来诊断疾病,仅是临床上的诊断方法之一,还必须结合阴阳、藏象、气血津液等其他辨证方法,才能真正把握住疾病的本质,作出正确的判断。

(四) 用于疾病的治疗

五行学说在疾病治疗方面的运用,主要体现在控制疾病的传变以及确定治疗原则两个方面。

1. 控制疾病的传变

根据五行相乘相侮和子母相及的理论,五脏之间的病变是可以相互影响和传变的,因此在临床治疗时,除了针对有病内脏进行直接治疗外,还要考虑到可能被影响的内脏,及早采取一些预防性的治疗措施,以控制疾病的传变。不过,在具体运用时,要注意以

select the viscera that are subject to transmission for treatment. For example, liver disease, according to the theory of five elements, tends to transmit to the heart, the lung, the spleen and the kidney. However, clinically the organ that is more frequently to be affected by liver disease is the spleen. So preventive measures should be taken in advance to protect the spleen in the treatment of liver disease. The other is that the treatment should be done according to the functional state of the viscera. Though liver disease tends to transmit to the spleen, the transmission usually results from the abnormal changes of spleen function. If the spleen is sufficient in qi, healthy in function and powerful in resistance, liver disease is difficult to transmit to the spleen and no measures need to be taken to deal with the spleen. If the spleen is too weak to resist attack of liver disease, it will be invaded by liver disease. In this case measures must be taken to prevent further transmission in treating the spleen.

2. Deciding therapeutic principles

Visceral diseases, according to the inter-promotion and inter-restraint relationships among the five elements, may affect each other. Clinically the theory of the five elements can be used to readjust the relationships among the five zang-organs to realize the aim of treatment. Usually the therapeutic principles are decided in the light of inter-promotion and inter-restraint relationships.

The therapeutic principle decided according to inter-promotion relationship is termed "tonifying the mother-organ and purging the child-organ".

Tonifying the mother-organ is a therapeutic principle used to treat deficiency syndrome. It is also known as

下两点：一是选择容易被传及的内脏进行治疗。例如按照五行理论来解释,肝脏有病是可以传及心、肺、脾、肾四脏的,但从临床实际情况来看,最容易受其影响的则是脾脏,所以应首先考虑对脾脏采取预防性的治疗措施。二是根据内脏的功能状态来进行治疗。虽说肝脏有病容易传及于脾,但最终能否传变,还取决于脾脏本身的功能状态。如果脾气充足,功能健全,抵抗力强盛,则肝病不易传脾,也不需治脾;若脾脏虚弱,不能抵御肝传来的病邪的侵袭,就会导致疾病的传变,此时就必须配合健脾法治疗以防止传变。

2. 确定治疗原则

根据五行理论,五脏之间是有相互资生和克制关系的,五脏病变也可因这些关系而相互影响,从而在临床上就可以根据五行理论来调整五脏之间的关系来达到治疗疾病的目的。根据五行理论确定治疗原则,可从相生与相克两个方面进行。

根据相生关系确定的治疗原则,称为"补母泻子"。

补母,是应用于虚证时的治疗原则,故又称为"虚则补

"tonifying the mother-organ in the treatment of deficiency syndrome". This principle is mainly used to treat deficiency syndrome due to failure of the mother-organ to promote the child-organ. The aim of this principle is to strengthen the weakened child-organ by tonifying the mother-organ. Take insufficiency of liver-yin for example. Since it results from malnutrition of liver-wood due to insufficiency of kidney-yin, it can be treated by nourishing kidney-yin. Since the kidney is the mother-organ of the liver, tonifying kidney-water can promote liver-wood. That is why this therapy is called "enriching water to nourish wood."

Purging the child-organ is a therapeutic principle used to treat excess syndrome, also known as "purging the child-organ in treating excess syndrome". This principle is mainly used to treat excess syndrome resulting from disorder of the mother-organ by reducing exuberant pathogenic factors through purging the child-organ. For example, superabundance of heart-fire due to hyperactivity of liver-fire can be treated by purging the heart because the heart is the child-organ of the liver. That is why liver-fire can be reduced by purging heart-fire.

The principle decided according to inter-restraint relationship is called "inhibiting the strong organ and supporting the weak organ".

The abnormal states of inter-restraint among the five elements are over restraint and reverse restraint. In visceral disease, the manifestations of such abnormal relationships are signified by a series of pathological changes resulting from visceral imbalance. The principle of inhibiting the strong organ and supporting the weak organ means to correct visceral imbalance and restore visceral harmony in function. Inhibiting the strong organ and supporting the weak organ, two different sides of a thera-

其母"。补母的治则主要应用于因母不生子而出现的虚证,通过补其"母"的方法使虚损的"子"得到资助而由弱转强。如肾阴不足,肝木失于滋养,而致肝阴不足者,可用补肾阴的方法以滋养肝阴,因为肾为肝之母,通过补肾水可达到生肝木的目的,故称此治法为"滋水涵木法"。

泻子,是应用于实证时的治疗原则,故又称为"实则泻其子"。泻子的治则主要应用于因母病及子所出现的实证,通过泻子的方法使偏盛的邪气顺势而泄去。如肝火上炎,心火无制,而致心火亢盛者,可采取泻心法,因为心为肝之子,通过泻心火可达到降肝火的目的。

根据相克关系确定的治疗原则,称为"抑强扶弱"。

相克关系的异常,表现为相乘与相侮,在五脏病变中是由于五脏强弱不和而出现的一类病理变化。抑强扶弱,就是消除强弱不和的力量悬殊状态,引导五脏恢复平衡协调关系。抑强与扶弱是不同作用的两个方面,但二者之间是相互关联的。只有通过抑强,

peutic principle, are closely related to each other. The purpose of inhibiting the strong organ is to prevent it from bullying the weak organ while the aim of supporting the weak organ is to correct its deficiency so as to free it from the domination of the strong organ. Inhibiting the strong organ and supporting the weak organ can be used singly. However, they are frequently used in combination in order to quickly correct visceral imbalance. For inhibiting the strong organ, purging therapy is usually used; for supporting the weak organ, nourishing therapy is frequently resorted to. The application of this principle is often marked by simultaneous application of attack and tonification. For example, adverse flow of liver-qi tends to invade the spleen, but deficiency of spleen-qi also makes it easy for liver-qi to attack the spleen. Thus disease resulting from liver-qi attacking the spleen can be treated by inhibiting wood and supporting earth (also known as inhibiting the liver and strengthening the spleen), simultaneously reducing liver-qi and strengthening spleen-qi. With the regulation of both the spleen and the liver, there will be no difficulty in curing spleen disease.

才能纠正其太过之气而不致对弱者进行欺侮；只有通过扶弱，才能纠正其不及之气而不受强者的克制。抑强和扶弱可以单独使用，但大多数情形下宜联合使用，可使不平衡的脏腑关系迅速恢复正常。抑强，主要是采用泻法；扶弱，主要是采用补法。所以抑强扶弱原则在运用时往往采用攻补兼施的方法。如肝气横逆则易乘犯脾土，而脾气虚弱也易受肝气的乘袭，所以对于肝气犯脾的病证，就可采取抑木扶土(也称抑肝扶脾)的方法，一方面泻肝气，一方面补脾气，肝脾同调，则脾病可愈。

2 Zangxiang (viscera and their manifestations)

第二章 藏象

The term zangxiang first appeared in *Huangdi Neijing*. Zang, sharing the same pronunciation with viscera in Chinese, refers to internal organs inside the body; xiang means image or phenomenon. When used together, zangxiang, as analyzed above, simply refers to internal organs and the external manifestations of their physiological and pathological states. Obviously zang is the intrinsic base of xiang and xiang is the external manifestations of zang.

The content of zangxiang theory is composed of three parts: the physiological functions and pathological changes of the viscera, the description of which mainly focuses on the physiological functions; the relationships between the five zang-organs and the body, organs and orifices, including the relationships between the five zang-organs and the five constituents (namely vessels, tendons, muscles, skin and bones), the five sensory organs and the nine orifices (namely the tongue, eyes, mouth, nose, ears, external genitals and anus); the relationships between the zang-organs and the fu-organs, including the relationships among the five zang-organs, among the six fu-organs and the relationships between the zang-organs and the fu-organs.

The theory of zangxiang mainly studies the zang-organs and the fu-organs. That is why it is also known as "the theory of zang-fu organs". Zang-fu is a collective term for internal organs which are divided into two major categories, namely the five zang-organs and the six fu-

"藏象"一词,首先见于《黄帝内经》。藏,通"脏",是指隐藏于体内的内脏;象,是指形象或现象。藏象,即指藏于体内的内脏及其表现于外的生理、病理现象。可见,"藏"是"象"的内在根据,"象"是"藏"的外在反映。

藏象学说的内容主要有三个部分:一是内脏的生理功能和病理变化,其中重点阐述五脏的生理功能;二是五脏与形体官窍之间的关系,包括五脏与五体(脉、筋、肉、皮、骨)及五官九窍(舌、目、口、鼻、耳、二阴)之间的联系等;三是脏腑之间的关系,包括五脏之间、六腑之间以及五脏与六腑之间的多种联系。

藏象学说,主要以脏腑为基础,所以有时也称其为"脏腑学说"。脏腑是内脏的总称,主要有五脏与六腑两类。五脏,即心、肝、脾、肺、肾;六

organs. The five zang-organs include the heart, the liver, the spleen, the lung and the kidney; the six fu-organs include the gallbladder, the stomach, the small intestine, the large intestine, the urinary bladder and sanjiao (the triple energizer). Besides, there is another group of tissues and organs, similar to the zang-organs in function and the fu-organs in form, which are termed the extraordinary fu-organs, including the brain, the marrow, the bones, the vessels, the gallbladder and the uterus.

Though all pertain to the internal organs, the five zang-organs and the six fu-organs are different from each other in functions and characteristics. The common function of the five zang-organs is "to store jing-qi (essence)" which is refined food nutrient responsible for maintenance of life activities. The common function of the six fu-organs is "to transport and transform food". That means to receive and digest food, absorbing the nutrients and discharging the waste. That is why TCM has divided the internal organs into two distinct categories: the zang-organs and the fu-organs.

Zang-fu is the core of life activities. The substantial bases responsible for the physiological functions of the five zang-organs and the six fu-organs come from two aspects: one is morphological structure in anatomy and the other is the refined nutrient like qi, blood, yin and yang. Different morphological structure bears certain relationship with the physiological functions of certain internal organs. Take the heart and the stomach for example. Since the heart is directly connected with the vessels, it bears the function of propelling blood to flow in the vessels. Since the stomach is connected with the esophagus and the small intestine, it can receive and digest food. Thus the morphological structure of the internal organs is one of the substantial bases for maintaining their physiological functions. In TCM

腑，即胆、胃、小肠、大肠、膀胱、三焦。此外，还有一类组织器官，由于其功能类似于脏，形态相似于腑，中医学把它们称为"奇恒之腑"。奇恒之腑包括脑、髓、骨、脉、胆、女子胞。

五脏与六腑虽同为内脏，但各自的功能特点是不同的。五脏共同的功能特点是"藏精气"，即贮藏人体维持生命活动所需要的精微物质；六腑共同的功能特点是"传化物"，即受纳、消化饮食物，并吸收其精微，排泄其糟粕。正因为这两者总的功能特点不一样，所以将它们划分为脏与腑两类。

脏腑是人体生命活动的核心。维持五脏六腑生理功能的物质基础有两方面：一是解剖形态结构。不同的形态结构与内脏的某些生理功能有着一定的联系，如心脏与脉管直接相连，故心有推动血液在脉管内循行的功能；胃与食道、小肠相通，故胃有受纳、腐熟饮食的作用。所以内脏的形态结构，是维持其生理功能的物质基础之一。中医学早在2 000多年前就进行过人体解剖学的观察与研究，在《黄

anatomy was done over two thousand years ago. In *Huangdi Neijing* and *Nanjing* there are detailed records about the length of bones as well as the length, size and capacity of the stomach and the intestines. However, TCM pays more attention to the synthetic manifestations of the holistic functions of the body and is more sophisticated in cognizing the intrinsic nature of life from the external manifestations. Zangxiang theory holds that qi, blood, yin and yang are the essential substances for constituting and maintaining the physiological functions of the zang-fu organs. All the pathological changes result from deficiency or disturbance of these substances. Substantially, these refined substances are fine and minute. Though invisible to the eyes, they can still be understood and distinguished according to their physiological functions and pathologic changes. Generally speaking, qi and yang all have the functions of warming, propelling and fixating. However, qi mainly functions to propel and fixate while yang mainly functions to warm. Both blood and yin have the functions of nourishing and moistening. However, blood mainly functions to nourish while yin mainly functions to moisten. Qi, blood, yin and yang differ in qihua (qi-transformation). That is why they bear different physiological functions.

On the whole, zangxiang theory focuses on the study of physiological functions and pathological changes of the zang-fu organs, somatic tissues and organs as well as the mutual relationships among them. So it is the core of the

帝内经》、《难经》等古医籍中,有关于骨骼的长短,以及胃肠等脏器的大小、长短、容量等均有详细记载。但是,由于中医学更强调人体整体功能的综合表现,更善于从外部现象推测生命的内在本质,从而在不受解剖形态限制的前提下形成了关于人体生理病理的庞大理论体系。二是气、血、阴、阳等精微物质。藏象学说认为,构成脏腑并维持其生理功能的主要物质基础是气、血、阴、阳等精微物质,一切病理变化也都以这些精微物质的不足或紊乱为条件。从形质上讲,这些精微物质是极其精细而微小的,不能用肉眼直接观察,但可以从其生理功能及其病理变化方面来认识它们的本质并加以区分。一般来说,气与阳均具有温煦、推动和固摄作用,而气以推动、固摄作用为主,阳以温煦作用为主;血与阴均具有营养和滋润作用,而血以营养作用为主,阴以滋润作用为主。由于各脏腑器官气血阴阳的气化形式不同,因此不同的脏腑就具有各自不同的生理功能。

总之,中医藏象学说是研究脏腑和躯体组织器官的生理功能、病理变化及其相互关系的学说,是中医学理论体系

theoretical system of TCM. Though terminologically identical with some of the organs in modern medicine, the zang-fu organs in zangxiang theory are quite different in physiological functions. Because the zangxiang theory was established mainly on the basis of life experience and clinical practice. That is to say that TCM understands the internal organs through observing the physiological and pathological phenomena as well as therapeutic effect. Thus the conceptions of zang-fu organs in TCM are quite beyond the range of anatomical morphology. It is generally believed that the functions of the zang-fu organs in TCM are extensive, not only including part of the functions of the organs with the same names in modern medicine, but also covering certain functions of other related organs. Obviously the zang-fu organs in TCM are not just the conceptions of anatomy, but synthetic functional units.

的核心。虽然其脏腑名称与现代医学某些器官的名称相同,但生理功能却不完全相同。因为藏象学说的形成,主要是通过生活体验和临床实践,即对生理病理现象和治疗效应的观察等方面来认识内脏的,所以中医学脏腑的概念就大大超越了解剖形态的范围。一般认为,中医学所述的脏腑功能范围较广,不仅包含着西医同一脏器的部分功能,而且还概括了其他相关器官的某些功能在内。因此,中医学的脏腑不单纯是解剖学的概念,更重要的是一些综合性的功能单位。

2.1 The five zang-organs

The five zang-organs include the heart, the lung, the liver, the spleen and the kidney. The following is a brief description of the physiological functions of the five zang-organs and their relationships with the body, the organs and the orifices. The latter includes three aspects, i. e. the relationships of the five zang-organs with the five constituents, the organs that the five zang-organs open into and the focal external manifestations of the five zang-organs.

The five constituents include the vessels, the skin, the tendons, the muscles and the bones that are dominated by the five zang-organs respectively.

The orifices, simplification for "the five sensory organs and the nine orifices", include the tongue, the nose,

第一节 五脏

五脏,是心、肺、肝、脾、肾的合称。本节主要介绍五脏的生理功能、五脏与形体官窍的关系。五脏与形体官窍的关系,又包括五脏主五体、五脏开窍和五脏外华三个方面。

五体,即脉、皮、筋、肉、骨五种形体组织,五脏各主其一。

窍,是"五官九窍"的简称,包括舌、鼻、目、口、耳及二

the eyes, the mouth, the ears, the external genitals and the anus. The heart, the lung, the liver and the spleen govern one orifice respectively. But the kidney opens into the ears, the external genitals and the anus.

The focal external manifestations of the five zang-organs refer to five special areas (i. e. the face, the body hair, the nails, the lips and the hair) on the surface of the body on which the essence of the five zang-organs displays.

2.1.1 The heart

The heart is located in the chest between the two lobes of the lung. The heart occupies the first place among the five zang-organs and governs the life activities of the whole body. That is why it is said that the heart is "an organ of monarch" in *Huangdi Neijing*.

2.1.1.1 The physiological functions of the heart

The physiological functions of the heart are mainly to govern blood and to control the mind.

1. Governing blood

The function of the heart to govern blood means that the heart propels blood to circulate in the vessels and that the heart is related to the production of blood.

Blood circulates inside the vessels. Since the heart is connected directly with the vessels, its beat is the motive power to propel blood to flow in the vessels. Thus a relatively independent blood circulation system is formed with the heart, the vessels and blood. Only under the propelling of the heart beat and the control of the vessels can blood normally circulate all through the body, in which the heart beat is key to blood circulation.

阴。心、肺、肝、脾各主一窍，肾开窍于耳及二阴。

五脏外华，简称"五华"，是五脏精气显露于外的五个特殊部位，即面、毛、爪、唇、发。

一、心

心位于胸中，居两肺叶之间。心在五脏六腑中居于首要的地位，对全身生命活动起着主宰的作用，故《黄帝内经》称其为"君主之官"。

（一）心的生理功能

心的生理功能有两方面，一是主血，一是主神志。

1. 主血

心主血的功能，主要指心脏能够推动血液在脉管中运行，其次指心脏与血液的生成有关。

血液运行于脉管之中。由于心与脉管相连，心的搏动具有鼓动血液运行的能力，所以心是推动血液在脉管中运行的动力所在，由心、脉管、血液三者构成了一个相对独立的血液循环系统。血液只有在心的搏动与脉管约束的共同作用下，才能正常地运行于

The reason that the heart propels blood to circulate within the vessels lies in the propelling and warming functions of heart-qi and heart-yang as well as the nourishing and moistening functions of heart-yin and heart-blood. Sufficiency of heart-qi, heart-blood, heart-yin and heart-yang guarantee normal beat of the heart and continuous circulation of blood to nourish all parts of the body, thus maintaining the normal physiological functions of all tissues and organs with the manifestations of full vitality, ruddy complexion and normal pulse. However, if heart-qi, heart-blood, heart-yin and heart-yang are insufficient or in disturbance, the function of the heart to govern the vessels will be affected, leading to a series of pathological changes such as pale complexion and thin and weak pulse due to insufficiency of heart-qi as well as cyanotic complexion and unsmooth pulse or slow pulse with irregular intervals or slow regular intermittent pulse due to stagnation of heart-blood.

The heart also plays a role in the production of blood, known as "reddening" in TCM. After digestion and absorption of food by the spleen and stomach, the refined nutrients are transported up to the heart and the lung. Combined with the fresh air inhaled into the lung, warmed and steamed by heart-yang, these refined nutrients are transformed into red blood.

Besides, TCM believes that "the heart controls blood vessels", a combination of the ideas that "the heart governs blood" and "the heart controls the vessels". The idea that "the heart controls blood and vessels" is described in the section of "the relationship between the heart and the body, the sensory organs and the orifices."

周身,而其中心脏的搏动是维持血液运行的关键,起着主导作用。

心之所以能够推动血液在脉管内运行,是依赖于心气、心阳的推动和温煦作用,以及心阴、心血的营养和滋润作用。心之气血阴阳充足,心的搏动就正常,人体的血液循环不息,营养周身五脏六腑、四肢百骸,使各组织器官的生理功能正常,从而表现出精力充沛、面色红润光泽、脉象和缓有力等现象。如心之气血阴阳不足或失调,就会影响心主血脉的功能而出现一系列病理表现,如心气不足,可见面色苍白、脉细弱无力;心血瘀阻,可见面色青紫、脉涩结代等。

同时,心对血液的生成具有"化赤"的作用。饮食物经过脾胃的消化吸收之后,将其中的精微物质上输于心肺,在肺部结合自然界之清气,又在心阳的温煦蒸腾作用下,化生为红色的血液。

另外,中医学有"心主血脉"之说,即将"心主血"与"心主脉"合并起来形成的一个专用术语。有关"心主脉"的内容,请参见"心与形体官窍的关系"一节。

2. Controlling the mind

The function of the heart to control the mind is also known as "the heart storing spirit". In a broad sense, spirit refers to the supreme dominator of life activities in the whole body. In a narrow sense, spirit is a collective term for cognition, thinking, consciousness and mental states. The idea that the heart controls the mind means that the heart governs the mental activities.

The mental activities are closely related to the response of the brain to the external environment and certain intrinsic functions of the brain. Centering around the five zang-organs, TCM attributes the motivation of mental activities to the heart. It is obviously that the conception of the heart in TCM includes certain functions of the brain.

The normal function of the heart to control the mind depends on the nourishing and moistening functions of heart-blood and heart-yin which are the essential substantial bases for mental activities. Heart-qi and heart-yang function to activate and stimulate heart-spirit, which also plays an important role in ensuring the normal function of the heart to control the mind. If the function of the heart to control the mind is normal, people will be full of vigor, conscious in mind, agile in thinking and keen in response. If the function of the heart to control the mind is abnormal due to insufficiency or disturbance of heart-qi, heart-blood, heart-yin and heart-yang, it will inevitably lead to palpitation, insomnia, dreaminess, or even coma, delirium and unconsciousness.

2.1.1.2 The relationships between the heart and the body, the sensory organs and the orifices

1. The heart governs the vessels

The vessels, the routes for blood circulation, keep

2. 主神志

心主神志的功能,又称"心藏神"。神有广义和狭义之分。广义之神,是指整个人体生命活动的最高主宰。狭义之神,是对人的认知、思维、意识、情志等精神活动的总称。心主神志,即指心有主管人的精神活动的功能。

人的精神活动,与大脑对客观外界事物的反映及其固有的某些功能活动有关,但中医藏象学从以五脏为中心的理论出发,把精神活动的根本归属于心的范畴。因此中医学所讲的心,实际上也概括了大脑的某些功能活动。

心主神志功能的正常发挥,主要依赖心血、心阴对心神的营养及滋润作用,这是精神活动的重要物质基础,其次也与心气、心阳对心神的鼓舞及振奋作用有关。心主神志功能正常,则人的精神振奋,神志清晰,思维敏捷,反应灵敏。若心之气血阴阳不足或失调,使心主神明的功能异常,可出现心悸、失眠、多梦、健忘,甚至神昏、谵语、不省人事等症。

(二) 心与形体官窍的关系

1. 心主脉

脉管是血液流通的道路,

blood to circulate normally inside the vessels all through the body. The heart governing the vessels means that the heart bears close relationship with the vessels in structure, function and pathology. In structure, the heart is directly connected with the vessels. In function, the heart propels blood to flow inside the vessels by beating. In fact normal blood circulation is maintained by the heart and vessels working together. Thus normal function of the heart ensures smoothness of the vessels which is prerequisite to the normal flow of blood and the normal state of the pulse. However, abnormal function of the heart or unsmoothness of the vessels will disturb blood circulation and affect the state of the pulse. For example, insufficiency of heart-blood and emptiness of blood vessels will lead to thin and weak pulse; insufficiency of heart-yang will bring on deep and indistinct pulse.

2. The heart opens into the tongue

The idea that the heart opens into the tongue indicates that there is a special relationship between the heart and the tongue. For example, the state of the tongue can reflect the physiological functions and pathological changes of the heart because a branch of the heart meridian runs into the tongue. So the condition of heart-blood displays itself on the tongue. On the other hand, heart-spirit directly influences the sensation and the movement of the tongue. Thus whether the heart functions well in governing the vessels or in controlling the mind can be understood from the color and shape of the tongue. That is why it is said that "the tongue is the sprout of the heart" in TCM. If heart-qi, heart-blood, heart-yin and heart-yang are normal, the tongue is ruddy and lustrous in appearance, agile in movement, soft in texture, keen in taste and fluent in speaking. So insufficiency of heart-blood leads to lightly whitish tongue without taste; up-flaming of

它能够约束血液,使其正常地循行于周身。心主脉,是指心与脉在结构、功能以及病理上都有着密切的关系。在结构上,心与脉管直接相连;在功能上,心脏的搏动推动着血液在脉管中运行,由于心与脉的共同作用,才保证了血液的正常循环。因此,心的功能正常,脉道通利,则血液流畅,脉象和缓而有力;心的功能异常,或脉道不利,则血行障碍,脉象也会出现相应的异常反应。如心血不足,血脉空虚,可出现脉细弱;心阳不足,鼓动无力,可出现脉象沉微等。

2. 心开窍于舌

心开窍于舌,是说心与舌有着某种特定的联系,心的生理病理表现都可通过舌特异性地反映出来。这是由于,手少阴心经的别络上行联系到舌,心血的充足与否显露于舌,心神也直接影响着舌的感觉与运动。因此,无论是心主血脉还是心主神志的功能正常与否,都可从舌的色泽形态上反映出来,故中医学又有"舌为心之苗"之说。如心的气血阴阳正常,则舌质红润,舌体柔软灵活,味觉灵敏,语言流利。若心血不足,可见舌质淡白,食不知味;心火上炎,可见舌质红绛,或舌上生疮;

heart-fire brings on deep colored tongue or ulcerated tongue; abnormal heart-spirit results in curled tongue, stiff tongue and dysphasia.

3. External manifestation on the face

Since the condition of heart-qi, heart-blood, heart-yin and heart-yang mainly display on the face, observation of facial color and shape can enable one to know whether heart-qi, heart-blood, heart-yin and heart-yang are normal or not. If heart-blood is sufficient and flows smoothly, the face is ruddy and lustrous; if heart-qi is insufficient and heart-blood is deficient, the face is pale and lusterless; if heart-blood is stagnated, the face is cyanotic.

Appendix: The pericardium

The pericardium is a tissue surrounding the heart to protect the heart. Zangxiang theory holds that the heart is the monarch-organ and cannot be directly attacked by pathogenic factors. If pathogenic factors directly invade the heart, it will disturb heart-spirit and threaten life. So when pathogenic factors invade the heart, they first attack the pericardium. For example, the symptoms of high fever, coma and delirium in exogenous febrile diseases are described as "invasion of pathogenic factors into the pericardium" in TCM.

2.1.2   The lung

The lung is located in the chest. Since its location is the highest among the internal organs, it is compared to a "canopy". The lung is delicate, intolerable to cold and heat, and is easy to be attacked by pathogenic factors. That is why it is called "a delicate organ".

The function of the lung mainly depends on the propelling and fixating functions of lung-qi and, secondly, is

心神失常,可见舌卷、舌强、语言謇涩等。

3. 心华在面

华,有光华外现之义。心华在面,是说心的气血阴阳,可特异性地表露于面部,观察面部的色泽形态,可以判断心的气血阴阳正常与否。如心血充足,运行通畅,则面部红润有光泽;如心气不足,心血亏少,可见面白而无华;心血瘀阻,又可见面色青紫等。

附:心包

心包,又称"心包络",为心的外围结构,有保护心脏的作用。藏象学说认为,心为君主之官,不能轻易地被邪气所侵犯,若邪气直接侵犯于心,使心神失常,容易发生生命危险。所以外邪犯心,一般都首先由心包代其受邪,例如外感热病中出现高热、神昏、谵语等症,就称为"邪入心包"。

二、肺

肺位于胸中,位置最高,故有"华盖"之称。又因为肺脏娇嫩,不耐寒热,容易被邪气侵犯而发病,故又叫做"娇脏"。

肺的功能主要依赖于肺气的推动和固摄作用,其次与

related to the moistening function of lung-yin. The movement of lung-qi is characterized by dispersion and descent which are all reflected in the physiological functions of the lung.

Dispersion means to diffuse, dredge and spread upwards and outwards. Descent means the downward cleaning and clearing downwards and inwards.

Since the lung assists the heart to promote blood circulation, it is said in *Huangdi Neijing* that the lung is an "assistance-organ".

2.1.2.1 The physiological functions of the lung

The main physiological functions of the lung are dominating qi and managing the regulation of water passage.

1. Dominating qi

The physiological function of the lung to dominate qi covers two aspects: to dominate respiration and to control qi through out the body.

(1) Dominating respiration: The function of the lung to dominate respiration means that the lung controls the respiratory movement.

The lung is the main organ involved in respiratory movement and the place where air in and out of the body exchanges. The body inhales fresh air and exhales waste air through the respiratory movement of the lung so as to maintain the normal activities of life.

The normal function of the lung to dominate respiration, apart from the moistening function of lung-yin, mainly relies on the dispersing and descending functions of lung-qi. Waste air is exhaled out of the body by means of the dispersing function of lung-qi and fresh air is inhaled

肺阴的滋润作用也有关。肺气运动的特点有宣发和肃降两方面。宣发,是指向上向外的宣通发散;肃降,是指向下向内的清肃下行。这两方面的特点都体现在肺的生理功能之中。

由于肺具有辅心行血的作用,所以《黄帝内经》称肺为"相辅之官"。

(一)肺的生理功能

肺具有主气和主通调水道两方面的生理功能。

1. 主气

肺主气的功能包括主呼吸之气和主一身之气两个方面。

(1) 主呼吸之气 肺主呼吸之气,也称"肺司呼吸",是指肺具有主持呼吸运动的功能。

肺是人体呼吸运动的主要器官,是体内外气体交换的场所。通过肺的呼吸运动,吸入自然界的清气,呼出体内的浊气,如此不断地吐故纳新维持着人体生命活动的正常进行。

肺司呼吸功能的正常发挥,除了肺阴的滋润作用以外,主要依赖于肺气的宣发和肃降作用。通过肺气向上向外的宣通发散,呼出体内的浊

into the body through the descending function of lung-qi. Thus the dispersing function and descending function of lung-qi depend on each other and restrict each other to maintain the normal respiratory function of the body. Physiologically, harmonious dispersing and descending functions of lung-qi ensures smooth and regular respiration. If lung-qi fails to disperse and descend, it will affect respiration, leading to chest oppression, cough and dyspnea.

(2) Dominating qi through out the body: The function of the lung to dominate qi all through the body means that the lung controls and regulates qi in the whole body. Such a function is reflected in the following three aspects:

The first aspect is the production of the pectoral qi (or thoracic qi). The pectoral qi, part of qi in the body, is synthesized with the nutrients of food refined by the spleen and fresh air inhaled by the lung. When it is produced, the pectoral qi is transported and distributed, by means of the dispersing and descending functions of the lung as well as the function of the heart to control blood, to the whole body to warm and nourish the internal organs and tissues to maintain their normal physiological functions. Since fresh air in the natural world is a necessary condition for the production of the pectoral qi and is inhaled into the body by the lung, the respiratory function of the lung directly influences the production of the pectoral qi and qi in the whole body.

The second aspect is the regulation of qi activity. Qi is flowing constantly in the body. The movement of qi is characterized by ascending, descending, going-out and entering. The lung functions to disperse and descend,

气;通过肺气向下向内的清肃下行,吸入自然界的清气。因此,肺气的宣发和肃降,既相互制约,又相互依存,共同维持人体正常的呼吸功能。在生理情况下,肺气的宣降保持协调,则气道通畅,呼吸调匀。如肺失宣降,影响其呼吸功能,则出现胸闷、咳嗽、气喘等呼吸不利的症状。

(2) 主一身之气 肺主一身之气,是指肺有主持、调节周身之气的功能。其具体体现在如下三个方面:

一是宗气的生成。宗气是人体气的一部分,它是由脾通过消化饮食物,吸收其中的精微物质而上输于胸中,与肺吸入的自然界之清气互相结合而生成的。宗气生成后,再通过肺的宣发肃降及心主血的功能而布散于全身,以温养各脏腑组织,维持其正常的生理功能。由于自然界之清气是生成宗气的必要条件,它是依靠肺的呼吸功能来吸入的,所以肺司呼吸功能的正常与否,直接影响着人体宗气的生成,也影响着全身之气的生成。

二是气机的调节。人体之气是运行不息的,其基本的形式是升降出入。肺具有宣发肃降的功能,直接影响着全

directly influencing the activity of qi. The respiratory function of the lung, reflecting the ascending, descending, going-out and entering activities of qi, also exerts great effect on the movement of qi in the whole body. If the lung is normal in dispersion and descent as well as respiration, the visceral qi and the meridian qi in the whole body will be normal in ascending, descending, going-out and entering. It is clear that the lung regulates the activities of qi in the whole body.

The third aspect is to assist the heart to promote blood circulation. The heart controls blood vessels and the heart beat is the basic motive power to propel blood to circulate in the vessels. Besides, the lung is closely related to the vessels in the whole body. Because through the vessels blood from the whole body converges in the lung and then is distributed to all parts of the body. That is why it is said in *Huangdi Neijing* that "the lung is connected with all the vessels". It is just the convergence of blood from the whole body in the lung that makes it possible for the lung to assist the heart to promote blood circulation and to accomplish the activity of respiration.

As it is mentioned above, the function of the lung to govern qi in the whole body is closely related to the function of the lung to control respiration. The latter is the base of the former and the former is the aim of the latter. If the lung is abnormal in governing respiration, it will affect the production of the pectoral qi, the regulation of qi activity and the circulation of blood, leading to insufficiency of the pectoral qi, disturbance of qi activity and disorder of

身的气机运动,而肺之呼吸也体现出升降出入的特点,对全身之气的运动有重要影响。所以,全身之气的运行调畅与否,与肺气的宣发肃降和肺的呼吸功能都有密切关系。如肺气宣发肃降及呼吸功能正常,则周身各脏腑经络之气就随着肺气的运动而正常地升降出入。可见,肺对全身气的升降出入运动起着重要的调节作用。

三是辅心行血。心主血脉,心脏的搏动是推动血液运行的基本动力。同时,由于肺与周身的血脉都有密切的联系,血液一方面通过血脉从全身会聚于肺,另一方面又通过血脉从肺散行于全身,这就表现出辅心行血的作用。《黄帝内经》中有"肺朝百脉"的理论,"朝"是"会聚"的意思,周身血脉皆会聚于肺,是肺辅心行血的结构基础。只有通过这一形式,肺司呼吸的功能才得以实现。

从以上三个方面的内容可以看出,肺主一身之气的功能正常与否,与肺司呼吸的功能有密切关系。一方面,肺司呼吸是肺主一身之气的基础和前提;另一方面,肺主一身之气是肺司呼吸功能的目的和意义所在。如果肺司呼吸

qi and blood. The function of the lung to govern respiration will be affected if the production of the pectoral qi is insufficient or if the lung is abnormal in dispersion and descent or if blood circulation is in disorder.

功能失常,必然会影响到宗气的生成、气机的调节和心血的运行,可出现宗气不足、气机失调以及血行失常等相应的病变;反之,如果宗气生成不足,或宣发肃降失职,或血行失常,也会影响肺司呼吸的功能。

2. The regulation of water passage

Regulation here means dredging and readjusting. Water passage refers to the route for transmitting and discharging water. The lung governing the regulation of water passage refers to the function of the lung in propelling, adjusting and discharging water.

After taken into the body, water is absorbed by means of transportation and transformation of the spleen, and then transmitted upwards to the lung. On the one hand, lung-qi, by means of dispersing to the upper and external, transmits water to the surface of the body and transforms it into sweat to be discharged. At the same time, part of the water is excreted through respiration. On the other hand, lung-qi, by means of descending to the lower and the internal, transmits water to the viscera and then to the kidney where it is transformed into urine to be excreted out of the body. Besides, the descending function of the lung assists the large intestine in transmission, through which part of the water is discharged in defecation. Since the location of the lung is supreme, like a canopy, and because it also participates in the metabolism of water, the lung is called "the upper source of water" in TCM. If the lung fails to regulate water passage due to its disorder in dispersion and descent, it will affect the distribution and discharge of water, leading to production of phlegm, rheum, edema and disorder of urination.

2. 主通调水道

通调,是疏通、调节的意思。水道,指水液输布和排泄的道路。肺主通调水道,即指肺具有推动、调节水液输布和排泄的功能。

摄入体内的水液,经脾的运化功能吸收后,上输于肺。肺气一方面通过其向上向外的宣发作用,将水液输布到体表,经利用后化为汗液而排出体外,同时呼气中也排出了部分水分;另一方面通过其向下向内的肃降作用,将水液输布至内脏,经利用后下行于肾,在肾的气化作用下生成尿液,下输膀胱而排出体外。另外,肺气的肃降有助于大肠的传导功能,大便中也排出了部分水分。由于肺为华盖,位置最高,而肺又参与了体内水液代谢的过程,所以中医学又称肺为"水之上源"。如果肺失宣降,导致肺主通调水道的功能失常,影响水液的输布和排泄,便可出现痰饮、水肿及小

2.1.2.2　The relationships between the lung and the body, the sensory organs and the orifices

1. The lung governing the skin

The function of the skin is to protect the body, excrete sweat and adjust body temperature. The relationship between the lung and the skin can be understood from the following two aspects. One is that the lung can disperse and transport the wei-qi (defensive qi) and body fluid to the skin to warm, nourish and moisten the skin so as to maintain the normal functions of the skin. The other is that the normal opening and closing activities of the sweat pores on the skin can excrete sweat, adjust body temperature, assist the lung to respire and discharge the turbid qi. That is why sweat pores are also called "qi gate" in TCM. If the functions of the lung are normal, the skin will be well nourished, manifesting as fine and close skin, appropriate excretion of sweat and strong power in resisting exogenous pathogenic factors. If lung-qi and lung-yin are deficient, it will lead to dry skin, profuse sweat and susceptibility to cold. When exogenous pathogenic factors invade the body, they usually attack the skin first and then affect the lung, stagnating lung-qi and leading to such symptoms as aversion to cold, fever, stuffy nose and cough. Besides, TCM also holds that "the lung governs the skin and hair", a combination of the terms "the lung governing the skin" and "the lung having its external manifestion on the hair". The idea will be described in following section.

2. The lung opening into the nose

The nose, an organ for smelling, is a route for air to be breathed in and out of the body. Since the lung controls respiration and dominates qi in the whole body, so the nose is regarded as the orifice into which the lung opens.

便异常等病症。

（二）肺与形体官窍的关系

1. 肺主皮

皮，即皮肤，具有保护人体、排泄汗液及调节体温等功能。肺与皮肤的关系，可从两方面来理解：一是肺可以宣发输布卫气和津液至皮肤，以温养、滋润皮肤，维持皮肤正常的生理功能。二是皮肤汗孔开合有度，既可排泄汗液，调节体温，又可协助肺的呼吸功能，排出部分浊气，所以汗孔又叫做"气门"。如肺的功能正常，皮肤得养，则皮肤致密，汗液排泄适度，抵御外邪的能力亦强。如肺之气阴不足，皮肤失养，可见皮肤干燥枯槁、多汗而易于感冒；而外邪侵袭人体，也常从皮肤影响及肺，引起肺气不宣，出现恶寒、发热、鼻塞、咳嗽等症状。此外，中医学还有"肺主皮毛"的说法，即将"肺主皮"与"肺华在毛"合而为一的专用术语。关于"肺华在毛"，请参见下文。

2. 肺开窍于鼻

鼻是嗅觉器官，为呼吸之气出入的通道，而肺司呼吸，主一身之气，故称"鼻为肺之窍"。鼻的嗅觉和通气功能与

In fact the smelling and ventilating functions of the lung are closely related to the function of lung-qi. Only when lung-qi is harmonious and respiration is smooth can the nose be sensitive in smelling. For example, failure of lung-qi to disperse leads to stuffy nose, running nose and hyposmia; insufficiency of lung-qi brings on unsmooth respiration with the nose.

The throat, located posterior and inferior to the nose, is an organ in charge of vocalization and serves as the gate of respiration. Since the lung meridian runs across the throat and the lung itself governs respiration, the ventilation and vocalization are closely related to the functions of the lung. If lung-qi and lung-yin are deficient or if lung-qi fails to disperse, it will not only lead to unsmoothness of the throat in ventilation, but also bring on changes of vocalization, consequently resulting in pruritus in the throat, sore throat, hoarse voice or aphonia.

3. External manifestation on the body hair

Since the lung dominates the skin, the defensive qi and body fluid dispersed by the lung nourish the skin and the body hair. With proper nourishment of the defensive qi and body fluid, the body hair appears lustrous and is not easy to lose. Thus the condition of the body hair reflects the functional states of the lung. If lung-qi and lung-yin are insufficient, the body hair cannot get enough nourishment, making the body hair dry and easy to break and lose.

2.1.3 The liver

The liver is located below the diaphragm and in the right rib-side. The liver "pertains to yin in entity and yang in function". This is the physiological characteristics of the liver. As one of the five zang-organs, the liver pertains to yin because it stores yin-blood. However in function the liver pertains to yang because yang-qi in the liver

肺气的作用紧密相关。肺气调和,呼吸通畅,鼻的嗅觉才能灵敏。如肺气不宣,可见鼻塞流涕,嗅觉减退;如肺气不足,可致鼻息不利等。

鼻之后下方为喉。喉主发音,也是呼吸的门户。肺的经脉经过喉部,肺主呼吸,故喉的通气与发音也与肺的功能有关。如果肺之气阴不足,或肺气失宣,不但可造成喉咙的通气不利,还会使声音发生变化,出现喉痒、喉痛、声音嘶哑或失音等。

3. 肺华在毛

由于肺主皮肤,肺宣发的卫气和津液可以通过皮肤而滋养毫毛,使毫毛具有光泽而不易脱落,故毫毛的荣枯可反映出肺的功能正常与否。如肺之气阴不足,毫毛失养,则出现毫毛干燥枯槁,并容易折断或脱落等。

三、肝

肝位于横膈之下,右胁之内。肝的生理特性是"体阴用阳"。"体阴",是指肝为阴脏而内藏阴血;"用阳",是指肝之阳气活泼好动,易升发,性刚强。由于肝具有刚强的特

is very active and resolute, tending to disperse. That is why the liver is described as "a general-organ".

2.1.3.1 The physiological functions of the liver

The liver possesses two physiological functions: to govern shu-xie (dredging and regulating) and to store blood.

1. To dredge and regulate

Shu-xie in Chinese means to dredge and smooth the route of something. The liver governing shu-xie actually means that the liver dredges the routes and regulates the movement of qi so as to ensure smooth flow of qi in the body. The movement of qi is described as qi-ji (qi activity) in TCM. So to regulate the movement of qi means to regulate the activity of qi. The physiological activities of all the internal organs and tissues depend on the normal movement of qi. Since the liver can regulate the activity of qi, it plays an important role in regulating the physiological functions of all the internal organs and tissues. The function of the liver to regulate qi activity is demonstrated in the following aspects:

(1) To promote circulation of blood and metabolism of body fluid: Blood circulation and body fluid metabolism all depend on the propelling function of the visceral qi, the normal flow of which relies on the regulating and dredging function of the liver which are prerequisite to constant blood circulation and normal metabolism of body fluid. If the movement of qi is abnormal due to failure of the liver to dredge and regulate, it may affect blood circulation and body fluid metabolism, bringing on corresponding pathologic changes. For example, if the liver is weak in dredging and regulating, the activity of qi will be stagnated and blood circulation will be obstructed, leading to blood stasis; or if the liver is hyperactive in dredging and regu-

性,所以《黄帝内经》称肝为"将军之官"。

(一) 肝的生理功能

肝具有主疏泄和主藏血两方面的功能。

1. 主疏泄

疏泄,即疏通畅达的意思。肝主疏泄,是指肝可以疏通、调节人体气的运动,从而使气的运动保持通畅。气的运动过程中医称之为"气机",因此调节气的运动也就是调节气机。人体各脏腑组织的生理活动,都有赖于气的正常运动;肝主疏泄,能够调畅气机,从而对各脏腑组织的生理功能发挥着重要的调节作用。肝主疏泄调节气机的功能,主要表现在以下四个方面。

(1) 促进血液运行和津液代谢 血液的运行和津液的代谢,都有赖于有关脏腑之气的推动作用,而脏腑之气的正常运行,又必须依靠肝气的疏通才能保持调畅。故肝的疏泄功能正常,是促进血液循环不息和津液代谢正常的必要条件。若肝失疏泄,气的运行失常,就可影响血液运行和津液代谢,出现相应的病变。如肝疏泄不及而气机郁结,血行不畅,可形成瘀血;或肝疏泄

lating, blood will flow adversely with qi, causing haematemesis; or if qi activity is obstructed, water passage will be stagnated, leading to phlegm, rheum and edema.

(2) To assist the spleen and the stomach to digest food: The digestion and absorption of food are accomplished by the spleen and the stomach. However, the dredging and regulating functions of the liver play an important role in the process of digestion. Because the liver regulates the activity of spleen-qi and stomach-qi with its dredging and regulating functions, ensuring a harmonious balance between the function of spleen-qi to elevate the lucid and the function of the stomach-qi to descend the turbid so as to guarantee a normal process of digestion. Besides, the bile, accumulation of surplus liver-qi, comes from the liver and excretes into the small intestine to assist digestion. The normal secretion and excretion of the bile are closely relatcd to the dredging and regulating functions of the liver. If the dredging and regulating functions of the liver are abnormal, the activity of spleen-qi, stomach-qi and gallbladder-qi will be affected, leading to disturbance in digesting and absorbing food. If liver-qi attacks the spleen and the stomach, the activities of spleen-qi and stomach-qi will be affected, subsequently leading to abdominal distension, abdominal pain and diarrhea due to failure of spleen-qi to ascend on the one hand, and gastric distension and pain, vomiting and hiccup due to failure of stomach-qi to descend on the other. If failure of the liver to dredge and regulate affects the secretion and excretion of the bile, it will also bring on symptoms due to disharmony between the liver and gallbladder, such as hypochondriac pain, jaundice and anorexia.

(3) To regulate mental activity: Mental activity refers to psychological activities such as joy, anger, anxiety and contemplation, etc. Mental activity, part of spiritual

（2）协助脾胃消化 人体对饮食物的消化吸收，是由脾胃来完成的，而肝的疏泄功能对消化过程起着十分重要的协助作用。这种协助作用主要表现在，肝通过疏泄来调畅脾胃的气机运动，使脾气之升清与胃气之降浊得以协调配合，从而保证消化过程的正常进行；同时，由于胆汁来源于肝，是肝之余气积聚而成，贮存于胆，并排出于小肠而发挥其帮助消化的作用，而胆汁的正常分泌与排泄，与肝的疏泄功能有密切关系。如果肝失疏泄，影响到脾、胃、胆的气机，必会引起饮食的消化吸收障碍。若肝气侵犯脾胃，使脾胃气机升降失常，既可出现腹胀、腹痛、腹泻等脾气不升的病变，也可出现胃部胀痛、呕吐、嗳气等胃气不降的症状。若肝失疏泄，影响到胆汁的分泌与排泄，还可出现胁痛、黄疸、食欲不振等肝胆不和的症状。

（3）调畅情志活动 情志，是指人的喜、怒、忧、思等心理活动。情志活动是精神

activity, is dominated by the heart and closely related to the dredging and regulating functions of the liver. The normal mental activity depends on sufficiency of blood and smooth activity of qi which can be promoted by the liver. With the normal functions of the heart and the liver, qi and blood will flow harmoniously and smoothly, making it better for people to regulate their mental activities and enjoy happiness and pleasure. If qi activity is in disorder due to failure of the liver to dredge and regulate, it will lead to abnormal changes of mental activities, such as heavy heart, melancholy, sentimentality, hiccup and sigh due to stagnation of liver-qi. If liver-qi flows adversely, qi will stagnate and transform into fire, bringing on symptoms of irascibility, susceptibility to rage, reddish complexion and eyes, head distension and headache due to hyperactivity of liver-qi.

(4) To regulate menstruation: The physiological characteristics of women, such as menstruation, pregnancy and delivery, are closely related to blood. The liver regulates the activity of qi to enable blood to flow downward into the uterus to meet the need for menstruation, pregnancy and delivery. That is why it was said in ancient times that "the congenital base for women is the liver". If the liver fails to dredge and regulate, it will clinically lead to various women diseases, such as irregular menstruation, dysmenorrhea, amenorrhea and sterility.

2. To store blood

The liver storing blood refers to the function of the

活动的一部分,它固然属心所主管,同时也与肝的疏泄功能密切相关。因为正常的情志活动有赖于血液的充足、气机的调畅,而肝能疏通气机,促进血行,使气血调和,这样人就可较好地协调自身的情志活动,表现出精神愉快、心情舒畅、乐观开朗等情绪反应;肝失疏泄,气机不调,便可导致情志活动的异常。如肝失疏泄而气机不畅,可表现为心情不舒、郁郁寡欢、多愁善虑、嗳气太息等肝气抑郁的证候;若肝气横逆而气郁化火,可表现为性情急躁、容易发怒、面红目赤、头胀头痛等肝气亢奋的证候。

（4）调理妇女月经 妇女的生理特点是以血为用,如行经耗血、妊娠血聚养胎、分娩出血等,都与血液的充盈及运行有着密切的关系。而肝主疏泄,调畅气机,使血脉流通,下注胞宫,对维持妇女月经、生育等特殊的生理活动起着非常重要的作用,所以古人有"女子以肝为先天"的说法。如肝的疏泄功能失常,临床上可出现多种妇产科病症,如月经不调、痛经、闭经、不孕、不育等。

2. 主藏血

肝主藏血,是指肝具有贮

liver to store blood and regulate the volume of blood.

The physiological significance of the liver to store blood lies in the fact that liver-blood nourishes the liver itself. With the nourishment of blood, the liver will have sufficient yin-fluid to prevent liver-yang from becoming hyperactive. Besides, in the course of regulating blood volume, liver-blood can nourish the tissues and organs in the whole body to sustain their physiological activities.

The liver storing blood is a course in which blood enters the liver and comes out of the liver. Under physiological condition, the volume of blood in different parts of the body varies due to the difference of their physiological activities. Generally speaking, the organs in the body comparatively need less blood when the body is in a quiet state, the rest of blood flows into the liver. When the body takes strenuous activities or when people become excited, the organs in the body comparatively need more blood. In this case, the liver transports blood stored to other parts of the body to meet the need of their physiological activities. If physiological activities are different, the volume of blood needed is also different. In fact the blood needed by different organs and tissues constantly varies with the change of physiological activities. Such a constant variation is also closely related to the function of the liver to store blood. That is to say that the liver, based on its function to store blood, adjusts the volume of blood to meet the need of different physiological activities.

If the function of the liver to store blood is in disorder, it may lead to two kinds of pathological changes. One is insufficiency of liver-blood. In this case the body cannot get enough nourishment, leading to dizziness, vertigo,

藏血液和调节血量的功能。

肝藏血的生理意义在于,肝血可以濡养自身,肝得血养则阴液充足,肝阴足则能制约肝阳而不致过亢;同时在调节血量的过程中,肝血能滋养全身组织器官以适应其生理活动的需要。

肝藏血的过程是一个血液出入于肝的过程。在生理状态下,人体各部分的血液量随着其生理活动的不同状态而有所不同。一般地说,安静状态下人体各器官血液的需要量较小,其有余的血液就回流入肝,贮藏起来。当人体在剧烈活动或情绪激动时,各器官血液的需要量就较大,此时肝就把所贮藏的血液输送出来,以满足机体生理活动的需要。在不同的生理活动中,各器官所需要的血量互有差异。因此,随着生理活动的变化,血液在各组织器官之间重新分配着,这种重新分配也与肝藏血的功能密切相关。也就是说,肝脏在贮藏血液的基础上,能根据机体生理活动的不同状态来调节各部分的血量,以适应不同生理活动的需要。

肝主藏血功能失常,可引起两方面的病变。一是藏血不足,也叫做肝血不足。由于肝血虚少,周身失养,可出现

weakness of limbs, scanty and light-colored menses or a-menorrhea. The other is failure of the liver to store blood which may lead to abnormal flow of blood, causing various symptoms such as haematemesis, epistaxis, hematochezia and profuse menorrhea, or even constant haematemesis or sudden profuse uterine bleeding in severe cases.

2.1.3.2　The relationships between the liver and the body, the sensory organs and the orifices

1. The liver governing the tendons

The tendons are the tissues that connect the muscles, the skeleton and the joints. The contraction and relaxation of the tendons maintain the flexion and extension or lateral rotation of the joints.

The liver governing the tendons means that the physiological functions of the tendons depend on liver-blood to nourish and liver-yin to moisten. Only when liver-yin and liver-blood are sufficient can the tendons get enough nourishment and the joints move flexibly and powerfully. If liver-yin and liver-blood are deficient, the tendons cannot get enough nourishment, leading to unsmooth movement of the joints, tremor of hands and feet, numbness of the limbs or susceptibility to fatigue.

2. The liver opening into the eyes

The liver meridian runs upward into the eyes. So the eyes are nourished by liver-yin and liver-blood. Besides, the liver can regulate the activities of the eyes with its dredging and regulating functions. Thus eyesight is closely related to the liver. The conditions of the liver can be observed from the manifestations of the eyes. That is why it is said that "the liver opens into the eyes". For example, insufficiency of liver-yin and liver-blood may lead to

头昏、目眩、肢体乏力、妇女月经量少色淡或闭经等症状。二是藏血失职,也叫做肝不藏血。由于血液不能归藏于肝而妄行,可出现吐血、衄血、便血、妇女月经量多等症状,严重时可导致呕血不止,或崩漏下血量多等症。

(二)肝与形体官窍的关系

1. 肝主筋

筋,是联结肌肉、骨骼和关节的一种组织。筋的收缩和弛张,维持着人体关节运动的屈伸或转侧。

肝主筋,是指筋有赖于肝血的营养和肝阴的滋润,才能保持正常的功能。肝阴肝血充足,筋得其养,关节运动便灵活而有力。如果肝之阴血不足,血不养筋,可出现关节活动不利、手足震颤、肢体麻木或容易疲劳等症状。

2. 肝开窍于目

目即眼睛,中医学也称"精明"。由于肝的经脉上连于目,肝之阴血营养于目,肝之疏泄调节于目,故目的视觉功能与肝密切相关,而肝的功能正常与否,也往往从目反映出来,所以说"肝开窍于目"。如肝阴肝血不足,可见两目干

dryness of the eyes and blurred vision; failure of the liver to dredge and regulate may lead to up-flaming of liver-fire, consequently bringing on redness, swelling and pain of the eyes and cataract.

Besides, the essence of the five zang-organs and six fu-organs all flows into the eyes. So the eyes are not only related to the liver, but also to the other viscera. For example, the white part of the eyes pertains to the lung that governs qi, so it is termed qi-wheel; the black part of the eyes pertains to the liver that governs wind, so it is termed wind-wheel; the internal and external canthi pertain to the heart that governs blood, so they are termed blood-wheel; the upper and lower eyelids pertain to the spleen, so they are termed muscle-wheels; the pupil pertains to the kidney that governs water, so it is termed water-wheel. Altogether they are called "five wheels".

3. The external manifestation of the liver on the nails

The nails here include both the nails of fingers and toes. TCM believes that the nails are the extensions of the tendons. The nails, like the tendons, depend on liver-blood to nourish. Thus deficiency of liver-blood often affects the color and quality of the nails. For example, if liver-blood is sufficient, the nails are firm and bright, ruddy and lustrous; if liver-blood is insufficient, the nails are soft and thin, or even deformed or brittle.

2.1.4 The spleen

The spleen, located in the abdomen, governs digestion and absorption. As the source of qi, blood and body fluid, the spleen plays a vital role in maintaining life activities. Such a function of the spleen only comes into play

涩、视物模糊；肝失疏泄，肝火上炎，可见目赤肿痛、目睛生翳等。

另外，由于五脏六腑之精气皆上注于目，所以目不仅与肝有关，而且与其他脏腑都有内在的联系。如白睛属肺，因肺主气，故称白睛为气轮；黑睛属肝，因肝主风，故称黑睛为风轮；内、外眦属心，因心主血，故称内、外眦为血轮；上、下眼胞属脾，因脾主肉，故称上、下眼胞为肉轮；瞳孔属肾，因肾主水，故称瞳孔为水轮。以上合称"五轮"。

3. 肝华在爪

爪即爪甲，包括手指甲和脚趾甲。中医学认为爪是筋延续在外的部分，故称"爪为筋之余"。爪与筋一样，也要依赖肝血的濡养，所以肝血的盈亏，往往可以影响爪甲的荣枯。如肝血充足，则爪甲坚韧明亮，红润而有光泽；若肝血不足，则爪甲软薄，甚至变形或脆裂。

四、脾

脾位于腹中，主管消化吸收，是化生气血津液的源泉，对维持生命活动起着根本的作用，而这种作用是人体出生

after birth. That is why it is said that "the spleen is the acquired base of life" and "the source of qi, blood and body fluid".

2.1.4.1 The physiological functions of the spleen

To govern transportation and transformation and to command blood are two major physiological functions of the spleen.

1. To govern the transportation and transformation

The function of the spleen to govern transportation and transformation means that the spleen can digest food, absorb nutrients of food and water, and then transport them to the heart and the lung.

When taken into the stomach, food is digested and absorbed by the stomach and the small intestine. But it must depend on the transporting and transforming functions of the spleen to transform into nutrients which, relying on the functions of the spleen to transmit and dispersing essence, are distributed to the four limbs and the other parts of the body. The rest of the water absorbed from the food nutrients is transported to the lung and the kidney and, by means of qi transformation taking place in the lung and the kidney, transformed into sweat and urine to be excreted out of the body. So the transporting and transforming functions of the spleen are usually divided into two parts: transporting and transforming food nutrients, and transporting and transforming water. Since the transporting and transforming of food nutrients and water take place at the same time in the process of digesting, absorbing and transmitting food, they are closely related to each other and pathologically affect each other.

The transporting and transforming functions of the

以后才体现出来的,所以称脾为"后天之本"、"气血生化之源"。

(一) 脾的生理功能

脾的生理功能包括主运化和主统血两方面。

1. 主运化

脾主运化,是指脾能够消化饮食,吸收其中的精微物质和水液,然后再转输至心肺的功能。

饮食入胃后,对饮食物的消化和吸收,实际上是在胃和小肠内进行的。但是,必须依赖于脾的运化功能,才能将水谷化为精微。同样,也有赖于脾的转输和散精功能,才能把水谷精微"灌溉四旁"和布散至全身。另一方面,对被吸收的水谷精微中多余水分,能及时转输至肺和肾,通过肺、肾的气化功能,化为汗和尿排出体外。因此一般将脾主运化的功能分为运化精微和运化水液两个方面。但是,由于在脾的消化、吸收和转输过程中,运化精微和运化水液是同时进行的,所以,这两方面的功能之间有着密切的联系,病理上也往往相互影响。

脾主运化的功能,除了与

spleen are mainly concerned with, apart from the warming function of spleen-yang, the propelling function of spleen-qi. The movement of spleen-qi is marked mainly by elevation. That is why it is said in TCM that "the spleen governs the activity of elevating the lucid". To elevate means to ascend and transmit; the lucid refers to the food nutrients. The idea that "the spleen governs the activity of elevating the lucid" indicates that the function of spleen-qi is to transmit food nutrients to the heart and the lung. If the function of the spleen to elevate the lucid is normal, qi and blood will be sufficient, and there will be exuberant vitality in the activities of life. Besides, to elevate also means to lift and fixate. The elevation of spleen-qi can also fixate the viscera and prevent them from prolapse.

The normal state of the functions of the spleen to transport and transform is called healthy transformation of spleen-qi while the abnormal state of the functions of the spleen to transport and transform is called unhealthy transformation of spleen-qi. The main clinical manifestations of the latter can be divided into four groups: anorexia, abdominal distension, abdominal pain and loose stool if the digesting and absorbing functions are weak; phlegm, rheum and edema if dampness and water are retained due to disturbance of water metabolism; dizziness and spiritual lassitude if the spleen fails to elevate the lucid; visceroptosis, prolonged diarrhea and proctoptosis if spleen-qi sinks.

2. To command blood

To command means to control. To command blood means that the spleen controls blood circulation inside the vessels and prevent it from flowing out of the vessels.

The spleen commands blood with its fixating function. If

脾阳的温煦作用有关外,主要依赖于脾气的推动作用。脾气的运动特点,是以上升为主,故中医学有"脾主升清"的说法。升,指上升和输布;清,指饮食中的精微物质。脾主升清,即通过脾气的作用将饮食中的精微物质上输于心肺。因此,脾主升清功能正常,气血化生充足,人体的生命活动就能保持旺盛的生机。另一方面,"升"还具有升提、托举之意。脾气上升,还能固摄内脏,维持内脏恒定的位置而不致下垂。

脾的运化功能正常,称为脾气健运;脾的运化功能失常,称为脾失健运。其临床表现主要有:消化吸收功能减弱,表现为食欲不振、腹胀、腹痛、便溏等症;水液代谢障碍,引起水湿内停,可出现痰饮、水肿等症;如脾不升清,可见头晕目眩、神疲乏力;如脾气下陷,可见内脏下垂、久泻脱肛等。

2. 主统血

统,是统摄、控制的意思。脾主统血,指脾能够统摄血液在脉管中运行,使其不致逸出脉外。

脾统血,主要依赖于脾气

spleen-qi is sufficient, it can control blood and directs
blood to circulate inside the vessels. Such a function of the
spleen is also related to spleen-yang. Thus deficiency of
spleen-qi and spleen-yang will impair the function of the
spleen to command blood, leading to hematochezia, hematuria, sudden profuse uterine bleeding and subcutaneous
purpura.

2. 1. 4. 2　The relationships between the spleen and the body, the sensory organs and the orifices

1. The spleen governing the muscles and the four limbs

The idea that the spleen governs the muscles and the
four limbs means that the muscles and the four limbs depend on the nutrients transported and transformed by the
spleen to nourish. With the normal function of the spleen,
sufficient qi and blood will be transformed from food nutrients; with sufficient nourishment, both the muscles and
the limbs will become strong. If he function of the spleen
is abnormal, the absorption of food nutrients will be reduced, leading to insufficient production of qi and blood
and bringing on malnutrition of the muscles and the limbs
with the symptoms of emaciation, lassitude of the limbs or
even atrophy of the limbs.

2. The spleen opening into the mouth

The mouth is the starting point of the digestive canal. Since digestion is governed by the spleen, the mouth
is the orifice into which the spleen opens. The idea that
the spleen opens into the mouth means that the functional
states of the spleen can be observed from the manifestations on the mouth. If the spleen is normal in function,
the appetite and taste in the mouth will be normal; if the

对血液的固摄作用。脾气充足,就能将周身血液控制、约束在脉管中循行,从而防止其逸出于脉外。其次,脾统血的功能与脾阳也有关。因此脾气脾阳虚弱,导致统血功能失常,血液不循常道,就会出现便血、尿血、崩漏、皮下紫斑等多种出血病证。

(二) 脾与形体官窍的关系

1. 脾主肌肉、四肢

脾主肌肉、四肢,是指肌肉与四肢的营养均来自脾运化的水谷精微。脾气健运,水谷精微化生气血充足,肌肉四肢得其营养,则肌肉丰满壮实,四肢强劲有力。若脾失健运,水谷精微吸收减少,气血化生不足,肌肉四肢失养,则肌肉消瘦软弱、四肢倦怠乏力,甚至痿废不用。

2. 脾开窍于口

口为消化道的开端。由于消化功能由脾所主,所以口成为脾之"窍"。脾开窍于口,是指脾的运化功能正常与否,可从口的某些方面表现出来。如脾运强健,则食欲旺盛,口味正常;如脾运失健,可见食

spleen is abnormal in function, it will lead to anorexia, no taste in the mouth, or greasy and sweet taste in the mouth.

3. The external manifestation on the lips

The spleen opens into the mouth and the lips are the external parts of the mouth. So the functional states of the spleen can be observed from the color and shape of the lips. If the spleen is normal in function, qi and blood will be sufficient, and the lips will be ruddy and lustrous; if the spleen is abnormal in function, qi and blood will become scanty, and the lips will be pale, lusterless or even sallow.

2.1.5 The kidney

The kidney is located in the waist. That is why it is said in *Huangdi Neijing* that "the waist is the house of the kidney". The kidney stores essence and the essence transforms qi and produces blood. Besides, the kidney is the source of genuine yin and genuine yang. So the kidney is closely related with the essence, qi, blood, yin and yang. Since the kidney-essence comes from parents and is the primary substance for constituting human body and conceiving new life, TCM regards the kidney as "the prenatal base of life".

2.1.5.1 The physiological functions of the kidney

The physiological functions of the kidney are composed of six parts: to govern growth and development, to govern reproduction, to govern water, to govern reception of qi, to produce marrow to enrich the brain and transform blood and to nourish and warm the internal organs.

1. To govern growth and development

The kidney stores essence, qi, yin and yang. The

欲减退,口淡乏味,或口腻、口甜等。

3. 脾华在唇

脾开窍于口,而唇为口之外露部分,脾的功能状况,可从唇的色泽、形态反映出来。如脾气健运,气血充足,口唇红润而有光泽;如脾失健运,气血衰少,则口唇淡白无华,或萎黄不泽。

五、肾

肾位于腰部,所以《黄帝内经》说"腰为肾之府"。肾藏精,精能化气、生血;肾又为人体真阴、真阳之根本,所以肾与精、气、血、阴、阳等重要生命物质都有密切关系。由于肾精禀受于父母,来源于先天,是构成人体及养育新的生命体的原始物质,所以中医学认为肾为人体的"先天之本"。

(一)肾的生理功能

肾具有主生长发育、主生殖、主水、主纳气、生髓充脑化血及濡养温煦各脏腑等六个方面的功能。

1. 主生长发育

肾中藏有精、气、阴、阳,

growth and development of the body mainly depend on the kidney-essence, kidney-yin and kidney-yang. After birth, the kidney-essence gradually becomes abundant with the development of the body. During the childhood, the abundance of the kidney-essence is marked by dental transition, growth of hair and body. During youth period, the kidney-essence is further enriched, marked by full development of all organs and maturity of reproductive function. During the mid-age and prime period of life, the kidney-essence has developed to its peak, characterized by sturdy build, rich vitality and strong tendons and bones. After the mid-age and during the old-age, the kidney-essence gradually declines, and so are the functions of the five zang-organs and six fu-organs, leading to a series of signs of senility, such as loss of hair and teeth, hunchback, poor hearing and gradual loss of reproductive function. At different stages of life process, the body and its physiological functions vary with the changes of the essence in the kidney. That is to say that the essence, qi, yin and yang in the kidney decide the growth and development of the body. If these substances in the kidney are deficient, the growth and development of the body will be affected, leading to a series of pathological manifestations, such as hypoevolutism, feeblemindedness, atrophy and flaccidity of tendons and bones as well as senilism.

2. To govern reproduction

The reproductive function includes the development of sex organs, maturity and maintenance of sex as well as fertility which are all closely related with the kidney-essence, kidney-yin and kidney-yang. When the body develops to the period of youth, the essence in the kidney enriches

人的生长发育过程,主要依靠肾中精气及其阴精与阳气的作用。人出生以后,随着生长发育而肾中精气也逐渐充盛,在少年时期首先表现出更换牙齿、头发变长、身体增高等形体变化;到青年时期,肾中精气更加充盛,各器官发育逐渐成熟,并逐渐有生殖功能;中壮年时期,由于肾中精气最为充盛,所以身体壮实,精力充沛,筋骨强健;中年以后至老年时期,肾中精气日渐减少,五脏六腑的功能也日益衰退,就出现发脱、齿落、背驼、耳聋等一派衰老的现象,生殖功能也逐渐丧失。在整个人体生命过程的生、长、壮、老的各个阶段中,其形体和生理功能随着肾中精气的盛衰变化而变化。也就是说,肾中精气以及阴阳决定着机体的生长发育,是一生盛衰之根本。如果肾精肾气或肾阴肾阳不足,影响了人体的生长发育,就可引起小儿发育迟缓、智力低下、筋骨萎软以及成人早衰等一系列病理表现。

2. 主生殖

人的生殖功能,包括生殖器官的发育情况、性功能的成熟与维持及生育能力等,都与肾中精气以及阴阳的盛衰密切相关。当人体生长发育至

to a certain degree and produces a kind of reproductive substance known as tiankui which can promote the development of sex organs and maintain normal sex function. Consequently man has sperm and experiences seminal emission, and woman has menarche. These physiological changes indicate genitality. Man and woman maintain such a sex function and genitality after their middle age. At the period of old age, the kidney-essence gradually declines. Subsequently tiankui becomes exhausted and, accordingly, genitality declines and disappears in the end. This shows that the essence, qi, yin and yang in the kidney play a key role in the genitality and reproduction. If these vital substances are deficient, the genitality and reproduction will inevitably be affected, leading to maldevelopment of sex organs, weakness of sex function and sterility.

3. To govern water

To govern water means that the kidney controls the metabolism of water.

The metabolism of water is related to many organs like the lung that regulates water passage, the spleen that transports and transforms water, the liver that promotes the metabolism of water and the triple energizer that serves as the passage of water. However, the function of the kidney to govern water is key to the metabolism of water. When taken into the stomach, the water is transmitted to the kidney with the collective action of the spleen, the lung, the liver and the triple energizer. The kidney regulates the whole process of transporting and excreting water, playing a very important role in maintaining a

青年时期,由于肾中精气充盛到一定程度,体内就产生了一种叫"天癸"的物质。天癸可促进人体生殖器官的发育成熟,并维持正常的性功能。因此,男子便产生精液而能排精,女子便有月经来潮,开始具有生殖能力。这种性功能与生殖能力一直维持到中年以后。到了老年时期,随着肾中精气的减少,天癸逐渐耗竭,生殖功能也随之衰退,直至完全丧失。这说明肾中精气以及阴阳对人的生殖功能起着决定性的作用,是生殖繁衍之根本。若肾中精气以及阴阳不足,人的生殖功能就必然会受到影响,出现生殖器官发育不良、性功能低下,以及不孕不育等病变。

3. 主水

肾主水,指肾具有主管人体水液代谢的功能。

人体的水液代谢,与许多脏腑都有关系,如肺主通调水道、脾主运化水液、肝促进津液代谢、三焦为水道等,而肾主水的功能则是调节水液代谢的中心环节。水液经饮食进入于胃,再经脾、肺、肝、三焦等脏腑的作用而下归于肾,肾主水则能调节水液输布和排泄的全过程,对维持体内水液代谢的整体平衡发挥着重

holistic balance of water metabolism. It is said in *Huang-di Neijing* that "the kidney is the door of the stomach. If the door is not properly closed, water will be accumulated inside the body."

The function of the kidney to govern water is accomplished with its function of qi-hua (qi-transformation). After absorbed by the spleen, the water is transported to the lung and distributed to all parts of the body with the dispersing and descending functions of the lung. After being used by all the tissues and organs in the body, the water is collected into the kidney. With its function of qi-transformation, the kidney separates the lucid part from the water and elevates it again to the lung to keep certain amount of water inside the body on the one hand, and transforms the rest part into urine to be transported to the bladder and excreted out of the body on the other.

The kidney depends on kidney-yang and kidney-qi to transform water. With the steaming and fixating functions of kidney-yang and kidney-qi, the kidney elevates the lucid part of water to the heart and the lung. With the warming function of kidney-yang and propelling function of kidney-qi, the kidney descends the turbid part of water and transforms it into urine to be excreted out of the body. So deficiency of kidney-yang and dysfunction of qi-transformation of the kidney will lead to profuse urine, enuresis and incontinence of urine due to weakness in steaming and fixating on the one hand, and scanty urine, anuria and edema due to weakness in warming and propelling on the other.

4. To govern reception of qi

Reception means acceptance and storage. To govern reception of qi means that the kidney can receive fresh air inhaled by the lung to assist the lung to govern respiration.

要作用,所以《黄帝内经》说:"肾者,胃之关也,关门不利,故聚水而从其类也。"

肾主水的功能是依靠肾的气化作用来实现的。水液经脾吸收而上输于肺,通过肺气的宣发肃降输布至全身,全身各组织器官利用以后,又汇聚于肾。肾通过气化作用,一方面将其中的清者分别出来,再上升于肺,以保持体内一定量的水液;另一方面,将其中的浊者生成尿液,下输膀胱而排出体外。

肾对水的气化作用,是依靠肾阳与肾气来完成的。由肾阳的蒸腾和肾气的固摄作用,促使水液之清者上升,复归于心肺;由肾阳的温化和肾气的推动作用,促使水液之浊者下降,形成小便而排出于体外。因此,肾之阳气虚弱,气化作用失常,既可出现尿多、遗尿、尿失禁等蒸腾固摄无力的症状,也可产生尿少、尿闭、水肿等温化推动失常的病变。

4. 主纳气

纳,有接受、藏入之义。肾主纳气,是指肾能够受纳肺所吸入的清气,以协助肺司呼吸的功能。

The respiratory activity is controlled by the lung. But the fresh air inhaled by the lung from the natural world has to be descended into the kidney to ensure free and smooth respiration and keep the respiration into a certain depth so as to meet the need of various viscera and tissues for fresh air. There is a close relationship between the function of the lung to govern respiration and the function of the kidney to receive qi. The former is prerequisite to the latter and the latter is the basic condition of the former. Normal respiration is accomplished by coordinative action of both the lung and the kidney.

The function of the kidney to receive qi is accomplished with the fixating function of kidney-qi. Only when kidney-qi is abundant and normal in receiving qi can the lung respire evenly and the air passage be clear. If kidney-qi is deficient and the function of the kidney to receive qi is weak, the fresh air inhaled by the lung cannot be descended to the kidney, bringing on various pathological changes like more exhalation and less inhalation, shortness of breath and frequent asthma.

5. To produce marrow to enrich the brain and transform blood

The kidney stores essence and the essence stored in the kidney can produce marrow. The marrow includes cerebral marrow, spinal cord and bone marrow. When transported into the bones, the marrow can nourish the bones. That is why TCM believes that "the kidney governs the bones". The spinal cord is connected with the brain, nourishes the brain and maintains the physiological functions of the brain together with the cerebral marrow. That is why the brain is called "the sea of marrow" in TCM. If the kidney-essence is insufficient, the production of cerebral marrow will be reduced, leading to various

人体的呼吸运动,是肺脏所主管的,而肺吸入的自然界之清气,又必须下达于肾,由肾为之受纳,这样呼吸运动才能通畅、调匀,并保持一定的深度,从而满足各脏腑组织对清气的需求。所以,肺司呼吸是肾主纳气的前提条件,而肾主纳气则是肺司呼吸的根本条件,正常呼吸运动正是由肺、肾两脏功能互相配合协调而共同完成的。

肾主纳气的功能,是依靠肾气的固摄作用来进行的。只有肾气充沛,摄纳正常,才能使肺的呼吸均匀,气道通畅。如果肾气虚弱,纳气功能减退,吸入之气不能归藏于肾,就会出现呼多吸少、气短、动则气喘等肾不纳气的病理变化。

5. 生髓、充脑、化血

肾藏精,肾精又能化生髓。髓包括脑髓、脊髓和骨髓。髓充于骨,则能滋养骨骼,所以中医学有"肾主骨"的理论。脊髓上通于脑,与脑髓共同濡养脑,维持脑的生理功能,故称脑为"髓海"。若肾精不足,脑髓化生减少,髓海空虚,就可出现头痛、眩晕、健忘、反应迟钝等脑功能失常的病变。

pathological changes, such as headache, dizziness, amnesia and retard response.

The production of blood, apart from the transformation of food nutrients by the spleen and stomach, is related to the kidney-essence. Physiologically the kidney-essence and blood promote each other and transform into
each other. So sufficient kidney-essence ensures abundant
production of blood while deficient kidney-essence leads to
insufficient production of blood. Clinically blood deficiency
syndrome due to deficiency of kidney-essence must be
treated by the therapy for nourishing the kidney and enriching the essence.

6. To nourish and warm the viscera

Kidney-yin and kidney-yang restrain each other and
depend on each other, playing an important role in maintaining the normal functions of the kidney. Kidney-yin,
also known as primordial yin or genuine yin, can nourish
yin in all the viscera, serving as the source of yin-fluid in
the body. Kidney-yang, also known as primordial yang or
genuine yang, can warm yang in all the viscera, serving
as the source of yang-qi in the whole body. Since kidney-
yin and kidney-yang are the sources of yin and yang in the
other viscera, the deficiency of kidney-yin and kidney-
yang may lead to deficiency of yin and yang in the other
viscera. Clinically, deficiency of kidney-yin mainly leads
to deficiency of liver-yin, heart-yin and lung-yin; deficiency of kidney-yang mainly brings on deficiency of
spleen-yang and heart-yang. On the other hand, yin-essence and yang-qi in the kidney depend on the essence,
yin and yang in the other organ to nourish and foster.
Thus insufficiency of yin-essence or yang-qi in the other
viscera will eventually involve the kidney or consume yin-
essence or yang-qi in the kidney, or prevent the kidney
from storing essence, consequently leading to deficiency

血液的生成,除来源于脾
胃化生的水谷精微之外,还与
肾精有关。肾精与血液之间
存在着相互资生和相互转化
的关系。故肾精充足,则血液
化生充盛;肾精亏虚,则血液
化生不足。临床上对肾精亏
虚所致的血虚证,必须采用补
肾填精的方法治疗才能收效。

6. 濡养和温煦诸脏腑

肾阴和肾阳之间,既互相
制约,又互相依存,对保持肾
的正常功能起着重要的作用。
肾阴又叫"元阴"、"真阴",能
够濡养各脏腑之阴,为一身阴
液之本;肾阳又叫"元阳"、"真
阳",能够温煦各脏腑之阳,为
一身阳气之本。由于肾阴肾
阳是人体各脏腑阴阳的根本,
所以肾阴虚可引发其他有关
脏腑的阴虚,肾阳虚可导致其
他有关脏腑的阳虚。从临床
实际来看,肾阴虚主要是引起
肝阴虚、心阴虚和肺阴虚;肾
阳虚主要是引起脾阳虚和心
阳虚。反之,肾中阴精与阳气
也要依赖其他脏腑精气阴阳
的滋生和化育,才能保持充盛
而不衰。因此,其他脏腑的阴
精或阳气不足,日久也必累及
于肾,或耗损肾中的阴精或阳

of essence, yin and yang in the kidney. This is what "impairment of the five zang-organs inevitably exhausting the kidney" means.

气,或使肾无所藏而精气自亏,从而导致肾中精气阴阳的亏损,这就是"五脏之伤,穷必及肾"的道理。

2.1.5.2 The relationships between the kidney and the body, the sensory organs and the orifices

(二) 肾与形体官窍的关系

1. The kidney governing the bones

The kidney governing the bones means that the development and functions of the bones depend on the kidney-essence. The kidney stores essence and the essence can transform into bone marrow to nourish the bones, promote the growth and repair of the skeleton and strengthen the skeleton. If kidney-essence is deficient, it will affect the production of bone marrow, leading to flaccidity of the skeleton and hypoevolutism in infants as well as brittleness of bones and susceptibility to fracture in the aged.

The teeth are the extensions of the bones. Both the bones and teeth need kidney-essence to nourish. If kidney-essence is abundant, the teeth are firm and not easy to lose. If kidney-essence is deficient, the teeth will grow slowly in infants and tend to become loose or even lose in adults.

2. The kidney opening into the ears, the external genitals and the anus

Kidney-essence produces marrow and the ears are connected with the cerebral marrow. Thus the functional states of the ears are closely related with kidney-essence. When the kidney-essence is sufficient, the cerebral marrow will be sufficient and the ears will be keen in hearing. If kidney-essence is insufficient, the cerebral marrow will be deficient and the ears will become weak in hearing, leading to tinnitus and deafness. The reason that old people

1. 肾主骨

肾主骨,是指骨骼的生长发育和功能的发挥,都有赖于肾精的充养。肾藏精,精可以化生骨髓,骨髓可以滋养骨骼,促进骨骼的生长、修复,使骨骼强劲而坚固。如果肾精亏少,骨髓空虚,骨骼失去营养,则出现小儿骨骼软弱无力,发育迟缓,以及老年人骨质脆弱,易于骨折等。

齿为骨之余,两者都需要得到肾精的滋养。肾精充盛,则牙齿坚固而不易脱落。肾精亏虚,则小儿牙齿生长缓慢,成人牙齿易于松动,甚至早脱。

2. 肾开窍于耳及二阴

由于肾精生髓,耳与脑髓相通,故耳的功能正常与否,也与肾精有密切关系。肾精充足,髓海满盈,耳窍得养,则听觉灵敏;反之,肾精不足,髓海空虚,耳窍失养,则听力减退,或出现耳鸣、耳聋等。人到老年听力每多下降,就是因

tend to be poor in hearing lies in the fact that kidney-essence declines naturally when people are growing old.

The relationship between the kidney and the external genitals can be understood from the functions of the kidney to govern water and reproduction. For example, the excretion of urine must depend on the function of the kidney to transform qi. So the symptoms of frequent urination, enuresis, incontinence of urine and anuria are usually caused by failure of the kidney to govern water. Besides, the function of the kidney to govern reproduction also covers the function of the external genitals. Thus failure of the kidney to govern reproduction may lead to impotence, premature ejaculation and seminal emission, or leukorrhea.

The relationship between the kidney and the anus refers to the fact that the kidney influences the functions of the spleen, the large intestine and the anus to control defecation through kidney-yin and kidney-yang. The function of kidney-yang is to absorb water by warming to promote the formation of feces. The function of kidney-yin is to moisten the intestines and the anus to smooth defecation. So insufficiency of kidney-yin and kidney-yang all lead to disorder of defecation. For example, insufficiency of kidney-yin leads to constipation due to intestinal dryness; deficiency of kidney-yang brings on insufficiency of spleen-yang, consequently causing diarrhea due to disorder in transportation and transformation.

3. External manifestation on the hair

The hair depends on blood to nourish. That is why it is said that "the hair is the extension of blood." Since the kidney stores essence which can transform into blood, exuberance of essence and blood will make the hair appear thick and lustrous. If the kidney-essence is insufficient

为肾精自然衰减的缘故。

二阴,即前阴和后阴。前阴包括尿道和外生殖器,后阴指肛门。肾与前阴的关系,可联系肾主水及肾主生殖的功能来理解。如尿液的排泄,必须依赖于肾的气化作用,因此尿频、遗尿、尿失禁、尿闭等病变,大多与肾主水的功能失常有关。另外,肾主生殖,也涵盖了外生殖器的功能,所以肾主生殖的功能失常,可出现男子阳痿、早泄、遗精,或女子白带过多等病变。

肾与后阴的关系,主要是指肾通过其阴、阳来影响脾、大肠及肛门的功能,从而决定大便的排泄状况。肾阳的作用是通过温化而吸收水液,促使大便成形;肾阴的作用是滋润肠腑及肛门,使大便排出顺畅。故肾阴肾阳不足,都可引起大便的排泄异常。如肾阴亏虚,可导致肠液枯涸而发生便秘;肾阳虚弱,可导致脾阳不足,运化失常而产生腹泻等。

3. 肾华在发

头发的营养来源于血液,故称"发为血之余"。由于肾藏精,肾精可化生血液,精血旺盛,头发得养,则生长浓密而有光泽。如肾精不足,血液

and blood is deficient, the hair will appear thin, dry, white and easy to lose. So the state of the hair is closely related to the kidney-essence. That is why it is said that "the kidney focally manifests itself on the hair".

Appendix: Mingmen (life-gate)

Life-gate refers to the root and foundation of life. Though there are different ideas about the location and functions of life-gate in history, it is generally believed that it is related closely with the kidney. Since the kidney is the foundation of the whole body and the essence stored in the kidney is key to the conception and development of life as well as the control of senility, it is quite similar to the function of life-gate. Though the kidney has various functions, TCM regards one of them as the most important and terms it life-gate. In fact, life-gate is included in the concept of the kidney. It is believed that life-gate contains both water and fire. The water and fire in life-gate actually refer to kidney-yin and kidney-yang. But now life-gate is expounded according to the importance of kidney-yang. Clinically disease due to decline of life-gate-fire is basically the same as that due to insufficiency of kidney-yang. Therapeutically, the therapy for reinforcing life-gate-fire is identical with that for invigorating kidney-yang.

2.2 The six fu-organs

The six fu-organs refer to the gallbladder, the stomach, the small intestine, the large intestine, the bladder and the triple energizer. The common physiological func-

亏虚,头发失养,则头发稀疏、枯槁、易白,并容易脱落。所以头发的生长及荣枯状态,与肾精的关系极为密切,因此说"肾华在发"。

附:命门

命门,本意指生命的关键、根本。关于命门的部位和功能,历来有许多不同的见解,但大多确认命门与肾有密切关系。由于肾为人体一身之根本,肾中所藏的精气是生命产生、发育成长的关键,也是控制衰老进程的关键,这一意义本身就具有"命门"的含义。也就是说,中医学把肾的各种功能作用中最重要的一部分单独提出,取名为"命门",而实际上命门仍属于"肾"的范畴。命门之中有水也有火,命门之水火实际上就是肾阴和肾阳,但现在人们主要是从强调肾阳的重要性方面来阐发"命门"理论。从临床上来看,命门火衰的病证与肾阳不足基本一致,补命门之火与补肾阳也没有根本的差别。

第二节 六腑

六腑,是指胆、胃、小肠、大肠、膀胱和三焦。六腑的共同生理功能是"传化物",即受

tion of the six fu-organs is "to transmit and transform food", i. e. receiving and digesting food, absorbing the nutrients and excreting the waste. Since the six fu-organs should be clear in order to transmit and transform food, it is said that "the six fu-organs function to descend" and "the six fu-organs function well if they are unobstructed".

2.2.1 The gallbladder

The gallbladder is connected with the liver and contains bile. The bile comes from the liver and is the accumulation of the surplus part of liver-qi. The bile is yellow in color and bitter in taste, playing an important role in assisting the absorption of food. That is why the bile is called "the essential juice" or "the lucid juice" and the gallbladder is called "the fu-organ of essential juice" or "the fu-organ of lucid juice" in TCM.

The physiological function of the gallbladder is to store and excrete the bile. The gallbladder itself is empty. After produced by the liver, the bile is stored in the gallbladder and directed by the dredging and dispersing functions of the liver, excreted into the small intestine to participate in the process of digestion and absorption of food and promote the small intestine to separate the lucid from the turbid.

Whether the excretion of the bile is normal or not is concerned with the dredging and dispersing functions of the liver on the one hand and the unobstructed condition of the gallbladder on the other. Failure of the liver to dredge and disperse or obstruction of the gallbladder itself will affect the excretion of the bile and disturb digestion and absorption, frequently leading to anorexia, abdominal distension, vomiting, hypochondriac pain or even jaundice if the bile is extravasated in the muscles and skin.

纳、消化饮食物,吸收其精微、排泄其糟粕。由于六腑传化水谷,须保持通畅下行,故有六腑"以降为顺"、"以通为用"的说法。

一、胆

胆与肝相连,附于肝下,内贮胆汁。胆汁来源于肝,是肝之余气溢入于胆积聚而成。胆汁味苦色黄,对帮助某些食物的消化具有重要的生理作用。由于胆汁清净,所以中医学又将胆汁称为"精汁"、"清汁",而将胆称为"中精之腑"、"中清之腑"。

胆的生理功能是贮存胆汁和排泄胆汁。胆腑中空,胆汁由肝生成后贮存于胆,然后在肝气疏泄的作用下排泄入小肠,参与消化吸收过程,并促进小肠分别清浊功能的正常进行。

胆汁排泄正常与否,一方面与肝气的疏泄有关;另一方面与胆腑的通畅与否有关。肝气疏泄失职,或胆腑失于畅通,都会使胆失于疏泄。若胆失疏泄,胆汁排泄不畅,引起消化吸收功能障碍,可出现食欲不振、腹胀、呕吐、胁痛等症状,若胆汁泛溢于肌肤,则出

2.2.2   The stomach

The stomach is connected with the esophagus in the upper and the small intestine in the lower, usually divided into three parts, namely shangwan (the upper part of the stomach and cardia), zhongwan (the middle part of the stomach) and xiawan (the lower part of the stomach and pylorus).

The physiological function of the stomach is to receive and digest food. The chyme transformed in the stomach is then transmitted to the small intestine. Since the stomach is big and can contain large amount of food, it is called "the sea of food and water" in *Huangdi Neijing*.

The stomach depends on the propelling of stomach-qi to perform its function. Stomach-qi is the basic motive power for transmitting food and water in the stomach downwards. The canal connecting the stomach and the small intestine must be kept unobstructed so that the chyme can smoothly be transmitted from the stomach to the small intestine. That is why the physiological function of the stomach is often described as "the stomach functions to descend" and "the unobstructed condition is prerequisite to the normal function of the stomach" in TCM, usually abbreviated as "the stomach governing descent". Dysfunction of the stomach will lead to distending stomach-ache and poor appetite due to disharmony of stomach-qi, or belching, vomiting, nausea and hiccup due to failure of stomach-qi to descend or upward flow of stomach-qi.

现黄疸。

二、胃

胃又称为胃脘,上连食道,下通小肠。胃脘分为上脘、中脘、下脘三个部分,胃的上部及贲门部分称上脘,胃的中部称中脘,胃的下部及幽门部分称下脘。

胃的生理功能是受纳和腐熟水谷,具有对饮食物进行初步消化并形成食糜的作用。饮食经口,下入于胃中。胃接受容纳了饮食物之后,经过初步的腐熟消化,形成食糜,然后向下传入小肠。由于胃的容量很大,能容纳较多的饮食物,故《黄帝内经》称胃为"水谷之海"。

胃的功能主要依赖于胃气的推动。胃气是胃中水谷运行的根本动力,其运动特点是以降为主。同时,胃与小肠之间的道路必须保持畅通,这是维持"降"的基本条件,只有通降无阻,形成食糜状的饮食才能依次进入小肠。所以中医学常用"以降为顺"、"以通为和"来说明胃的正常生理功能,简称为"胃主通降"。胃的功能失常,可引起胃气不和,出现胃脘胀痛、食少等症;亦可导致胃气不降或上逆,出现嗳气、恶心、呕吐、呃逆等症。

Since the food received and digested by the stomach is the main substance for producing qi and blood, the stomach is called "the sea of food".

2.2.3　The small intestine

The small intestine is located in the middle of the abdomen, connected with the stomach at the pylorus in the upper and the large intestine at ileocecal junction in the lower. The physiological function of the small intestine is to receive the chyle and separate the lucid from the turbid.

1. To receive the chyle

The small intestine receives the chyme from the stomach and keeps for a certain period of time in order to further digest it.

2. To separate the lucid from the turbid

The lucid refers to food nutrients and the turbid refers to the waste of food. After further digestion and absorption of the nutrients and part of the water, the small intestine transmits the waste to the large intestine. This process is called "to separate the lucid from the turbid" in TCM.

In fact, to receive the chyme and to separate the lucid from the turbid are two aspects in the digesting and absorbing process. There is a close relationship between these two aspects. The former is the condition of the latter and the latter is the result of the former.

TCM emphasizes the functions of the five zang-organs, so the digesting function of the small intestine is attributed to the transporting and transforming function of

因为胃受纳腐熟的饮食物,是化生气血的主要物质基础,所以又称胃为"水谷气血之海"。

三、小肠

小肠盘踞于腹中,上以幽门与胃连接,下以阑门与大肠相通。小肠的生理功能有两个方面:一是受盛化物;二是分别清浊。

1. 受盛化物

受盛化物指小肠接受由胃初步消化而下输的食糜,贮盛容纳相当长的时间,以进行充分的消化。

2. 分别清浊

清指水谷精微,浊指食物糟粕。小肠在对由胃传来的饮食物进行充分消化的基础上,吸收其中的精微物质及部分水液,并将食物残渣继续向下传送至大肠,中医学把这一过程称为"分别清浊"。

实际上,小肠受盛化物和分别清浊的功能,是同一消化吸收过程的两个方面,受盛化物是分别清浊的前提,分别清浊是受盛化物的结果,两者有着密切的内在联系。

由于藏象学强调以五脏为中心,所以中医学往往把小肠消化吸收的功能归属脾主

the spleen. That is why clinically diseases due to disorder of the small intestine in digestion and absorption, such as anorexia, abdominal distension and loose stool, are differentiated as "dysfunction of the spleen" and treated from the aspect of the spleen.

　　The function of the small intestine to absorb water decides the quantity of urine. If the small intestine absorbs water normally and the water is fully absorbed and distributed to all parts of the body, the stool will appear in normal form and the urination will be smooth. If the small intestine is abnormal in absorbing water and the water is kept in the intestines and moves downward with the waste, then the stool will be sloppy and the urine will become scanty. Such a condition is usually differentiated as "dysfunction of the spleen". If the small intestine absorbs too much water, the urine will become profuse and the stool will become retained. Such a condition is called "constipation due to spleen deficiency and scanty fluid", indicating the relationship between the small intestine and the spleen. Clinically diarrhea in some cases is treated by the therapy "for promoting urination to consolidate the stool", focusing on promoting urination to reinforce the function of the small intestine to absorb water. The syndrome of "constipation due to spleen deficiency and scanty fluid" can be treated by slowing down the descending activity to reduce the speed of the small intestine in absorbing water.

2.2.4　The large intestine

　　The large intestine is connected with the small intestine in the upper and the anus in the lower. The physiological function of the large intestine is mainly to receive the waste of food transmitted down from the small intestine. After absorbing part of the water in it, the large intestine

运化的范畴。因此,临床上常将小肠消化吸收失常的病变,如食欲不佳、腹胀、便溏等,辨证为"脾失健运"而从脾治疗。

　　另外,小肠吸收水分的功能与尿量的多少有一定关系。若小肠吸收功能良好,水液被充分吸收而布散周身,则大便成形,小便畅利。若小肠吸收功能不良,水液居于肠内而随糟粕下行,则大便稀薄,小便偏少,辨证为"脾失健运";反之,如果小肠吸收水液过多,则使小便增多而大便秘结,中医学称之为"脾约",这正是小肠与脾有特殊的功能联系的缘故。所以临床上对某些腹泻患者,采用"利小便即所以实大便"的治法,其意就在于通过加强利尿来促进小肠的吸收功能;而对于"脾约"症,则采用缓下的方法来减少小肠对水液的吸收。

四、大肠

　　大肠上连小肠,下为肛门,与外界相通。大肠的生理功能,主要是接受小肠下输的食物残渣,再继续向外传送,在此运行过程中,又吸收了其

transmits the waste downward and transforms it into stool to be excreted from the anus.

The function of the large intestine to transmit the waste of food is described in *Huangdi Neijing* as "transmission and excretion", the activities of which are accomplished by the propelling function of the large intestinal qi. If the large intestine is abnormal in function, it will lead to constipation due to improper transmission and diarrhea due to insufficient absorption of water.

2.2.5 The bladder

The bladder, located in the lower abdomen, is responsible for storing and discharging urine.

The water and turbid qi produced in the process of metabolism are changed into urine through qi-transforming function of the kidney and transmitted to the bladder. When certain amount of urine is accumulated in the bladder, it is excreted naturally out of the body through the action of qi-transformation. The storage and excretion of urine by the bladder result from the fixating and qi-transforming functions of qi. Since bladder-qi is controlled by the kidney-qi, the fixating and qi-transforming functions of kidney-qi is key to the storage of urine in the bladder and excretion of urine out of the bladder. Generally speaking, failure of kidney-qi to fixate and transform qi due to deficiency affects the function of the bladder to excrete urine. If the bladder is attacked by exogenous pathogenic factors, qi-transformation activity will be affected, also leading to disorder in excreting urine. But the syndrome in the former case is deficiency and the syndrome in the latter case is excess. Deficiency of bladder-qi usually leads to symptoms of polyuria, enuresis and incontinence of urine. Obstructed transformation of qi often brings on

中的部分水分,形成粪便而排出体外。

大肠传送食物残渣的功能,《黄帝内经》概括为"传导"作用,这是依赖于大肠之气的推动而实现的。如大肠功能失常,一是传导不利可出现便秘;二是吸收功能减退可出现腹泻等。

五、膀胱

膀胱位于小腹部,为贮尿的器官,其功能是贮存小便和排泄小便。

人体在新陈代谢过程中形成的水液及浊气,经肾的气化作用而生成小便,下输于膀胱暂时贮存,当膀胱内小便积存到一定量时,就通过气化作用而自然地排出体外。膀胱的贮尿和排尿功能,是气的固摄作用和气化作用相互协调的结果,而膀胱之气的运动受肾气的主宰,肾气的固摄和气化作用是膀胱贮存和排泄小便的决定性因素。一般来说,肾气虚而固摄、气化失常时,可导致膀胱排尿异常;若膀胱本身感受外邪,使气化不利,也会导致排尿异常。但前者形成的是虚证,后者形成的是实证。凡膀胱气虚不固,可见尿多、遗尿、尿失禁等症;若膀胱气化不利,可见小便不利、

symptoms of unsmooth urination, dripping urination and anuria.

淋漓不爽、尿闭等症。

2.2.6 Sanjiao (the triple energizer)

六、三焦

2.2.6.1 The conception of the triple energizer

（一）三焦的概念

The triple energizer is a special fu-organ, serving to divide the internal organs in the chest and abdomen and generalize certain functional systems of the body.

三焦是一个特殊的腑，它既是对人体胸腹部位及其所藏脏腑器官的划分，又是对人体某些功能系统的概括。

The triple energizer is composed of three parts, i.e. the upper energizer, middle energizer and lower energizer. The diaphragm and the navel are regarded as the lines to divide the triple energizer. The part above the diaphragm is the upper energizer, the part below the diaphragm and above the navel is the middle energizer, and the part below the navel is the lower energizer. The upper energizer includes the thorax, the heart and the lung; the middle energizer includes the upper abdomen, the spleen, the stomach, the liver, the gallbladder and the small intestine; the lower energizer includes the lower abdomen, the kidney, the bladder and the large intestine.

三焦，可分为上焦、中焦、下焦三部。对于三焦部位的划分，通常以横膈和脐为界线，横膈以上为上焦，横膈以下、脐以上为中焦，脐以下为下焦。上焦主要包括胸部和心、肺，中焦主要包括上腹部和脾、胃、肝、胆、小肠，下焦主要包括下腹部和肾、膀胱、大肠等。

2.2.6.2 The physiological function of the triple energizer

（二）三焦的生理功能

The triple energizer is an independent functional system which is based on the morphological structure of the internal organs and tissues. In fact it is a generalization of the physiological functions of the internal organs. The physiological functions of the triple energizer include the following two aspects:

三焦作为一个独立的功能系统，是以人体各脏腑组织的形态结构为基础的，因而它实际上是对各脏腑生理功能的高度综合和概括。三焦的生理功能可包括如下两个方面。

1. A generalization of yuan-qi (primordial qi) and water passage

1. 三焦是对元气和水液运行通道的概括

The triple energizer serves as a transmitting system, through which substances like the primordial qi and water

三焦是人体主要的输导系统，人体的某些物质如元

are transported and transmitted.

The primordial qi, the root source of qi, comes from congenital essence and nourishes the acquired base of life. It is the primary motivation of life activity. The primordial qi originates from the kidney and, through the transportation and transmission of the triple energizer, is distributed to all parts of the body for warming and nourishing the viscera and the tissues so as to activate and promote the physiological functions of the other viscera and tissues. If the primordial qi is deficient and the transportation of the triple energizer is not smooth, it will lead to qi deficiency in certain areas in the body.

When taken into the stomach and transported and transformed by the spleen, the water is transmitted upwards to the lung which, by means of regulating the water passage, transmits the water downwards to the kidney. The kidney separates the lucid from the turbid with its function of transforming qi. Such a continuous circulation maintains normal metabolism of water inside the body. The lung is located in the upper energizer, the spleen in the middle energizer and the kidney in the lower energizer. It is the triple energizer that organizes these three organs into a system for transmitting and metabolizing water. That is why triple energizer is regarded as a very important passage of water. If the triple energizer is obstructed, the functions of the lung, the spleen and the kidney will certainly be affected, leading to oliguria and edema.

2. A generalization of the physiological functions of certain internal organs

The generalization of the physiological functions of certain viscera with the triple energizer is mainly concerned with the digestion and absorption of food, distribu-

气、水液等的运输和传导，是以三焦作为道路的。

元气是人体的根本之气，其来自于先天，充养于后天，是人体生命活动的原动力。元气的根源在于肾，并可通过三焦而输布周身内外上下，温养脏腑组织，以激发和推动各脏腑组织的生理功能。如果元气虚弱，三焦通道运行不畅，便可引起某些部位的气虚现象。

水液由口摄入，经脾的运化功能，上输于肺，肺主通调水道，又下降于肾，肾再通过气化作用而分别清浊，如此不断循环上下，维持着人体的水液代谢。其中，肺居上焦，脾居中焦，肾居下焦，正是三焦将肺、脾、肾三脏联结成一个水液输布、代谢的系统，所以说三焦也是水液运行的重要通道。如果三焦水道不利，影响肺、脾、肾等脏的相应功能，就会产生尿少、水肿等病变。

2. 三焦是对人体某些内脏功能系统的概括

用三焦来概括相应部位的某些内脏的部分生理功能，主要是针对饮食的消化吸收、

tion of food nutrients and metabolism of water. *Huangdi Neijing* used three similes to describe the functions of the triple energizer: the upper energizer is like fog, the middle energizer is like maceration and the lower energizer is like sewer.

(1) The upper energizer is like fog: The heart and the lung are located in the upper energizer. This simile describes the functions of the heart and the lung to distribute essence. That is to say that the function of the heart and the lung to distribute food nutrients is just like fog permeating everywhere. When exogenous pathogenic factors invade the upper energizer, it not only affects the dispersion and distribution of essence, but also leads to the symptoms of dysphoria, palpitation, cough and chest oppression due to dysfunction of the heart and lung.

(2) The middle energizer is like maceration: This simile describes the digestion and absorption of food by the spleen and the stomach. In fact the digestion and absorption of food are not only related to the spleen and the stomach, but also to the liver and the gallbladder. The stomach governs reception and digestion of food; the spleen governs transportation and transformation of food nutrients; the liver and the gallbladder smooth the activity of qi, excrete the bile and promote digestion. Since the spleen, the stomach, the liver and the gallbladder are located in the upper abdomen, this simile is actually a generalization of the digesting and absorbing functions of these organs. If pathogenic factors are retained in the middle energizer, the digesting and absorbing functions will be affected, leading to distending fullness of the upper abdomen, vomiting, diarrhea and jaundice.

(3) The lower energizer is like sewer: This simile describes the functions of the kidney and the bladder that

水谷精微的输布和津液的代谢而言的,《黄帝内经》把这一过程归纳为三句话:上焦如雾,中焦如沤,下焦如渎。

(1) 上焦如雾　上焦为心、肺两脏所居之处。上焦如雾,是以"雾"的弥漫状态来形容心肺宣发输布精气的功能。也就是说,心肺将精微物质输布于周身,状如雾露般弥漫,无处不到。如果外邪侵犯上焦,不但影响精气的正常宣发和输布,还可见心烦、心悸、咳嗽、胸闷等心肺功能失常的病变。

(2) 中焦如沤　沤,是久浸的意思,物经久浸则易腐变。中焦如沤,是以"沤"来形容脾胃等对饮食物的消化吸收状态。食物的消化吸收功能,不仅与脾胃有关,与肝胆也密切相关。胃主受纳、腐熟水谷,脾主运化精微,肝胆则疏利气机,排泄胆汁,促进消化,而脾胃肝胆皆居于上腹部,所以中焦如沤,是概括了脾胃肝胆在消化吸收方面的功能。如果邪聚中焦,影响消化吸收功能的正常发挥,可见脘腹胀满、呕吐、腹泻、黄疸等脾胃肝胆的病变。

(3) 下焦如渎　渎,是水道的意思。下焦如渎,是以

move the turbid liquid downward and discharge it out of the body. This is in fact a generalization of the functions of the kidney and the bladder in producing and excreting urine. If pathogenic factors invade the lower energizer, the excretion of urine will be affected, leading to oliguria, frequent urination, urgent urination and pain in urination.

2.3 The extraordinary fu-organs

The extraordinary fu-organs refer to another group of tissues and organs.

2.3.1 The characteristics of the extraordinary fu-organs

The extraordinary fu-organs are characterized by hollowness, similar to the six fu-organs in morphology, and storage of essence, similar to the five zang-organs in function. That is why this group of tissues and organs are called the extraordinary fu-organs, including the brain, the marrow, the bones, the vessels, the gallbladder and the uterus. Among the extraordinary fu-organs, the gallbladder is a special one. It is hollow inside and excretes bile to promote digestion, similar to the functions of the six fu-organs, but it also stores bile which is part of the essence, similar to the functions of the five zang-organs. That is why the gallbladder belongs both to the six fu-organs and the extraordinary fu-organs.

2.3.2 The physiological functions of the extraordinary fu-organs

The following paragraphs are only devoted to the

"渎"来形容肾与膀胱将水浊不断地向下疏通、向外排泄的状态,亦即概括了肾与膀胱在生成和排泄小便方面的功能。如果邪侵下焦,主要是影响小便的正常排泄,可见尿少、尿频、尿急、尿痛等肾与膀胱的病变。

第三节 奇恒之腑

奇,异的意思;恒,常的意思。奇恒之腑,是指不同于一般脏腑的另一类组织器官。

一、奇恒之腑的特点

奇恒之腑的特点是,其形态多中空,与六腑相似,而其功能则是贮藏精气,又与五脏类同,故称之为"奇恒之腑"。奇恒之腑,包括脑、髓、骨、脉、胆、女子胞六种组织器官,其中胆是一个比较特殊的器官。其形态中空,可排泄胆汁以助消化,与六腑的功能特点一致,但它所贮藏的胆汁称为"精汁",也是人体精气的一部分,又与五脏的功能特点相似,因而胆既是六腑之一,又把它归属奇恒之腑。

二、奇恒之腑的功能

本节主要介绍脑与女子

functions of the brain and the uterus. The physiological functions of the rest extraordinary fu-organs are already introduced in the other chapters and sections.

2.3.2.1 The brain

The brain is located in the skull and is composed of marrow. That is why the brain is called "the sea of marrow" in *Huangdi Neijing*. The physiological functions of the brain include the following aspects:

1. The center of life activities

The brain plays a very important role in life activities. It governs the five zang-organs and six fu-organs and regulates life activities. Impairment of the brain will threaten life. That is why it is said in *Huangdi Neijing* that "stabbing the brain will cause immediate death."

2. Governing the mental activities

The brain is an organ responsible for cognition and thinking. All the mental activities result from the reflection of things in the objective world. Though zangxiang theory attributes the mental activities to the heart, it never neglects the role of the brain. For example, it is said in *Huangdi Neijing* that "the head is the place where mental activities take place". Li Shizhen, a great doctor in the Ming Dynasty, pointed out that "the brain is the place where the primordial spirit is kept". When the brain is normal in function, people will be full of vigor, clear in thinking, fluent in speaking and strong in memory. If the brain is abnormal in function, it will lead to dispiritedness, retard thinking, dizziness, poor memory or mental disorder.

胞的功能,其余内容在其他章节中已有叙述,此处不再重复。

(一) 脑

脑位于头颅之内,由髓汇聚而成,所以《黄帝内经》称之为"髓海"。脑的生理功能主要有如下几方面。

1. 生命活动的中枢

脑在人体生命活动中具有十分重要的作用,主要表现在主宰五脏六腑的功能、调节一身的生命活动方面。如果脑受到损伤,就会危及生命。所以《黄帝内经》说:"刺头中脑户,入脑立死。"

2. 主管精神活动

脑是认识和思维的器官,人的各种思维意识及情志活动,都是客观外界事物反映到脑的结果。虽然藏象学说将脑主管精神活动的作用归属于心主神明的功能,但也已认识到脑在精神活动方面的重要作用。《黄帝内经》有"头者,精明之府"的说法。明代李时珍曾指出"脑为元神之府",即指脑是人的精神活动的重要器官。脑主管精神活动的功能正常,则精神振奋,意识清楚,语言清晰,记忆力强;若脑的功能失常,则可出现精神委靡,思维迟钝,头晕目眩,记忆力下降等症,或发

3. Governing sensation and motion

There are various sensory organs in the body, such as the eyes, ears, nose, tongue and skin that respectively receive sound, light and flavor as well as the stimulation of pain, cold and heat. The brain receives such stimulation through the meridians. The brain also governs the limbs. The brain transmits the order to move through the meridians to the limbs. The brain also constantly regulates the movement of the limbs. That is why the movement of the limbs is rhythmical and accurate. If the brain is abnormal in governing and regulating the limbs, it will cause bradyesthesia and dyskinesia.

The zangxiang theory emphasizes the importance of the five zang-organs, so the functions of the brain are attributed to the five zang-organs respectively. For example, the mental activities are divided into shen (spirit), po (superior soul), hun (inferior soul), yi (memory) and zhi (conception) which are attributed to the five zang-organs respectively, i. e. the heart storing spirit, the lung storing superior soul, the liver storing inferior soul, the spleen storing memory and the kidney storing conception. Clinically mental activities are most closely related to the heart, the liver and the kidney. Because the heart governs the mind and all mental activities; the liver governs dredging and dispersing and regulates mental activities; and the kidney stores yin-essence in order to produce marrow to enrich the brain. That is why mental diseases are clinically treated from the heart, the liver and the kidney.

2.3.2.2　The uterus

The uterus is located in the lower abdomen. The

生精神异常方面的病症。

3. 主管感觉和运动

人身有各种感官,如眼、耳、鼻、舌、身(皮肤)等,可分别接受外来的声、光、味以及疼痛、寒热等刺激,脑通过经脉接受这些刺激而产生感觉。脑又是肢体运动的主宰。人先在脑中产生运动的意念,意念信号通过经脉传向肢体,肢体就发生运动。脑对肢体运动还能持续进行调节,使运动具有一定的节奏和精确度,以达到脑中意念所规定的目的。因此,脑主管感觉和运动的功能失常,就会出现感觉迟钝,运动失调等病变。

由于藏象学说是强调以五脏为中心的,所以在中医学理论体系中,多将脑的这些重要功能分属于五脏。如将人的精神活动分为神、魄、魂、意、志五个方面,而分别归之于五脏,即心藏神,肺藏魄,肝藏魂,脾藏意,肾藏志。但从临床实际来看,精神活动与心、肝、肾三脏的关系最为密切。这是因为心主神明,主管整个精神活动;肝主疏泄,调节人的情志活动;肾藏阴精,可生髓充养于脑。所以,临床上精神情志活动异常的疾病,往往从心、肝、肾三脏论治。

(二) 女子胞

女子胞又名胞宫,即子宫,

physiological function of the uterus is to produce menses and conceive fetus.

The uterus usually maturates at the age of 14 and begins to produce menses, a periodic phenomenon of uterine bleeding. In adult women, blood is periodically accumulated in the uterus for conceiving and nourishing fetus. If pregnancy does not take place, the accumulated blood will be excreted out of the body. Such an excretion of blood from the uterus is known as menstruation. After excretion of the accumulated blood, the uterus begins to accumulate blood again for another periodic menstruation. Menstruation takes place once a month regularly like morning and evening tides. That is why menstruation is also called "monthly tide" in Chinese medicine.

After pregnancy, the uterus is the place to nourish the fetus. There is no menstruation during pregnancy. But great quantity of blood is constantly transported to the uterus to nourish the fetus. The uterus becomes larger and larger with the development of the fetus. After delivery there is still no menses because blood is transported upwards and transformed into milk. After weaning, milk gradually stops secreting. Then blood is transported downward into the uterus and menses begins to occur again.

The function of the uterus to produce menses and to conceive fetus is a complicated process and depends on the nourishment and coordination of other viscera. Often the following three factors are involved in this process.

1. Essence stored in the kidney

When essence, yin and yang stored in the kidney

位于小腹部,是女性独有的器官。女子胞具有发生月经和孕育胎儿两方面的生理功能。

女性从十四岁左右开始,女子胞发育渐趋成熟,开始有月经来潮。月经,是子宫周期性出血的现象。成年女性的子宫在月经周期内有一个积蓄血液的过程,这是受孕和养育胎儿的前提。如果在一个周期之内没有受孕,积蓄的血液就排出体外,从而发生月经来潮。积蓄的血液排尽之后,又进入下一个周期的血液积蓄过程。月经以月为周期,按时而来,按时而去,如同潮汐一样,故称"月经来潮"。

受孕以后,子宫就成了孕育胎儿的场所。这时,月经停止,大量的血液不断地灌注于子宫,以滋养胎儿。随着胎儿的逐渐长大,子宫也日益增大直至分娩。分娩后的哺乳期间,血液化为乳汁而上行,此时仍无月经来潮,要等到断乳之后,乳汁渐收,血液下行,才会恢复正常的月经周期。

女子胞发生月经和孕育胎儿的功能,是一个复杂的生理活动过程,有赖于其他脏腑的充养与协调。主要有如下三方面因素。

1. 肾中精气的作用

肾中藏有精气阴阳,当精

develop to a certain level, tiankui (reproductive substance) occurs. Tiankui can promote the development and maturation of the genitals, including the uterus. When the uterus becomes maturated, it is ready to produce menses and conceive fetus. When a woman becomes old, essence, yin and yang stored in the kidney are gradually reduced, and so is tiankui. Eventually menstruation stops and the uterus can no longer conceive fetus.

2. The function of liver-qi and liver-blood

The liver plays a very important role in the physiological functions of the uterus. On the one hand, the liver governs dredging and dispersing activities and regulates the movement of qi. With the assistance of the liver, the uterus functions normally, producing menses and conceiving fetus. On the other hand, the liver stores blood and regulates the volume of blood. Such a function of the liver is closely related to the quantity of menses and nourishment of the fetus. Since the function of the uterus is closely related to liver-qi and liver-blood, there is an old saying that "the liver is the congenital base of life for women".

3. The functions of the thoroughfare and conception vessels

The thoroughfare and conception vessels start from the uterus. The thoroughfare vessel is the sea of blood and regulates qi and blood in the twelve regular meridians. The conception vessel governs the uterus and pregnancy. If these two vessels function well, blood will be transported smoothly into the uterus to ensure regular menses and conception of fetus. The functions of these two vessels are assisted and regulated by the kidney and

气阴阳充盛到一定程度时，就产生天癸。天癸生成后，能促进生殖器官的发育并使之成熟。女子胞在天癸的作用下发育成熟之后，就具备了发生月经和孕育胎儿的条件。到了老年，由于肾中精气阴阳日趋减少，天癸亦随之衰减，因此月经逐渐停止，并失去了孕育胎儿的能力。

2. 肝气肝血的作用

肝对女子胞的生理功能，起着十分重要的调节作用。一方面肝主疏泄，调畅气机，使女子胞的功能正常，则能发生月经及受孕；另一方面肝主藏血，能贮藏血液和调节血量，影响女子胞血液的充盈和正常运行，从而与月经量的多少和养育胎儿的功能有着紧密的联系。由于女子胞的功能与肝气肝血的作用密切相关，所以前人有"女子以肝为先天"的说法。

3. 冲任二脉的作用

冲任二脉同起于胞中，在女子即起于女子胞中。冲为血海，能调节十二经脉之气血；任主胞胎，与女子妊娠有关。所以冲任二脉通利，血液下注于女子胞，平时可产生月经，孕时则养育胎儿。当然，冲任二脉的盛衰，还要受到

the liver. In fact, the kidney, the liver, the thoroughfare and conception vessels physiologically coordinate with each other to influence the uterus.

Besides, the heart, the lung and the spleen also influence the functions of the uterus. Because the heart governs blood and propels the circulation of blood; the lung governs qi and directs the flow of blood; and the spleen commands blood, governs transportation and transformation and serves as the source of qi and blood.

2.4   The relationships among the zang-organs and the fu-organs

The human body is an organic whole, composed of the viscera, the meridians and many other tissues and organs. The relationships between the zang-organs and the fu-organs are a component part in the theory of zangxiang. The zang-organs and the fu-organs are connected with each other through the meridians in structure, coordinate with each other and differ from each other in physiology as well as affect each other and transmit to each other in pathology.

2.4.1   The relationships among the five zang-organs

2.4.1.1   The relationship between the heart and the lung

The relationship between the heart and the lung is signified by the inter-dependence between qi and blood. Physiologically, the lung dominates qi and assists the heart to propel blood circulation; the heart governs blood and blood nourishes the lung and maintains the respiratory function of the lung. Since the pectoral qi accumulates in

肾、肝两脏功能的调节,肾、肝、冲任二脉与女子胞是关系女子生殖生理功能并相互协调的统一整体。

此外,由于心主血、能推动血液运行,肺主气、气行则血行,脾统血、主运化而为气血生化之源,所以心、肺、脾三脏对女子胞的功能也有一定的影响。

第四节   脏腑之间的关系

人体是一个统一的有机整体,由脏腑、经络等许多组织器官所构成。脏腑之间的关系,是藏象学说中整体性联系的内容之一。人体各脏腑之间,在结构上通过经络而相互沟通,生理功能上既分工又合作,在病理变化上也可互相影响和传变。

一、五脏之间的关系

(一)心与肺

心与肺之间的关系,主要体现为气与血之间的相互依存。在生理方面,肺主气,辅心行血,可促进心脏推动血液运行;而心主血,营养于肺,可维持肺的呼吸功能。由于宗

the chest, by means of flowing in the heart vessels to propel qi and blood and running in the respiratory tract to regulate respiration, to warm the heart and the lung, it can strengthen the coordination between the heart and the lung in propelling blood circulation and governing respiration.

Pathologically, deficiency of lung-qi and disorder of the lung in dispersing and descending will affect the function of the heart to propel blood; insufficiency of heart-yang will weaken blood circulation, leading to disorder of lung in respiration with the symptoms of cough, asthma, chest oppression and palpitation.

2.4.1.2 The relationship between the heart and the spleen

The relationship between the heart and the spleen includes two aspects. On the one hand the heart governs blood and promotes blood circulation while the spleen commands blood to circulate in the vessels. The coordination of the heart and the spleen ensures the normal circulation of blood. On the other hand, the heart nourishes the spleen if there is sufficient blood in the heart and regulates the function of the spleen because the heart governs the mind; the spleen absorbs food nutrients and transforms them into blood for the heart if it functions well. So clinically insufficiency of heart-blood or disorder of heart-spirit affects the function of the spleen; dysfunction of the spleen or failure of the spleen to command blood also leads to disorder of the heart, bringing on simultaneous disorder of both the spleen and the heart with the symptoms of palpitation, insomnia, poor appetite and loose stool, etc.

2.4.1.3 The relationship between the heart and the liver

The relationship between the heart and the liver is signified by circulation of blood and regulation of mental

气积聚于胸中,温养心肺两脏,具有贯心脉以行气血和走息道以司呼吸的功能,所以能加强心血运行与肺司呼吸之间的协调平衡。

在病理方面,如肺气虚弱,宣降失常,可影响心的行血功能;而心之阳气不足,血行无力,也会导致肺的呼吸功能失常,从而出现咳嗽、气喘、胸闷、心悸等症。

(二) 心与脾

心与脾在生理上的关系,主要体现在两个方面。一是心主血而推动血液运行,脾统血而统摄血液循行于脉管,两者互相配合,共同维持血液的正常运行。二是心血充盈,可营养于脾,心主神明,可调节脾的运化功能;脾运化功能正常,吸收的水谷精微能化生心血并营养心神,两者有相互依存的关系。因此,当心血不足或心神失常时可引起脾失健运,脾运失常或脾不统血时亦可导致心的病变,都导致心脾同病,而出现心悸、失眠、食少、便溏等症。

(三) 心与肝

心与肝的关系,主要表现在血液的运行和精神情志活

activities. The heart governs blood and is the motivation of blood circulation; the liver stores blood and is a very important factor in the storage and regulation of blood. So the heart and the liver coordinate with each other in blood circulation. The heart governs the mind and regulates mental activities; the liver governs dredging and dispersing and adjusts emotional activities. They are closely related to each other in maintaining mental and emotional activities.

　　Clinically insufficiency of liver-blood and deficiency of heart-blood may affect each other, leading to deficiency of both liver-blood and heart-blood with the symptoms of pale complexion, palpitation and dizziness. Disorder of heart-spirit and failure of the liver to dredge and disperse and e-motional upset frequently affect each other, leading to dysphoria, insomnia, irritability and susceptibility to rage due to exuberance of heart-fire and liver-fire.

2.4.1.4 The relationship between the heart and the kidney

　　The relationship between the heart and the kidney is mainly signified by inter-dependence between heart-yin/heart-yang and kidney-yin/kidney-yang. The heart pertains to fire in the five elements and is located in the upper energizer; the kidney pertains to water in the five elements and is located in the lower energizer. Heart-fire (heart-yang) has to descend to the kidney to warm kidney-yang and prevent abnormal flow of water; kidney-water (kidney-yin) has to ascend to nourish heart-yin and prevent hyperactivity of heart-yang. Such a coordination between the upper and the lower is called "coordination between the heart and the kidney" or "coordination between water and fire". If kidney-yin fails to nourish heart-yin due to insufficiency, it will lead to deficiency of heart-yin and hyperactivity of heart-yang, bringing on

动的调节方面。心主血,是血液运行的原动力;肝藏血,是贮藏和调节血液的重要因素。因此,心、肝两脏在血液的运行方面是互相配合的。心主神明,主管人的精神活动;肝主疏泄,调节情志活动。也就是说,两者在维持精神情志活动方面有着密切的关系。

　　在临床上,心血不足与肝血不足的病变可互相影响,导致心肝血虚的病证,出现面色无华、心悸、头昏、目眩等症状。心神失常与肝失疏泄、情志失调也可互相累及,出现心烦、失眠、急躁易怒等心肝火旺的症状。

(四) 心与肾

　　心与肾之间,首先体现在心之阴阳与肾的阴阳之间的相互依存关系。心在五行属火,位于上焦;肾在五行属水,位于下焦。心火(阳)必须下降于肾,以温煦肾阳,使水液不致泛滥;而肾水(阴)必须上济于心,以滋养心阴,使心阳不致偏亢。这种阴阳上下交通的关系,就称为"心肾相交"或"水火既济"。如果肾阴不足,不能上滋心阴,导致心阴虚而心阳偏亢,可出现心烦、失眠、耳鸣、腰膝酸软等症;或心火不能下降,肾水独居于

dysphoria, insomnia, tinnitus and weakness of the waist and knees. If heart-fire fails to descend, it will cause heat in the upper and cold in the lower, leading to dysphoria, insomnia and cold sensation below the waist and knees. Such pathological cases are called "disharmony between the heart and the kidney".

Besides, the heart governs blood and the kidney stores essence. Blood and essence can transform into each other. So insufficiency of heart-blood will cause deficiency of kidney-essence and deficiency of kidney-essence, in turn, will result in insufficiency of heart-blood, consequently leading to disorder of both blood and essence with the symptoms of pale complexion, palpitation, tinnitus and weakness of the waist and knees.

2.4.1.5　The relationship between the lung and the liver

The relationship between the lung and the liver is signified by the regulation of qi activity. On the one hand, the lung and the liver coordinate with each other in regulating qi activity. The lung governs qi in the whole body, controls respiration and regulates qi activity; the liver governs dredging and dispersing and promotes qi to flow in the whole body. On the other hand, the lung and the liver adjust the movement of qi through the activities of ascent and descent. Lung-qi functions to descend and depurate while liver-qi functions to elevate and disperse. The liver and the lung, by means of ascent and descent, restrain each other and depend on each other so as to maintain the normal flow of qi in the whole body and avoid hyperactivity, adverse flow or sinking tendency. That is to say that the normal ascending and descending movement of qi depends on the coordination of the lung and the liver.

Besides, the lung and the liver affect each other

下,导致上热下寒,则表现为心烦、失眠、腰膝以下冷等症状。这两种情形,都叫做"心肾不交"。

其次心主血,肾藏精,精与血之间可以相互化生。故心血不足能引起肾精亏虚,肾精亏虚也能引起心血不足,出现面色无华、心悸、耳鸣、腰膝酸软等精血同病的现象。

(五) 肺与肝

肺与肝的关系,主要体现在气机的调节方面。一方面,肺与肝在功能上相互协同,参与对气机的调节。其中,肺主一身之气,司呼吸而调节气机;肝主疏泄,促进周身气机的通畅。另一方面,肺与肝通过升与降的相互作用来调节气的运动。肺气以肃降为顺,而肝气以升发为宜,肝升与肺降之间具有相互制约、相互为用的作用,能保证全身气机的正常运行,而不致有亢逆或下陷之虞。也就是说,全身气机升降运动的正常进行,离不开肺与肝两脏的密切配合与协调。

此外,肺与肝还可通过病

pathologically. For example, fire transformed from liver stagnation may lead to disorder of the lung in depuration and descent; lung-heat may invade the liver and lead to disorder of the liver in dredging and dispersing. In both cases simultaneous disorder of the liver and the lung will be caused, clinically leading to reddish complexion, redness of eyes, irritability, susceptibility to rage, cough and pain in the chest and hypochondria due to simultaneous appearance of fire-heat and adverse flow of qi.

2.4.1.6 The relationship between the lung and the spleen

Physiologically, two aspects are involved in the relationship between the lung and the spleen. One is the production of the pectoral qi. The lung is responsible for inhaling fresh air and the spleen for absorbing food nutrients through transportation and transformation. The accumulation of the fresh air and food nutrients in the chest eventually transforms into the pectoral qi. Thus the normal functions of the lung and the spleen are prerequisite to sufficient production of the pectoral qi. The other is the metabolism of fluid. The spleen absorbs and transports water and the lung distributes water to all parts of the body, both of which are important to the metabolism of water. If deficiency of spleen-qi or insufficiency of lung-qi affects the production of the pectoral qi, it will lead to shortness of breath, no desire to speak, chest oppression, poor appetite and loose stool. If it affects the metabolism of fluid, it will bring on cough, asthma, profuse phlegm, edema and oliguria.

2.4.1.7 The relationship between the lung and the kidney

The relationship between the lung and the kidney is

理变化来互相影响。如肝郁化火可以犯肺,导致肺的肃降失常;肺热也可以乘肝,导致肝的疏泄失职。两者都形成肝肺同病,临床可出现面红目赤、急躁易怒、咳嗽、胸胁痛等火热与气逆并见的病症。

(六) 肺与脾

肺与脾在生理上主要有两方面的关系。一是在宗气生成方面。肺通过司呼吸功能吸入自然之清气,脾通过主运化功能吸收水谷之精气,自然之清气与水谷之精气互相结合,积聚于胸中,才能形成宗气。所以,肺脾两脏功能正常,是保证宗气生成充足的必要条件。二是在津液代谢方面。脾通过主运化功能吸收和转输水液,肺通过主通调水道功能布散水液至全身,两者都是人体津液代谢不可缺少的重要环节。当脾气虚弱或肺气不足时,如影响到宗气的生成,可出现气短、懒言、胸闷、食少、便溏等症;如影响到津液的代谢,可出现咳喘、痰多、水肿、尿少等症。

(七) 肺与肾

肺与肾的关系,主要表现

signified by respiration and fluid metabolism. The lung regulates water passage and the kidney controls water. The coordination of the lung and the kidney maintains the normal distribution and excretion of water. Besides, the lung governs respiration and the kidney receives qi. The lung and the kidney work together to accomplish respiratory activity and ensure air exchange between the internal and the external. Pathologically, disorder of the lung in regulating water passage and weakness of the kidney in transforming qi affect each other and cause disturbance in water metabolism, leading to edema and oliguria; failure of the lung to disperse and descend and failure of the kidney to receive qi also affect each other and causes disorder in respiration, bringing on symptoms of cough, chest oppression, shortness of breath and frequent dyspnea, etc.

2.4.1.8　The relationship between the liver and the spleen

The relationship between the liver and the spleen involves two aspects: digestion and blood circulation. The liver governs dredging and dispersing and regulates the ascending and descending activities of spleen-qi and stomach-qi, which is beneficial to the transportation and transformation of the spleen. The spleen governs the transportation and transformation of food nutrients that are transformed into blood to nourish the liver, which is beneficial to the dredging and dispersing functions of the liver. If the liver fails to dredge and disperse and invades the spleen, it will cause dysfunction of the spleen, clinically leading to hypochondriac pain, abdominal distension and loose stool, etc.

2.4.1.9　The relationship between the liver and the kidney

The liver and the kidney depend on each other. That is why it is said that "the liver and the kidney share the

在呼吸运动和津液代谢方面。肺主通调水道,肾为主水之脏,肺肾配合,共同维持水液的正常输布与排泄。同时,肺司呼吸,肾主纳气,肺肾协作,共同完成人体的呼吸运动,保证体内外清浊之气的充分交换。在病理上,无论是肺之通调失常,还是肾之气化不利,皆可互相影响,导致水液代谢障碍,产生水肿、尿少等症;肺失宣降与肾不纳气,也可互相传变,导致呼吸运动异常,出现咳嗽、胸闷、气短、动辄喘息等症。

（八）肝与脾

肝与脾的关系,主要表现在消化功能方面与血液运行方面。肝主疏泄,调畅脾胃气机升降,有助于脾的运化功能;脾主运化水谷精微,化生气血濡养于肝,也有利于肝的疏泄。若肝失疏泄,横逆犯脾,易致脾运失健,临床表现为胁痛、腹胀、便溏等症。

（九）肝与肾

肝与肾之间存在着十分密切的相互依赖关系,所以历

same origin" and "yi and kui share the same origin". "Yi" pertains to wood in the five elements and refers to the liver here; and "kui" pertains to water in the five elements and refers to the kidney here.

There are two reasons to explain why "the liver and the kidney share the same origin". One is that essence and blood come from the same source. The liver stores blood and the kidney stores essence. Sufficient blood in the liver makes it possible for the kidney to store the essence and abundant essence in the kidney provides necessary nourishment for the liver. So blood and essence promote each other and transform into each other. The other is mutual promotion between yin-fluids. The kidney pertains to water and the liver to wood. Thus kidney-water nourishes liver-wood and liver-yin invigorates kidney-yin. The mutual promotion and transformation between liver-yin and kidney-yin maintain the coordination between them and the superabundance of them.

Pathologically, insufficiency of liver-blood may lead to deficiency of kidney-essence and deficiency of kidney-essence will, in turn, bring on insufficiency of liver-blood, consequently resulting in dizziness, tinnitus and weakness of the waist. Besides, insufficiency of kidney-yin may lead to deficiency of liver-yin or prolonged deficiency of liver-yin may cause insufficiency of kidney-yin, usually resulting in deficiency of both liver-yin and kidney-yin.

2. 4. 1. 10　The relationship between the spleen and kidney

The kidney is the congenital base of life while the spleen is the acquired base of life. The relationship between the spleen and the kidney is in fact the inter-dependence between the congenital and acquired bases of

来有"肝肾同源"、"乙癸同源"等说法。此处"乙"属木,代表肝;"癸"属水,代表肾。所以"乙癸同源"与"肝肾同源"具有相同含义。

"肝肾同源"可体现在两个方面:一是精血同源。因为肝藏血,肾藏精,肝血充盈则肾有所藏,肾精充足则肝有所养,所以血与精之间存在着相互滋生和相互转化的关系;二是阴液互通。因为肾属水,肝属木,肾水能资生肝木,肝阴也能下济肾阴,肝阴与肾阴之间息息相通,相互化生,维持着协调与充盛。

在病理情况下,若肝血不足可导致肾精亏损,肾精亏损也可导致肝血不足,出现头昏、目眩、耳鸣、腰酸等症。若肾阴不足引起肝阴亏虚,或肝阴亏虚日久引起肾阴不足,则导致肝肾阴虚的病证。

(十) 脾与肾

肾为先天之本,脾为后天之本,脾与肾的关系主要表现为先天之本与后天之本之间的相互依存关系。脾气健运,

life. If the spleen is normal in function, it will absorb and transport food nutrients to nourish the kidney. If kidney-yang is sufficient, it will warm spleen-yang and promote the spleen to transport and transform. Thus the inter-pro-motion between the spleen and the kidney is vital to life activities. Besides, the spleen transports and transforms water while the kidney governs water metabolism. Both organs coordinate with each other in the process of water metabolism.

Pathologically, weakness of spleen-qi and dysfunction of the spleen in transportation and transformation will not provide the kidney with enough food nutrients, leading to insufficiency of kidney-essence with the manifestations of abdominal distension, loose stool, weakness of the waist and tinnitus. Failure of insufficient kidney-yang to warm spleen-yang causes deficiency of spleen-yang, leading to deficiency of both spleen-yang and kidney-yang with the manifestations of cold pain in the abdomen, diarrhea with undigested food or morning diarrhea and edema, etc.

2.4.2 The relationships among the six fu-organs

The relationships among the six fu-organs mainly in-volve the coordination in the process of digesting, absorb-ing and excreting food. After primary digestion in the stomach, food is transmitted to the small intestine where the chyme is further digested by separating the lucid from the turbid. At the same time the gallbladder excretes bile into the small intestine to promote digestion. After ab-sorption, the small intestine transports food nutrients up-wards to the heart and the lung to nourish the whole body. The rest of water is transformed by the kidney into urine and transmitted to the bladder. Thus the small intestine transmits the waste of food to the large intestine where

吸收转输的水谷精微可充养于肾;肾阳充足,温煦脾阳,能促进脾的运化功能。因此,脾与肾相互资助,相互促进,对维持人体生命活动都起着根本的作用。另外,脾运化水液,肾主管水液代谢,两脏在津液代谢过程中具有协同作用。

在病理上,如果脾气虚弱,运化不健,水谷精微不能充养于肾,可导致肾精不足,表现为腹胀、便溏、腰酸、耳鸣等症;肾阳不足,不能温煦脾阳,导致脾阳也虚,则形成脾肾阳虚,表现为腹部冷痛、下利清谷或五更泄泻、水肿等症。

二、六腑之间的关系

六腑之间的关系,主要体现在对水谷的消化、吸收和排泄过程中的分工协作和有序配合。饮食由口入胃,经过胃的受纳腐熟,下传于小肠。小肠接受胃初步消化后形成的食糜,通过分别清浊,进一步消化吸收;同时胆通过把胆汁排泄入小肠以帮助消化。小肠吸收水谷之精微,上输心肺以营养全身;其剩余的水液,经肾的气化作用生成尿液,下

part of the water in the waste is absorbed and the rest is transformed into feces to be excreted out of the body. The triple energizer, the passage of water with its qi flowing from the upper to the lower, is also involved in the digestion, absorption and excretion of food. Generally speaking, digestion is accomplished by coordinative action of the stomach, the gallbladder and the small intestine; absorption mainly takes place in the small intestine, but the large intestine also absorbs part of water; excretion is accomplished by the bladder and the large intestine.

The six fu-organs mainly function to transport and transform food and water. So they constantly receive, transmit and excrete. When food and water are transmitted from the upper to the lower, the stomach and the intestines alternate with the states of fullness and emptiness so as to keep an unobstructed condition. That is why it is said that "the six fu-organs function well when they are not obstructed" and that "the disorder of the fu-organs can be treated by dredging therapy". Clinically disorders of the six fu-organs tend to affect each other. For example, failure of the gallbladder to dredge and disperse will affect the stomach, leading to hypochondriac pain, jaundice, poor appetite and vomiting due to dysfunction of both the gallbladder and the stomach. Consumption of fluid by excess-heat in the stomach will obstruct the large intestine, causing constipation.

2.4.3 The relationship between the five zang-organs and the six fu-organs

The relationship between the five zang-organs and the six fu-organs, though complicated, can be summarized

归膀胱;最后小肠将食物残渣继续下传于大肠。大肠吸收食物残渣中剩余的部分水分,使大便成形而排出体外。三焦之气化贯通上下,为水液运行之道路,所以与消化、吸收和排泄的过程均有关。归纳起来说,人体的消化过程是由胃、胆、小肠三个器官密切协作而完成的,吸收过程主要在小肠,大肠也吸收了部分水分;排泄则是膀胱和大肠的作用。

由于六腑传化水谷,需要不断地受纳、传导和排泄,在水谷自上而下的过程中,胃与肠之间又必须虚实更替,保持宜通不宜滞的状态,所以前人有"六腑以通为用"、"腑病以通为补"的说法。临床上,六腑的病变也常常互相影响。如胆失疏泄,可影响到胃,出现胁痛、黄疸、食少、呕吐等胆胃同病的症状;而胃有实热,消灼津液,亦可使大肠腑气不通,出现大便秘结等症。

三、五脏与六腑之间的关系

五脏与六腑之间具有多种复杂的关系,其主要关系表

as "mutual internal and external relationship". The zang-organs pertain to yin while the fu-organs to yang. Yin controls the internal and yang manages the external. Such a coordination between yin and yang as well as the internal and external makes up a special mutual internal and external relationship between the zang-organs and the fu-organs.

This special mutual internal and external relationship between the zang-organs and fu-organs covers five aspects: the heart and the small intestine, the lung and the large intestine, the spleen and the stomach, the liver and the gallbladder as well as the kidney and the bladder. But no organ is internally and externally related to the triple energizer. That is why the triple energizer is called "a solitary fu-organ". However, it is said in *Huangdi Neijing* that "the kidney is externally and internally related to the triple energizer and the bladder."

The internal and external relationship between the zang-organs and the fu-organs is signified by mutual association with the meridians, mutual coordination in functions and mutual affection in pathology. The mutual association between the zang-organs and the fu-organs with the meridians is introduced in the chapter of the meridians and collaterals. The following discussion only focuses on the mutual coordination in functions and mutual affection in pathology.

2.4.3.1 The internal and external relationship between the heart and the small intestine

The heart governs blood vessels and propels blood to circulate in the whole body, also nourishing the small intestine. The small intestine receives chyme, absorbs food nutrients and transforms them into blood to enrich the heart. Physiologically they depend on each other; pathologically "the heart shifts heat to the small intestine" (that is to move exuberant heart-fire downward to the

现为"脏腑相合"。因为脏属阴,腑属阳,阴主里,阳主表,所以一脏一腑,一阴一阳,一表一里互相配合,就形成了脏腑相合的特殊联系。

脏腑相合包括五对表里相合关系,即心合小肠、肺合大肠、脾合胃、肝合胆、肾合膀胱。三焦没有相合的脏,故称为"孤府"。但《黄帝内经》中又把三焦寄合于肾,而提出"肾合三焦、膀胱"的概念。

脏腑相合,既有经脉上的相互络属,也有功能上的相互配合和病理上的相互影响。脏与腑在经脉上的相互络属,可参见"经络"章。以下讨论脏与腑在功能上的相互配合和病理上的相互影响。

(一) 心合小肠

心主血脉,运行血液于周身而能滋养小肠,小肠受盛化物,吸收的水谷精微能化生心血而充养于心,两者存在着相互依赖的关系。在病理方面,历来有"心移热于小肠"的说法,即心火亢盛,可循经下移

small intestine along the meridian), leading to dysphoria, reddish tongue, sores in the mouth, oliguria, brownish urine and painful urination.

2.4.3.2　The internal and external relationship between the lung and the large intestine

The lung governs depuration and descent while the large intestine controls transmission. Normal function of the lung will transmit fluid downward to moisten the large intestine and promote the transmission of the large intestine. Normal function of the large intestine will ensure smoothness of the large intestinal qi and promote depuration and descent of lung-qi. So physiologically the lung and the large intestine depend on each other. Pathologically, failure of the lung to depurate and descend and failure of the large intestine to transmit will affect each other, bringing on various symptoms due to disorder of both the lung and the large intestine, such as chest oppression, cough, retention of dry feces or constipation.

2.4.3.3　The internal and external relationship between the spleen and the stomach

The spleen and the stomach are all located in the abdomen and pertain to the middle energizer, together governing the digestion and absorption of food and serving as the source of qi, blood and body fluid. That is why the spleen and the stomach are regarded as the "acquired base of life" in all the classics of TCM, the theory about which is known as "the theory of the spleen and the stomach".

The physiological relationship between the spleen and the stomach covers the following three aspects.

1. Coordination in reception and transportation

The spleen governs transportation and transformation while the stomach controls reception and digestion. This

于小肠,出现心烦、舌红、口舌糜烂及尿少、尿赤、尿痛等症。

(二) 肺合大肠

肺气主肃降,大肠主传导。肺气肃降正常,津液下输大肠,肠腑濡润,可促进大肠传导下行;而大肠传导正常,腑气通利,也有利于肺气的肃降。所以肺之肃降与大肠的传导功能之间是互相协助的。在病理上,肺失肃降与大肠传导失司的病变往往相互影响,出现胸闷、咳喘、大便干结或便秘等肺与大肠同病的现象。

(三) 脾合胃

脾与胃同居于腹中,皆属于中焦,二者共同担负着人体的消化吸收功能,构成人体气血津液生化之源,所以历来的中医古典文献常将脾与胃合称"后天之本",有关的理论学说则被称为"脾胃学说"。也就是说,脾与胃在生理上有着非常密切的关系。

脾与胃的生理关系可以概括为以下三个方面。

1. 纳运协调

脾主运化,胃主受纳、腐熟,两者在消化功能上的密切

is what the coordination of the spleen and stomach in reception and transportation means. After being taken into the stomach, food is primarily digested in the stomach, making it possible for the transportation and transformation of the spleen; after being further digested in the spleen, food nutrients are absorbed by the spleen to meet the need of the stomach for further reception. Only when reception and transportation are well coordinated can normal digestion and absorption of food be ensured.

2. Mutual influence of ascent and descent

Spleen-qi governs the elevation of the lucid while stomach-qi controls the descent of the turbid, both of which restrict and assist each other. Through elevating the lucid the spleen transports food nutrients up to the heart and the lung; through descending the turbid the stomach moves the waste of food downwards. Without the descent of stomach-qi the waste of food will stagnate in the middle energizer, food nutrients cannot be transported to the other parts of the body and spleen-qi cannot rise; without the ascent of spleen-qi food nutrients cannot be transported upwards, leading to mixture of the lucid and the turbid in the abdomen and failure of stomach-qi to descend. Only when the ascent of spleen-qi and descent of stomach-qi coordinate with each other can digestion be normally carried on. That is why TCM holds that "ascent ensures normal function of the spleen and descent harmonizes the function of the stomach".

3. Mutual promotion between dryness and dampness

The spleen prefers dryness and dislikes dampness while the stomach prefers moisture and dislikes dryness. Mutual promotion between dryness and dampness indicates that the spleen and stomach physiologically promote each other. The preference and aversion of the spleen are just

配合,称为纳运协调。食物入胃,先由胃受纳和腐熟,这就为脾的运化奠定了基础;而脾主运化,进一步消化水谷,吸收并转输精微,又是适应胃继续受纳的需要。只有纳运协调配合,才能保证人体消化吸收功能的正常进行。

2. 升降相因

脾气主升清,胃气主降浊,两者互助互制,称为升降相因。脾主升清,能将水谷精微向上输送至心肺;胃主降浊,能使水谷浊气通降下行。没有胃气之降,水谷浊气壅塞于中焦,精微之气不能转输,脾气就不能升;没有脾气之升,水谷之清不能上行,则与浊气相混于腹中,胃气就不能正常地降。也就是说,脾升与胃降缺一不可,只有升降相互协调,消化过程才能正常地进行,所以中医学有"脾宜升则健,胃宜降则和"的理论。

3. 燥湿相济

脾喜燥恶湿,胃喜润恶燥,两者生理特性上的相互济助,称为燥湿相济。脾胃两脏在喜恶燥湿方面的特性正好相反。脾为脏,属阴,得阳燥

opposite to those of the stomach. The spleen is a zang-organ and pertains to yin in nature. It transports, transforms and elevates the lucid with the assistance of dryness of yang-qi. Dampness pertains to pathogenic factor of yin in nature, tending to encumbering the spleen and affecting the functions of the spleen to transport and transform food and elevate the lucid. That is why the spleen prefers dryness and dislikes dampness. The stomach is a fu-organ and pertains to yang in nature. With the moisture of yin-fluid the stomach digests and descends food. Dryness is a pathogenic factor of yang in nature, tending to damage stomach-fluid and affecting the functions of the spleen to digest and descend food. That is why the stomach prefers moisture and dislikes dryness. Physiologically yin-fluid in the spleen is beneficial to the digestion and downward transmission of food. Besides, dryness of yang-qi in the stomach is helpful to the spleen to transport and transform food and elevate the lucid. So the spleen and the stomach promote each other with dryness and dampness, playing a very important role in the digestion of food and absorption of food nutrients.

Since the spleen and the stomach are closely related to each other in physiology, clinically spleen disorder and stomach disorder tend to affect each other, frequently leading to spleen disorder involving the stomach and stomach disorder involving the spleen, consequently bringing on the symptoms of anorexia, stomach distension, abdominal distension, vomiting, belching and diarrhea, etc.

2.4.3.4 The internal and external relationship between the liver and the gallbladder

The internal and external relationship between the liver and the gallbladder lies in the fact that both the liver and the gallbladder govern dredging and dispersing. The liver secretes and excretes bile while the gallbladder, at-

之气始能运化升清,而湿属阴邪,容易困脾,阻碍其运化升清的功能,所以脾的特性是喜燥恶湿;胃为腑,属阳,得阴液滋润则能腐熟润降,而燥属阳邪,易伤胃津,不利于胃的腐熟润降功能,因此胃的特性是喜润恶燥。在生理情况下,脾的阴润之气有利于胃的腐熟润降,胃的阳燥之气有利于脾的运化升清,两者燥湿相济,各得其利,在消化吸收功能中发挥着非常重要的作用。

由于脾胃生理关系十分密切,因此临床上脾病与胃病最易互相影响,往往脾病则胃亦病,胃病则脾亦病,出现食欲不振、脘腹胀满、呕吐、嗳气、腹泻等脾胃同病的症状。

(四) 肝合胆

肝与胆在生理上的关系,主要表现为肝胆同主疏泄。肝主疏泄,分泌和排泄胆汁;胆附于肝,贮存和排泄胆汁。

tached to the liver, stores and excretes bile. The bile, coming from the liver and stored in the gallbladder, is excreted into the small intestine to assist digestion. Such a movement of the bile is accomplished by the free and smooth activity of qi to be ensured by the dredging and dispersing functions of the liver. However, the dredging and dispersing functions of the liver can be affected by the state of the gallbladder. The mutual action of the liver and the gallbladder on the flow of qi is due to the fact that both the liver and the gallbladder govern the activities of dredging and dispersing. For example, failure of the liver to dredge and disperse may lead to inhibited flow of gallbladder-qi and unsmooth excretion of the bile; stagnation of the bile may affect the functions of the liver to dredge and disperse, leading to stagnation of liver-qi. Furthermore, failure of both the liver and the gallbladder to dredge and disperse will inhibit the excretion of the bile, bringing on hypochondriac pain, jaundice and anorexia.

2.4.3.5　The internal and external relationship between the kidney and the bladder

　　The internal and external relationship between the kidney and the bladder lies in their dependence and mutual coordination in the excretion of urine. The turbid part of water in the body is transformed into urine by qi-transforming function of the kidney and transported down into the bladder to be discharged out of the body. The storage and excretion of urine by the bladder are accomplished by qi-transforming function of the kidney. Sufficiency of kidney-qi and normal qi-transformation will enable the bladder to open and close properly to excrete urine. Disorder of qi-transformation in the kidney will affect the function of the bladder, leading to dysuria or polyuria and enuresis, etc. If there is damp-heat in the bladder, it will inhibit the activity of qi, give rise to invasion of pathogenic

胆汁来源于肝,贮藏于胆。胆汁排泄入肠以助消化,离不开气机的调畅,而肝气疏泄是保证气机调畅的前提;同时,胆腑通畅与否,也能影响肝气的疏泄。肝胆之间在气的运行方面的相互作用,称为肝胆同主疏泄。如肝失疏泄,可导致胆气不舒,胆汁排泄不畅;反之,胆汁瘀阻,也可影响肝之疏泄,使肝气郁结而不畅。肝胆失疏,胆汁排泄不畅,可出现胁痛、黄疸、食欲不振等症。

(五) 肾合膀胱

　　肾与膀胱的关系,主要表现为在排泄小便方面的相互依赖和协同作用。人体的水液通过肾的气化作用,其浊者形成尿液,下输膀胱以暂时贮留,然后排出体外。膀胱贮尿和排尿的功能,是在肾的气化功能正常的前提下完成的。肾气充足,气化正常,则膀胱开合有度,尿液排泄正常。如肾的气化失常,影响膀胱的功能,可出现小便不利或尿多、遗尿等症。反之,如膀胱湿热,气机不通,邪气逆行于肾,

factors into the kidney and affect qi-transforming function of the kidney, consequently impairing the kidney and clinically bringing on the symptoms of frequent urination, urgent urination and painful urination due to inhibited qi-transformation in the bladder and unsmooth urination as well as aching waist and lumbago due to impairment of the kidney.

Besides, *Huangdi Neijing* holds that the kidney is externally and internally related not only to the bladder, but also to the triple energizer. Since the kidney governs water and the triple energizer is water passage, they coordinate with each other in the metabolism of water. The triple energizer is connected with the upper and lower parts of the body. It can transport water in the whole body to the kidney. If kidney-qi is in disorder, it will lead to abnormal flow of water and accumulation of water in the triple energizer, eventually causing edema. Furthermore, the triple energizer can transport the primordial qi from the kidney to the whole body.

也会影响肾的气化功能，日久使肾脏受损，临床除有尿频、尿急、尿痛等膀胱气化不利、排尿不畅的表现外，还可出现腰酸、腰痛等肾脏受损的症状。

此外，《黄帝内经》认为肾在合膀胱之外，又与三焦相合。因肾主水，三焦为水道，两者在水液代谢方面有相互配合协调关系。因三焦贯通上下，能将全身水液下归于肾；肾之气化功能失常，水气泛滥，则停积壅聚于三焦，而致水肿。三焦还能为肾运行元气至周身。

3 Qi, blood and body fluid

第三章 气血津液

Qi, blood and body fluid, the essential substances for life activities, flow constantly inside the body and all originate from the viscera. They are produced by qi-transforming activities of the viscera and infused into the viscera to nourish the organs and tissues of the body.

Among the three, qi is the most active but invisible substance; blood and body fluid are visible, but must depend on the propelling action of qi to circulate in the whole body.

气血津液是人体生命活动的基本物质,具有流动不息的特征。它们都发源于脏腑,是脏腑气化功能的产物,又滋养、灌注于脏腑等器官组织而起营养作用。

在气、血、津液三类精微物质中,气是具有能动作用的特殊物质,但它没有形质可见;血和津液皆有形质可见,但必须依赖气的推动才能运行于周身。

3.1 Qi

第一节 气

3.1.1 The basic concept of qi

一、气的基本概念

The classic Chinese philosophy believes that the primary state of the universe is qi, the constant movement of which produces all the things in the universe, including life. Thus people in ancient China thought that the accumulation of qi would produce life while the dispersion of qi would put an end to life.

Qi is very active and in constant motion. Qi is also extremely fine and invisible.

宇宙的原初状态是气,由气的不断运动变化,衍生出万事万物。生命也是在气的运动变化中产生出来的。因此,古代中国人认为一切生命的存亡在于气的聚散,气聚则生,气散则亡。

气的特征是活力很强,并处于不断运动之中。气的形质极其精微,用通常的方法是不能直接观察到气的。

Qi is the most essential substance that makes up the body and maintains life activities. All vital substances in the body are transformed by constant motion and change of qi. The viscera, the meridians, the five sensory organs, the nine orifices and the body itself are formed by the motion, transformation and accumulation of qi.

气是构成人体和维持人体生命活动的最基本物质。由气的不断运动、变化，衍生出人体的各种生命物质。人体有脏腑、经络、形体、五官九窍等，这些宏观的形态结构，也是由气的运动变化和交感聚合而形成的。

3.1.2 The production of qi

Qi exists right after the formation of individual life. This kind of qi is inherited from kidney-qi of the parents during pregnancy. So it is called "congenital qi" which is the foundation of the development of new life.

After birth, the human body keeps absorbing nutrients from the external world to nourish the congenital qi. This is the acquired source of qi, also known as "acquired qi". Acquired qi originates from food nutrients and fresh air inhaled into the body.

In fact, the "congenital qi" and "acquired qi" are just two material sources of qi. The process of qi production also involves the other viscera. The inter-transformation among essence, qi, blood and body fluid influences the production of qi.

3.1.3 The physiological functions of qi

Qi is the essential substance that makes up the body

二、气的生成

人类个体生命一出生就有气存在，这种气是在胚胎时期禀受于父母的肾气，由于它在出生前生成，所以称为"先天之气"。先天之气是新的生命体开始发育成长的基础。

出生以后，人体还要不断地从外界摄取营养物质，以充养先天之气，这是气生成的后天来源，所以把它叫作"后天之气"。后天之气有两种来源，一是从饮食中获得营养物质，一是从呼吸中获得自然之清气。

"先天之气"和"后天之气"只是气生成的两个物质来源，而气生成的具体过程还需要其他脏腑的参与和协同作用。精、气、血、津液等基本物质之间的相互转化，对气的生成也有重要影响。

三、气的生理作用

气是形成人体结构并维

and maintains various physiological activities. Qi in different viscera and organs functions differently. Generally speaking, there are five physiological functions of qi.

3.1.3.1　Propelling function

Qi is the motivation of the physiological functions of all the viscera and organs in the body. The propelling function of qi can stimulate and maintain the physiological functions of the viscera and other organs. That is why qi is called the root of life. Qi in different viscera and organs functions differently. For example, kidney-qi promotes the development of the body and reproduction, transform water and receive lung-qi; heart-qi promotes blood circulation; lung-qi governs respiration and regulates water passage; spleen-qi promotes digestion and absorption of food and commands blood; liver-qi regulates various functions by smoothing the activity of qi. Weakness of qi in promotion will lead to hypofunction of the viscera and other organs and cause various deficiency problems.

3.1.3.2　Warming function

Qi warms the body and is the source of heat energy in the body. It is very important in maintaining normal body temperature and ensuring the physiological functions of all the viscera and organs. Since qi can warm the body, it is similar to yang in nature. So the kind of qi that warms the body is called "yang-qi". All the five zang-organs have yang-qi respectively. For example, heart-yang warms and

持人体各种生理活动的基本物质。气在不同的脏腑、器官中发挥着多种多样的生理作用。归纳起来说,气主要具有以下五种生理作用。

(一) 推动作用

气具有推动的作用,是人体所有脏腑器官功能活动的原动力。气的推动作用能激发和维持脏腑器官的生理功能,所以气被称为人体生命之根本。随着气所在脏腑器官的不同,所发挥的生理作用也各不相同。如在肾的气(肾气)能推动人体的生长发育和生殖功能,并能气化水液、摄纳肺气;在心的气(心气)能推动血液运行;在肺的气(肺气)能司呼吸、主通调水道;在脾的气(脾气)能推动对饮食的消化吸收,并能统摄血液;在肝的气(肝气)能疏泄气机而发挥多种调节功能等。气的推动作用减弱,主要表现为脏腑器官的功能减退,出现各种虚弱性疾病。

(二) 温煦作用

气具有温煦的作用,是人体热能产生的来源,对于维持人体正常体温,保证各脏腑器官生理功能的发挥,具有十分重要的意义。气的温煦作用是一种属阳的功能表现,所以具有温煦作用时的气被称为

dredges blood vessels to promote blood circulation; lung-yang warms and nourishes skin and muscular interstices, preventing exogenous pathogenic factors from invading the body; spleen-yang warms and transforms food and water, promoting digestion and absorption; liver-yang steams and fumigates qi, promoting qi transformation in the five zang-organs and the six fu-organs; kidney-yang warms life-gate, stimulates reproduction and transforms water. If the warming function of qi is weakened, it will lead to stagnation of internal cold, unsmooth circulation of qi and blood and devitalization of the visceral functions.

3.1.3.3 Protecting function

Qi can protect the body, resisting the invasion of various pathogenic factors and preventing disease. As to pathogenic factors, the kind of qi that protects the body is called "healthy qi" or "genuine qi". healthy qi functions to protect the whole body against the invasion of pathogenic factors and, after the invasion of pathogenic factors into the body or onset of disease, to fight against the pathogenic factors to promote healing of disease. If the protecting function of qi is weakened, it mainly leads to decline of body resistance and susceptibility of the body to invasion of pathogenic factors.

3.1.3.4 Fixating function

Fixation of qi means that qi can astringe and control liquid substances, such as blood, body fluid and sperm, to prevent them from losing. To be specific, qi fixating blood means that qi keeps blood to flow inside the vessels and prevent it from flowing out of the vessels; qi fixating sweat, urine and saliva means that qi controls the secretion

"阳气"。五脏皆各有阳气。如心阳能温通血脉,促进血液的运行;肺阳能温养皮毛腠理,防御外邪的侵袭;脾阳能温化水谷饮食,促进消化吸收;肝阳能蒸蕴气机,鼓舞五脏六腑之气化;肾阳能温煦命门,激发生殖功能,同时对水液有蒸腾气化作用。气的温煦作用减弱,主要表现为内寒凝结,气血运行不畅,脏腑功能不振。

(三) 防御作用

气具有防御作用,是人体抵御各种邪气、预防疾病的根本条件。针对"邪气"而言,发挥防御作用的气被称为"正气",也叫"真气"。正气的防御作用具体表现在两方面:一是能护卫全身肌表,防御外邪的入侵;二是当邪气已经入侵或发生了疾病后,正气能与邪气进行斗争,将邪气消除或驱邪外出,促使疾病痊愈。气的防御作用减弱,主要表现为机体抵抗力下降,易受邪气侵袭而致病。

(四) 固摄作用

气具有固摄作用,主要是对血液、津液、精液等液态物质具有收敛、摄纳并防止其流失的功能。其具体表现是:固摄血液,使血液循脉而行,防止其逸出脉外;固摄汗液、尿

and excretion of these liquids so as to restrict the excretion and prevent loss; qi fixating sperm means that qi balances sex function and prevents seminal emission. Besides defecation and location of the viscera are under the influence of the fixating function of qi. If the fixating function of qi is weakened, it will lead to loss of blood, body fluid and sperm. The weakness of the qi fixation may also lead to protracted diarrhea, incontinence of urine and stool as well as proctoptosis and hysteroptosis.

3.1.3.5　Qi-transforming function

　　Qi-transformation means changes caused by the movement of qi, which is the essential cause of the conception, development, growth and decline of life. Life activities concerned with qi-transformation can be divided into three categories. Firstly, through food and respiration the body absorbs nutrients from the external world and transforms them into essence, qi, blood and body fluid essential to the body. Secondly, inter-promotion among the refined substances (essence, qi, blood and body fluid etc.) is the process of automatic regulation, improvement and balance of life. Thirdly, waste substance and turbid qi are excreted out of the body in the process of life. If qi-transformation is weakened, the whole process of life will be in disorder or decline, leading to various diseases. The declination of qi-transformation even leads to death.

3.1.4　The moving styles of qi

　　Qi in the body is a kind of very active and refined

液、唾液等,控制其分泌与排泄,使其有节制地排出,防止异常流失;固摄精液,使性功能协调,防止其无故流失。此外,大便的排泄和内脏位置的恒定也受气的固摄作用的影响。若气的固摄作用减弱,主要表现为血液、津液、精液等的异常流失。其次,可出现久泄、二便失禁,以及脱肛、子宫脱垂等。

(五) 气化作用

　　气化,泛指由气的运动而产生的变化。气具有气化作用,是生命产生、发育、成长、衰老等一系列过程的根本原因。气化所涉及的生命运动极其广泛,大体可以概括为三个方面:第一,人体通过饮食、呼吸等从外界摄取营养物质,并把它转化成人体自身所需要的精、气、血、津液等生命物质;第二,体内各种精微物质(精、气、血、津液等)之间的相互转化,是生命体自我调整、完善、平衡的内在过程;第三,在生命过程中产生废物、浊气,向体外排出。气的气化作用减弱,整个生命过程就会紊乱或衰退,导致各种疾病的产生。气化衰竭,则导致死亡。

四、气的运动形式

　　人体的气,是具有很强活

substance that is in constant movement. The moving styles of qi, though differing from organ to organ, can be classified into four kinds, namely ascending, descending, coming in and going out. These four styles can be synthesized into two major categories, namely ascending and descending, coming in and going out.

Upward movement of qi means ascending while downward movement of qi means descending. Though ascending and descending are opposite, they can be transformed into each other. When qi ascends to the supreme point, it begins to descend. Such a transformation is known as "extreme ascending changes into descending". When qi descends to the lowest point, it begins to ascend. Such a transformation is known as "extreme descending turns into ascending". This is the upward and downward movement of qi under normal conditions.

Coming in and going out, two opposite moving styles of qi, take place alternately. When qi disperses outward (going out) to a certain degree, it begins to restrain itself inward (coming in). When qi restrains itself inward (coming in) to a certain degree, it begins to disperse outward (going out). This is the external and internal movement of qi under normal conditions.

Ascending and descending, coming in and going out are two types of the motion of yin and yang, which coordinate with each other. For example, the activities of ascending and going out pertain to yang; the activities of descending and coming in pertain to yin. So ascending coordinates with going out while descending coordinates with

力的精微物质,其主要特征在于不断地运动。气的运动形式,随所在脏腑器官的不同而各异,但归纳起来说,不外乎升、降、出、入四种基本形式。由于升与降相反,出与入相反,所以也可以把它们综合为升降与出入两组运动形式。

升降是上下之间的运动,气向上行为升,气向下行为降。升与降虽然相反,但两者之间可以相互转化。当升到达极点时,就会转而下降,这叫做"升已而降";当降到达极点时,就会转而上升,这叫做"降已而升"。这是正常情况下气的上下循环运动。

出入是内外之间的运动,气向外行为出,气向内行为入。出与入虽然相反,但两者之间也是交替进行的。当气向外发散(出)进行到一定阶段,就会转而向内收敛(入);当气向内收敛(入)到一定阶段时,就会转而向外发散。这是正常情况下气的内外循环运动。

升降与出入实际上是阴阳运动的两种不同形式,两者具有某种相互协调作用。如升、出皆属阳,降、入皆属阴,所以升与出之间相互协调,降与入之间相互协调。也就是

coming in.

The ascending, descending, coming in and going out activities of qi are accomplished by the viscera and meridians. Each zang-organ or fu-organ may differ from others in the moving style of qi. For example, liver-qi is ascending, lung-qi is descending, spleen-qi is ascending and stomach-qi is descending, etc. The zang-organs and the fu-organs, though different from each other in the moving styles of qi, coordinate with each other and form a special system for regulating qi activity. For example, the liver and the lung restrict but coordinate with each other in ascending and descending; the spleen and the stomach associate and cooperate with each other in ascending and descending , etc. The meridians and collaterals are the important routes for qi to flow. With the different running directions of the meridians, the ascending and descending activities of qi also become different. The meridians of the viscera run from the internal to the external, qi in these meridians flows outward accordingly. If the meridians run from the external to the internal of the body, qi in these meridians will flow from the external to the internal. If the meridians run from the head to the lower part of the body, qi in these meridians will accordingly flow from the upper to the lower. If the meridians run from the feet upward, qi in these meridians will certainly flow upward.

The ascending, descending, coming in and going out activities of qi are very important to life. If these activities of qi are normal, the functions of the viscera and the meridians will be normal. If these activities are abnormal, the functions of the viscera and meridians will be in disorder. If these activities of qi stop, death will occur.

说，升降正常与否会影响到出入，出入正常与否也会影响到升降。

气的升降出入，是通过脏腑、经络来实现的。每一脏或腑都可以具有升降出入不同的运动方式，但各有侧重不同。如肝气以升为主；肺气以降为主；脾气以升为主，胃气以降为主，等等。脏腑之间有侧重的升降出入相互配合协调，形成了人体独特的气机调节方式。如肝与肺升降相互制约、协调；脾与胃升降相互关联与配合等。经络是气运行的重要通道，随着经络的走向不同，气的升降出入也不同。内脏的经络从里出表，气也随之向外运行；经络从外进入体内，气也随之向内运行。经脉从头向下走，气也随之下降；经脉从足向上行，气也随之向上升。

气的升降出入运动，对于人体生命是极其重要的。升降出入运动正常，脏腑、经络的功能才能正常；升降出入运动失常，脏腑、经络的功能就会紊乱；升降出入运动停止，生命就会死亡。

3.1.5 The classification of qi and its production, distribution and functional characteristics

There are various classifications and names of qi. Usually qi is classified into yuan-qi (the primordial qi), zong-qi (the pectoral qi), ying-qi (the nutrient qi) and wei-qi (the defensive qi).

3.1.5.1 Yuan-qi (primordial qi)

The primordial qi, also called primary qi or genuine qi, is the most essential qi in the body and the vital foundation of life.

1. The production of the primordial qi

The primordial qi mainly comes from kidney-qi of the parents during pregnancy. That is why TCM usually calls the primordial qi "the congenital qi". The power and quantity of the primordial qi are already fixed after birth. However, after birth the primordial qi still needs further nourishment and enrichment to enable it to be distributed to the whole body and to exert normal physiological effect. The primordial qi transformed from food nutrients provided by the spleen and stomach is called "acquired qi".

2. The distribution of the primordial qi

The primordial qi is stored in the kidney and distributed to all parts of the body through the triple energizer. The primordial qi transformed from food nutrients provided by the spleen and stomach must be stored in the kidney so that it can be distributed to the whole body. Though

五、气的分类及其生成、分布与功能特点

由于不同的分类方法,气的具体名称很多。通常我们把气分为元气、宗气、营气、卫气四种。

(一)元气

元气也称原气、真气等。元气是人体最根本的气。元,有本源、根本之义。人体生命力的根本,在于元气。

1. 元气的生成

元气首先来源于先天,是在胚胎时期禀受于父母的肾气。因此,中医常把这种元气称为"先天之气"。人出生以后,先天元气的强弱多少即已确定。但出生以后,元气还有一个充养的过程。人在后天主要通过饮食获取营养物质,以充养先天之元气,使元气进一步充实、丰沛,才能布散全身而发挥正常的生理效应。人体在后天通过脾胃运化获取营养物质而化生的元气,也称为"后天之气"。

2. 元气的分布

元气首先藏于肾中,然后通过三焦流布到全身。由脾胃运化水谷精微而化生的元气,也必归藏于肾中,才能转输至全身。所以,元气分布于

the primordial qi is distributed to all parts of the body, it originates from the kidney.

3. The functional characteristics of the primordial qi

The primordial qi shares the common functions of qi, such as propelling, warming, protecting, fixating and qi-transforming, etc. The functions of the primordial qi are different if its location is different. The characteristics of the primordial qi in the kidney include three aspects: to promote the growth and development of the body and maintain reproductive functions of the body; to promote qi transformation to regulate water metabolism and excretion of urine; to fixate sperm and inhaled fresh air to ensure the functions of the kidney to store essence and receive qi. The primordial qi distributed to all parts of the body warms and promotes all the viscera so as to bring their physiological functions into full play. For example, the spleen governs transportation and transformation; the lung governs respiration; the heart dominates blood; the liver controls dredging and dispersing; the stomach is responsible for reception and digestion, etc. These are all the concrete manifestations of the effect of the primordial qi on the viscera. Thus the primordial qi is the vital qi in the body and is the motivation of all life activities. The state of the primordial qi decides the state of life.

3.1.5.2 Zong-qi (the pectoral qi)

The pectoral qi is a kind of essential qi in the body. Since it is produced after birth, it is a kind of acquired essential qi.

The pectoral qi accumulates in the chest. When transported from the chest, it is divided into ying-qi (the nutrient qi) and wei-qi (the defensive qi) which are distributed to the whole body.

全身,但以肾为元气之根源。

3. 元气的功能特点

元气具有气的一般功能,即推动作用、温煦作用、防御作用、固摄作用、气化作用。元气随其所在不同而有不同的功能特点。在肾之元气的功能特点有三:一能推动人体的生长发育,维持人体的生殖功能;二能行气化而主管水液代谢,司小便开合;三能固摄精液、吸入之气,从而有藏精、纳气的功能。输布到全身的元气,具有温养和推动各脏腑并使之发挥正常功能的作用,如脾主运化,肺司呼吸,心主血,肝主疏泄,胃主受纳、腐熟,等等,都是元气在各脏腑器官发挥其作用的具体体现。由此可见,元气是人体的根本之气,是所有生命活动的原动力所在,元气的盛衰,直接决定生命的存亡。

(二) 宗气

宗气也是人体的根本之气。宗,义即"根本"。由于宗气是在后天生成的,所以它是一种后天的根本之气。

宗气积聚于胸中,输出胸中后分为营气和卫气,布散至全身。

1. The production of the pectoral qi

The pectoral qi is produced by combining the fresh air inhaled by the lung with the food nutrients absorbed and transported by the spleen. The respiratory function of the lung and the transporting and transforming functions of the spleen influence the production of the pectoral qi.

2. The distribution of the pectoral qi

Since the pectoral qi accumulates in the chest, the chest is called "the sea of qi". Because the heart and the lung are located in the chest, the pectoral qi infuses into the heart and the lung and flows in the vessels and respiratory tract. So the state of the pectoral qi influences the functions of the heart vessels, the lung and the respiratory tract.

3. The functional characteristics of the pectoral qi

The pectoral qi has two functions. One is to warm and nourish the heart vessels to maintain their functions in transporting qi and blood. The other is to warm and nourish the lung and the upper respiratory tract to maintain their functions in governing respiration and vocalization. If the pectoral qi is insufficient, it will lead to palpitation, shortness of breath and weak voice, etc.

3.1.5.3 Ying-qi (nutrient qi) and wei-qi (defensive qi)

The nutrient qi and the defensive qi all come from the pectoral qi and are closely related to each other in production and circulation.

The nutrient qi pertains to yin and the defensive qi pertains to yang. So the nutrient qi and the defensive qi are also called ying-yin (nutrient yin) and wei-yang (defensive yang).

1. 宗气的生成

宗气是由肺吸入的自然之清气和由脾吸收转输而来的水谷之精微相结合而生成。肺的呼吸功能和脾的运化功能正常与否,都能影响宗气的盛衰。

2. 宗气的分布

宗气积聚于胸中,故称胸中为"气海"。心肺居于胸中,故宗气能贯注于心肺,并能行于血脉和呼吸道。宗气的盛衰,可以影响心脉、肺及呼吸道的功能。

3. 宗气的功能特点

宗气的主要功能有二:一是温养心脉,以维持其运行气血的功能;二是温养肺和上呼吸道,以维持其司呼吸和发声的功能。因此,若宗气不足,可出现心悸、呼吸气短、声音低弱等症。

(三)营气与卫气

营气与卫气都是从宗气分化而来,二者在生成、运行等方面有十分密切的关系,所以将它们合并介绍。

营气属阴,卫气属阳,故又简称营阴、卫阳。

1. The production of the nutrient qi and the defensive qi

Both the nutrient qi and the defensive qi come from the pectoral qi. The pectoral qi flows to the whole body from the chest in the form of the nutrient qi and the defensive qi. In terms of the production, the nutrient qi and the defensive qi, just like the pectoral qi, is produced by combining the fresh air inhaled by the lung with the food nutrients absorbed and transported by the spleen. The only difference lies in food nutrients. The nutrient qi comes from the "most essential part" of the food nutrients while the defensive qi comes from "the most active and powerful part" of the food nutrients.

2. The distribution of the nutrient qi and the defensive qi

The nutrient qi and the defensive qi are different in nature. The former, pertaining to yin in nature, flows inside the vessels while the latter, pertaining to yin in nature, flows outside the vessels. That also explains why the nutrient qi distributes in the internal organs while the defensive qi distributes over the surface of the body. Certainly there is the defensive qi in the internal organs and there is the nutrient qi in the superficies. But the nutrient qi mainly flows inside the internal organs and the defensive qi mainly circulates in the superficies.

1. 营气与卫气的生成

营气与卫气皆由宗气分化而来。宗气从胸中流向全身,就分为两条道路,一为营气,一为卫气。因此,营气与卫气的生成和宗气是一样的,也是由肺吸入的自然之清气与脾所运化的水谷之精微相结合而成。其区别在于,二者所来源的水谷之精微是有所不同的。营气来源于水谷精微中的"精气",卫气来源于水谷精微中的"悍气"。"精气"是指水谷精微中最有营养的部分,"悍气"是指水谷精微中性猛而活力特强的部分。

2. 营气与卫气的分布

由于营气与卫气在性质上有阴、阳之区别,所以在运行径路上有脉内、脉外之不同。营气得水谷精微之精气,性质属阴,故运行于脉内;卫气得水谷精微之悍气,性质属阳,故运行于脉外。同时,由于营气属阴,卫气属阳,所以营气的分布偏于内脏,卫气的分布偏于体表。当然,内脏也有卫气,体表也有营气,只是营气与卫气的主要分布部分有所侧重而已。

3. The functional characteristics of the nutrient qi and the defensive qi

The nutrient qi and the defensive qi are different from each other in functional characteristics. The functional characteristics of the nutrient qi are marked by transformation into blood to nourish the whole body, especially nourishing the internal organs to maintain their physiological functions. The functional characteristics of the defensive qi are marked by warming and nourishing the body and protecting the body against pathogenic factors, especially warming and nourishing the muscles and superficies as well as regulating sweat so as to protect the body against pathogenic factors. The defensive qi pertains to yang. That is why it can warm the body. But it regulates sweat to excrete excessive yang-heat so as to maintain a constant body temperature.

3.2 Blood

3.2.1 The basic concept of blood

Blood, mainly composed of the nutrient qi and body fluid, circulates inside the vessels. It is red in color and sticky in texture. Blood functions to nourish and moisten the body. It is vital to the maintenance of life.

3. 营气与卫气的功能特点

营气与卫气的功能特点各不相同。营气的功能特点是化生血液、营养全身,其中尤以营养内脏并维持其生理功能为主。卫气的功能特点是温养肌体、防御外邪,其中尤以温养肌表、调节出汗,从而抗御外邪入侵为主。因卫气属阳,故能温煦肌体,同时又通过调节汗孔开合,排泄多余的阳热之气,以维持体温的恒定。

第二节 血

一、血的基本概念

血也称血液,主要由营气和津液所组成,运行于脉管之中,外观呈红色、粘稠的液体。血具有营养和滋润作用,对于维持人的生命具有极重要意义。

血与五脏的关系非常密切。五脏需要血的营养和滋润作用,才能发挥其正常的功能,血也需要五脏的共同作用,才能源源不断地化生和获得补充。

3.2.2　The production of blood

The basic substance for producing blood is essence, including the congenital essence (kidney-essence) and the acquired essence (food nutrients). The congenital essence is prerequisite to the production of blood. Only when the acquired essence has combined with the congenital essence can blood be produced. Thus deficiency of kidney-essence will make it difficult to produce blood. However, the congenital essence is already fixed after birth. In this case the acquired essence plays a key role in the production of blood. For this reason the functions of the spleen and stomach are key to the production of blood. If the spleen and the stomach are normal in functions, they can absorb sufficient food nutrients to produce blood. If the spleen and stomach are weak in absorbing food nutrients, the production of blood is inevitably reduced.

The transformation of the essence into blood is in fact a process of qi-transformation. The organs involved in such a process are the heart and the lung. The function of the heart in the process of blood production is called "reddening", because the heart pertains to fire in the five elements and red in the five colors. With the action of heart-fire blood becomes red. The lung participates in the production of the nutrient qi by inhaling fresh air from the outside. The nutrient qi is an important component of blood. So the functions of the lung directly influence the production of blood. Besides, the liver regulates qi activity and influences qi-transformation in the whole body with its dredging and dispersing functions, also exerting certain effect on the production of blood.

二、血的生成

血液生成的物质基础主要是精,包括先天之精(肾精)和后天之精(水谷之精)。其中,先天之精是血液生成的首要条件,后天之精必须与先天之精结合,才能生成血液。因此,先天之肾精不足,血液将无从化生。然而,人出生以后,其先天之精已经确定,而后天之精就起着决定性的作用。所以在一般情况下,对血液生成有决定性影响的是脾胃的功能。脾胃功能正常,能从饮食中吸收足够的水谷精微,从而化生血液。若脾胃功能减弱,吸收水谷精微不足,化生血液也就减少。

精化生血的过程,是一个气化过程,必须在气的作用下才能完成。参与这一气化过程的内脏主要是心肺。心在血液生成过程中的气化作用称为"化赤"。这是由于心在五行属火,其色为赤,在心火的特殊作用下,血液才能变成红色。肺通过吸入自然之清气参与营气的生成,而营气是血液的一个组成部分,所以肺的功能正常与否,可直接影响血液的生成。此外,肝主疏泄对气机有重要调节作用,能影响全身的气化功能,对血的化生过程也有一定影响。

3.2.3　The physiological functions of blood

The physiological functions of blood are to nourish and moisten the body as described in *Nanjing*. Since blood contains the nutrient qi, it can nourish all the organs in the body. Through the meridians, blood transports nutrient substances to all parts of the body to nourish the five zang-organs, the six fu-organs, the five constituents, the five sensory organs and the nine orifices. It should be noted that blood is also the important material base for mental activities. If blood is sufficient, there will be sufficient vitality; if blood is deficient, there will be dispiritedness; if blood is in disturbance, there will be mental disorder. Since blood contains fluid, it can moisten the viscera and the body. When the fluid flows out of the vessels, it moistens the orifices and lubricate the joints.

Besides, blood also transports the turbid qi. When the turbid qi is transported to the lung, it is excreted from respiration. When it is transported to the kidney, it is discharged from urination. When it is transported to the superficies, it is excreted from sweating.

3.2.4　The circulation of blood

The vessels in the whole body form a relatively close circulatory system for blood circulation. Such a system is known as blood vessels in TCM included in the concept of meridians and vessels. The minute capillaries are called blood collaterals.

三、血的生理作用

血液具有营养和滋润的生理作用,《难经》概括为"血主濡之"。由于血液中含有营气,所以能对周身各脏腑器官起营养作用。血液通过经络的运行,把营养物质输送到全身各处,营养五脏六腑、五体、五官九窍,使之发挥正常的功能。值得重视的是,血是产生精神的重要物质基础,血液充足而调和则精神健旺,若血液不足则精神不振,血行逆乱则精神异常。由于血液中含有津液,故能滋润脏腑形体,尤其是溢于脉外的津液能滋润孔窍,滑利关节。

此外,血液还有运输浊气的作用。浊气经血液运送至肺,则从呼气排出;浊气经血液运送至肾,则从小便排出;浊气经血液运送至体表,则从汗排出。

四、血的运行

血液在脉管内正常地运行,全身脉管形成一个相对密闭的循环性管道系统。这种管道系统实际上就是通常所说的血脉,血脉属于广义经脉的范畴,其中细小的血脉也称血络。

Blood is propelled by the heart to circulate in the vessels. In fact the heart is the center of the blood circulatory system. In structure, the heart is connected with the vessels. That is why the heart can propel blood to circulate in the vessels. Since the circulation of blood is a circulatory process, the directions of blood circulation is either centrifugal or axopetal. The former means that the blood is propelled by heart-qi to flow out from the heart to the whole body through large vessels into large collaterals and fine capillaries. In such a way blood enters the internal organs to nourish and moisten the body. The latter means that blood accumulates from the fine capillaries to the large collaterals and the vessels into the heart under the propelling action of the heart.

Apart from the heart, other internal organs are also involved in the circulation of blood, including the lung, the spleen and the liver. Structurally the lung is connected with all the vessels in the body, known as "the lung facing all the vessels". With the association with the vessels, the lung distributes nutrient substances, like the pectoral qi, to the whole body and accumulates qi and blood from the whole body to assist the heart to propel blood circulation. The spleen commands blood, making the vessels compact, directing blood to circulate normally in the vessels and preventing it from flowing out of the vessels. The liver stores blood and regulates the volume of blood. Besides, the liver also governs dredging and dispersing, thus smoothing the activity of qi to promote blood circulation.

血液运行的动力来自心，心是血液循环系统的中枢。心在结构上与脉管相连，所以血液经心的推动而进入脉管中运行。由于血液运行是一个循环过程，所以血液运行的方向分为"离心"和"向心"两个方面。"离心"是指血液由心气推动从心流出，经较大的脉管流向全身，并反复分支，进入较大的络脉、较小的络脉直至最细小的络脉，即进入脏腑器官而发挥其营养滋润作用。"向心"是指血液从最细小的络脉逐渐汇聚，经较大的络脉、更大的络脉、经脉，最后回到心脏。血液返回心脏也是在心的推动作用下进行的。

除了心的推动作用外，血液的运行还需要多个内脏的协同作用，这些内脏主要有肺、脾、肝等。肺在结构上与全身的脉管相连，这叫做"肺朝百脉"。肺通过百脉的联系，既能将宗气等营养物质输布于全身，又能汇聚全身气血，从而起到辅心行血的作用。脾有统摄血液的作用，能令血脉周密，血液正常地在脉管中运行，不致于逸出脉外。肝有藏血的功能，通过肝藏血而调节血流量；肝又主疏泄，使气机调畅，有利于促进血液的流行。

The factor that directly acts on blood circulation is qi. For example, heart-qi propels blood to circulate; lung-qi assists the heart to propel blood circulation; spleen-qi commands blood; and liver-qi regulates the circulation of blood by dredging and dispersing qi. If heart-qi is insufficient, blood will become too weak to circulate; if lung-qi is insufficient, there will be no opportunity for blood to disperse; if spleen-qi is insufficient, it will be difficult for the spleen to command blood; if liver-qi fails to dredge, it will lead to stagnation of qi and stasis of blood. Besides, visceral yang also plays an important role in the circulation of blood. For example, deficiency of yang will inevitably cause deficiency of qi, making it difficult for blood to circulate; deficiency of yin will bring on cold and exuberant cold will coagulate blood.

Other factors that may affect blood circulation are the state of the vessels and the changes of cold and heat. Generally speaking, phlegm, dampness, blood stasis, swelling and nodules can block or compress the vessels and obstruct blood circulation. Blood is characterized by preference for warmth and aversion to cold. So excessive cold slows down the circulation of blood or even causes blood stasis; excessive heat accelerates blood circulation and even leads to bleeding in severe cases.

3.3   Body fluid

3.3.1   The basic concept of body fluid

Body fluid is a basic substance that makes up the body and maintains life activities. The main component of body fluid is water, also including nutrient substance. Body fluid is also a component of blood when it flows inside the vessels. However, body fluid also flows outside the ves-

直接对血液运行产生作用的因素是气。如心气推动血液运行,肺气辅心行血,脾气统摄血液,肝气疏泄气机调节血行等。若心气不足,则血行无力;肺气不足,则血失宣散;脾气不足,则脾不统血;肝气失疏,则气滞血瘀。此外,脏腑之阳在血液运行中也有重要作用。若阳虚则气必虚,气虚则不能行血;阳虚则生寒,寒盛则血液凝滞。

其他影响血液运行的因素有脉管的通利情况及寒热的变化等。凡痰湿、瘀血、肿结之类可阻滞或压迫脉管,妨碍血液运行。血液的特性是喜温而恶寒,所以寒凉能使血行缓慢,甚至形成瘀血;过热又可使血行加速,严重时可导致出血。

第三节   津液

一、津液的基本概念

津液,是构成人体和维持人体生命活动的基本物质之一,其主要成分是水,其中也含有部分精微物质。津液在血脉中,成为血液的组成部

sels in the viscera and the body. If secreting or excreting from the five sensory organs and the nine orifices, body fluid becomes urine, sweating, tears, snivel, saliva and drool, etc.

Body fluid can be divided into two parts: thin fluid and thick fluid which are different from each other in property, location and functions. Generally speaking, thin fluid flows quickly and is distributed in the skin, muscles and orifices to moisten the related parts of the body. The thick fluid relatively flows slowly and is distributed in the viscera, cerebral marrow and joints to nourish the related parts of the body. Though different in texture and distribution, both the thin and thick fluids come from food and water transformed by the spleen and stomach, functionally flowing inside and outside the vessels to permeate and supplement each other. Physiologically they are not strictly separated from each other; pathologically "impairment of the thin fluid" is relatively light while "loss of the thick fluid" is relatively serious.

3.3.2　The production of body fluid

The digestive and absorbing functions of the stomach, the spleen and the large and small intestines play a key role in the production of body fluid. Body fluid comes from food, especially water and liquid diet. The production of body fluid comes through a series of physiological activities, including the functions of the stomach to receive and digest, the functions of the spleen to transport, transform and transmit, the functions of the small intestine to receive and digest, and the functions of the large intestine to transmit and change. Different viscera may exert different effect on the water taken into the body. So the metabolism of body fluid is accomplished under the co-

分;津液在血脉外,则遍布于脏腑形体之中。若津液从五官九窍中分泌或排泄出来,就成为尿、汗、泪、涕、唾、涎等。

津液是津与液的合称,而津与液在性状、分布部位和功能等方面还是有区别的。一般地说,性状较清稀,流动性较大,布散于皮肤、肌肉和孔窍之中,起滋润作用的,总称为津;性状较稠厚,流动性较小,灌注于脏腑、脑髓、骨节之中,起濡养作用的,总称为液。津与液虽有一定区别,但两者同源于水谷,生成于脾胃,流布于经脉内外,能相互渗透、补充,所以通常在生理上不予严格区分,而并称为"津液",只是在病理上有"伤津"轻而"脱液"重的区别。

二、津液的生成

津液是通过胃、脾及大小肠的消化吸收功能而产生的。津液来源于饮食物,尤以水饮流汁食物为主。饮食物经过胃的受纳腐熟、脾的运化转输、小肠的受盛化物与分别清浊、大肠的传导变化等生理活动而生成津液,不同脏腑对水饮的作用方式不同,津液就是在不同脏腑功能的密切配合、相互协作下完成其代谢过程的。

ordination of different viscera.

3.3.3 The physiological functions of body fluid

The physiological functions of body fluid includes the following three aspects.

3.3.3.1 Moistening and nourishing

Body fluid contains large quantity of water and nutrient substances to moisten and nourish the viscera and the body. To be specific, the thin fluid, distributed in the skin and orifices, mainly functions to moisten the body; the thick fluid, distributed in the viscera and cerebral marrow, mainly functions to nourish the body.

3.3.3.2 The transformation of blood

Body fluid not only flows outside the vessels, but also inside the vessels to participate in the production of blood. Blood is composed of two parts: body fluid and the nutrient qi. If body fluid is insufficient, the production of blood will be reduced, leading to blood deficiency.

3.3.3.3 The transportation of the turbid qi

Body fluid can hold various turbid qi and waste materials produced by qi-transformation and transport them to the concerned organs to be excreted out of the body through urination, sweating and respiration. The waste materials and the turbid qi are directly excreted in the form of fluid through urination and sweating. But the turbid qi excreted through respiration is transported to the lung first by body fluid and then exhaled out of the body. If body fluid is insufficient, the turbid qi cannot be quickly excreted out of the body, seriously affecting qi-transformation and causing various pathological changes.

三、津液的生理作用

津液的生理作用,主要包括以下三个方面。

(一)滋润与营养

津液中含有大量的水分和营养物质,所以对脏腑形体具有滋润和营养作用。其中津多输布于肌肤、孔窍,故以滋润作用为主;液多输布于脏腑、脑髓,故以营养作用为主。

(二)化生血液

津液不但能流布于脉外,而且能进入血脉之中,参与血液的生成。从血液的组成来看,是由津液和营气相结合而生成的。若津液不足,化生血液减少,则可导致血虚。

(三)运输浊气

津液能够容纳人体气化作用所产生的各种浊气、废物,并把它运送到有关脏腑器官排出体外。浊气、废物排出的途径主要有三,即尿液、汗液和呼吸。尿液、汗液都是以津液的形式直接排出废物、浊气,从呼吸排出的浊气是经血液中的津液首先运送到肺,然后再呼出的。若人体津液不足,浊气不能迅速排出,积蓄于体内,会严重干扰气化功能,产生多种病理变化。

3.3.4　The transportation and metabolism of body fluid

The transportation and metabolism of body fluid are complicated, involving the physiological activities of several viscera. Body fluid, produced by the spleen and the stomach to absorb water and nutrients from food, is transported to the heart and the lung by the spleen to start its metabolic process. The viscera concerned with the metabolism of body fluid mainly include the spleen, the lung and the kidney as well as the heart, the liver, the bladder, the large intestine and the triple energizer.

The spleen, the lung and the kidney play a key role in the transportation and distribution of body fluid. The spleen, governing transportation and transformation, transports body fluid to the heart and the lung; the lung, governing the regulation of water passage, transports body fluid to the whole body and down into the kidney; the kidney, governing water and separating the clear from the turbid, again transports body fluid that is steamed and qi-transformed during the formation of urine into the heart and the lung. In propelling the circulation of blood, the heart also promotes the flow of body fluid.

In this way body fluid is transported to the whole body to nourish the five zang-organs and the six fu-organs. After being used, the rest of water and the waste metabolic materials are excreted out of the body through certain routes. The excretion of body fluid involves the lung, the kidney, the bladder and the large intestine. Lung-qi, governing dispersion, depuration and descent, excretes the fluid from the skin and respiratory tract and excretes the fluid together with feces from the large intestine.

四、津液的运行代谢

津液的运行代谢是一个极其复杂的过程,它涉及到多个脏腑的一系列生理活动。津液由脾胃从饮食物中吸收水分和营养物质而产生后,即由脾的运化功能将津液向上输送到心肺,就开始了津液的运行代谢过程。与津液的运行代谢有密切关系的内脏主要是脾、肺、肾三脏,其次与心、肝、膀胱、大肠、三焦等脏腑有关。

在津液的运行输布过程中,脾、肺、肾三脏起着关键的作用。脾主运化,将津液转输至心肺;肺主通调水道,将津液输布至全身,最后下归于肾;肾主水,能分清泌浊,在形成小便的同时,将水液之清蒸腾气化使之上行,复归于心肺。心在推动血液运行的同时,也促进了津液的运行。

津液被运送到全身各处,滋养五脏六腑。津液被利用以后,剩余水分和代谢废物将通过一定途径排泄出去。在津液的排泄过程中,需要肺、肾、膀胱、大肠等脏腑的共同作用。肺气宣发,使津液从皮肤和呼吸道排出;肺气肃降,令水液随粪便从大肠排出;肾

Kidney-qi, governing water, transforms the fluid into urine to be excreted as urine from the bladder. Among these different routes, urination and sweating are the major ones for the excretion of the fluid. Only part of the fluid is excreted through defecation and respiration.

Besides, the liver and the triple energizer also play a certain role in the distribution and excretion of body fluid. Liver-qi, governing dredging and dispersing, promotes the flow and metabolism of body fluid by means of regulating the activity of qi; the triple energizer, serving as a water passage, directs body fluid to flow downward through it to the kidney. In the whole process of the flow and metabolism of body fluid, the triple energizer, connecting the upper with the lower, participates in the whole process of the production, distribution and excretion of body fluid. To be specific, the upper energizer participates in the distribution of body fluid as implied in the idea that "the upper energizer is like fog"; the middle energizer participates in the absorption of body fluid as implied in the idea that "the middle energizer is like maceration"; the lower energizer participates in the excretion of body fluid as implied in the idea that "the lower energizer is like a sewer".

On the whole, the flow and metabolism of body fluid involve several viscera, but the lung, the spleen and the kidney are the most important ones. So the dysfunction or hypofunction of these three organs will affect the flow and metabolism of body fluid, leading to phlegm, retention of fluid and edema.

Appendix: The five zang-organs transforming five kinds of liquids

The five kinds of liquids include sweat, snivel, tear,

主水,通过分清泌浊形成小便,从膀胱排出。其中,尿液与汗液是津液代谢排出体外的主要途径,从大便和呼吸中也能排出一部分水液。

此外,肝与三焦对津液的输布与排泄也有一定作用。肝气主疏泄,通过调畅气机,促进津液的运行与代谢;三焦为水道,津液必须通过三焦才能下行及肾。在整个津液的运行与代谢过程中,三焦贯通上下,参与了津液的生成、输布与排泄全过程。上焦参与津液的输布,即"上焦如雾";中焦参与津液的吸收,即"中焦如沤";下焦参与津液的排泄,即"下焦如渎"。

综上所述可见,津液的运行代谢过程关系到多个脏腑器官,而以肺、脾、肾三脏的作用为主。此三脏功能减退或失调,都将影响津液的运行和代谢,从而形成痰饮、水肿等病理变化。

附:五脏化五液

五液,是一类特殊的津

saliva and drool. TCM believes that these liquids are transformed by the five zang-organs.

The relationships between the five zang-organs and the five kinds of liquids are described this way: sweat is the liquid of the heart, snivel is the liquid of the lung, tear is the liquid of the liver, saliva is the liquid of the spleen and spittle is the liquid of the kidney.

(1) Sweat comes from body fluid and is excreted out of the body through sweat pores under the steaming of yang-qi. The heart pertains to fire in the five elements. Heart-fire transforms into yang-qi to steam body fluid which comes out of the skin and becomes sweat. Thus sweat is regarded as the fluid of the heart. Insufficiency of heart-yang results in oligohidrosis while superabundance of heart-fire brings on polyhidrosis.

(2) Snivel refers to the nasal mucus that can moisten the nostrils. Since the nose is the orifice of the lung, so snivel is the liquid of the lung. If lung-qi fails to disperse, the nose will become stuffy and running; if lung-heat impairs body fluid, the nose will be dry with scanty snivel.

(3) Tear comes from the eyes and can moisten the eyes. Since the eyes are the orifices of the liver, the tear is certainly the liquid of the liver. If there is wind-heat in the liver, the eyes will become tearing; if liver-yin is insufficient, the eyes will become dry because of scanty tear.

(4) Saliva refers to the thin part of the fluid in the mouth. It can promote the intake of food. Since the mouth is the orifice of the spleen, saliva is the liquid of the spleen. If the spleen is weak, there will be profuse of saliva running out of the mouth; if spleen-yin is insufficient, the mouth will be dry because of scanty saliva in the

液,包括汗、涕、泪、涎、唾。中医学认为这类津液由五脏所化生,所以称为"五脏化五液"。

五脏与五液的关系是:汗为心之液,涕为肺之液,泪为肝之液,涎为脾之液,唾为肾之液。

(1) 汗:汗来源于津液,津液之所以能排出于汗孔而形成汗液,是受阳气蒸腾作用的结果。心在五行属火,心火化为阳气而能蒸化其津液,外出于肌肤便形成汗,所以汗为心之液。心阳不足则汗少,心火亢盛则汗多。

(2) 涕:涕是鼻中分泌的粘液,能滋润鼻孔。鼻为肺之窍,所以涕为肺之液。肺气失宣则鼻塞而流涕,肺热伤津则鼻干而涕少。

(3) 泪:泪出于目,能滋润眼睛。目为肝之窍,所以泪为肝之液。肝有风热则流泪不止,肝阴不足则泪少目干。

(4) 涎:涎为口中津液之清稀者,能帮助进食。口为脾之窍,所以涎为脾之液。脾虚失于固摄则涎多而外溢,脾阴不足则涎少而口干。

mouth.

(5) Spittle refers to the thick part of the fluid in the mouth. It can moisten the mouth and the tongue. TCM believes that saliva is produced at the mouth corners and spittle is produced under the tongue. Since the sublingual vein is connected with the kidney meridian, spittle is the liquid of the kidney. In terms of life cultivation, TCM holds that spittle is transformed from kidney-essence. That is why masters of life cultivation advocate to swallow spittle in order to enrich kidney-essence and cultivate health. If kidney-essence is deficient, spittle will become scanty and the mouth will become dry.

3.4　The relationships among qi, blood and body fluid

Qi, blood and body fluid are the basic substances that maintain life activities. These three substances can transform into each other through qi-transforming activity and depend on each other in physiological functions. If one of them has changed, the other two will make corresponding reactions. Such an inter-dependent relationship among them is not only signified in physiology, but also in pathology. Clinically the regulation of this inter-dependent relationship among qi, blood and body fluid is very important in treating diseases.

3.4.1　The relationship between qi and blood

Qi is active and pertains to yang while blood is static and pertains to yin. So the relationship between qi and blood can be understood according to the relationship between yin and yang. In TCM the relationship between qi

（5）唾：唾为口中津液之稠厚者，能滋润口舌。中医学认为涎生于口角，唾生于舌下，而舌下为肾脉所系，所以唾为肾之液。中医养生理论认为唾为肾精所化，养生家主张常吞咽口中津液（唾）以还肾生精，从而达到健身的目的。若肾之阴精不足，则唾少而口干。

第四节　气血津液之间的关系

气、血、津液都是维持人体生命活动的基本物质，三者之间既存在着通过气化作用而相互转化的关系，也存在着生理上相互作用的关系。如果某一方面发生了变化，另外两个方面就可能出现相应的反应。这种气血津液之间的关系不仅表现在生理上，也表现在病理变化上，因此在临床治疗上，调理气血津液之间的关系就显得非常重要。

一、气与血的关系

由于气性动而属阳，血性静而属阴，所以气与血之间的关系可以从阴阳的相互关系来认识。中医学用这样一句

and blood is generalized as "qi is the marshal of blood and blood is the mother of qi". Here "marshal" means governing and "mother" means source and foundation. Since qi pertains to yang, it can govern the circulation of blood; because blood pertains to yin, it is the source for qi-transformation. However, the relationship between qi and blood is not so simple as mentioned above.

3.4.1.1　The effect of qi on blood

The effect of qi on blood is mainly demonstrated in three aspects, i. e. qi producing blood, qi promoting the circulation of blood and qi controlling blood.

1. Qi producing blood

Qi promotes the production of blood in various ways. In terms of the composition, the nutrient qi is the main component of blood, indicating that the nutrient qi produces blood. In terms of the transformation of blood, the production of blood depends on qi-transformation. The material needed for the production of blood is the food nutrient transformed and absorbed by the spleen and the stomach. The normal functions of the spleen and the stomach are directly related to spleen-qi and stomach-qi. If spleen-qi and stomach-qi are vigorous, blood-producing function will be vigorous too. If spleen-qi and stomach-qi are deficient, blood-producing function will be weakened. In fact the transformation of the food nutrients into blood still needs the transformation of other visceral qi. For example, only when the food nutrients has combined with kidney-essence can the process of transforming the nutrients into blood be accomplished; only when blood transformed from the food nutrients and the kidney-essence has been processed by the transforming activity of heart-qi and lung-qi, especially heart-qi, can blood become red. If the functions of the spleen and the stomach are weak due

话来概括气与血的关系：气为血帅，血为气母。帅，即统帅、主管之义；母，有源泉、根本之义。因气属阳，故能统管血的运行；血属阴，所以是化生气的根源。但是，气与血的具体关系表现在多方面，并不限于上述的概括。

（一）气对血的作用

气对血的作用，主要表现在气生血、气行血、气摄血三个方面。

1. 气生血

气对血的生成具有促进作用，这种促进作用表现在多方面。从血液的组成来看，营气是血液的主要成分之一，这是营气化生血液的作用方面。从血液的化生过程来看，血液的生成依赖于多个脏腑的气化作用。血液生成的物质来源是脾胃运化吸收而来的水谷精微，而脾胃的功能正常与否，与脾胃之气直接相关，脾胃气旺则生血功能也旺，脾胃气衰则生血功能也衰。水谷精微生血，还需要其他脏腑气化作用的参与、配合。如水谷精微必须与肾精相结合，在气的作用下完成精化血的过程；水谷精微与肾精所化之血，必须在心肺的气化作用尤其是心的化赤作用下，才能形成赤色的血液等。若气虚而脾胃

to qi deficiency or if the transforming activity of visceral qi becomes weak, the normal process of blood transformation will be affected, leading to blood deficiency.

2. Qi promoting the circulation of blood

Blood depends on the propelling function of qi to circulate. That is why TCM holds that "normal flow of qi ensures normal circulation of blood, stagnation of qi leads stasis of blood". In terms of visceral functions, heart-qi is the primary motivation of blood circulation; lung-qi assists the heart to propel blood to circulate; liver-qi promotes the circulation of blood. If qi is too weak to propel blood, blood will flow slowly; if qi activity is obstructed, blood will become stagnant; if qi activity is in disorder, blood will flow abnormally.

3. Qi controlling blood

Qi controlling blood means that qi directs blood to circulate inside the vessels and prevents it from flowing out of the vessels. The kind of qi that can control blood and direct it to flow inside the vessels is spleen-qi. That is why TCM holds that "the spleen commands blood". If qi fails to control blood due to deficiency, blood will flow out of the vessels, leading to bleeding.

3.4.1.2 The effect of blood on qi

The effect of blood on qi is demonstrated in two aspects: carrying qi and producing qi.

1. Blood carrying qi

Blood pertains to yin and is static, so it keeps on flowing inside. Qi pertains to yang and is active, so it tends to move to the outside. When qi and blood have combined with each other, blood has acquired a motivation to move and qi has obtained a carrier to attach to. That is

功能不足,或脏腑气化作用减弱,都会影响血的正常化生,从而导致血虚。

2. 气行血

血液的运行,必须依赖气的推动作用,故中医学有"气行则血行,气滞则血瘀"的说法。结合脏腑来说,心气是推动血液运行的基本动力来源,肺气能辅心行血,肝气主疏泄能促进血液的运行。如果气虚推动无力,则血行迟缓;或气机阻滞,则血液瘀滞;或气机逆乱,则血液妄行。

3. 气摄血

气具有固摄的作用,表现在对血液的作用方面就是气摄血。气摄血,是指通过气的摄纳、统管等的作用,使血液保持在脉管内运行,而不致逸出脉外。具有摄纳、统管血液作用的气,主要指脾气,所以藏象学有"脾统血"的理论。气虚而不能摄血,可致血逸于脉外,形成出血。

(二) 血对气的作用

血对气的作用,主要表现在血载气和血生气两个方面。

1. 血载气

血属阴而主静,则易固守于内;气属阳而主动,故常发散于外。气与血相合,一方面血有了运行的动力,另一方面气有了运行的载体,所以说血

why it is said that blood can carry qi. That is to say that only when qi has attached itself to blood can it avoid dispersion and loss. Clinically massive hemorrhage is usually accompanied by loss of qi. Therapeutically, apart from using the therapy for supplementing blood and stopping hemorrhage, other therapeutic methods for supplementing qi and stopping prostration must be resorted to.

2. Blood producing qi

Qi and blood, pertaining to yin and yang respectively, can transform into each other and produce each other. The primordial qi is produced by the congenital essence in the kidney and the food nutrients transformed by the spleen and the stomach. The normal functions of these organs all depend on nutrients provided by blood flowing in the vessels, and so do the other viscera and meridians. Thus the production of qi by blood is accomplished through its provision of nutrients for the viscera and meridians.

3.4.2　The relationship between qi and body fluid

The relationship between qi and body fluid is similar to the relationship between qi and blood, because body fluid is a component of blood. Besides, body fluid exists not only in the vessels, but also in all the tissues and organs in the body. In this sense, the relationship between qi and body fluid differs in some way from the relationship between qi and blood.

3.4.2.1　The effect of qi on body fluid

The effect of qi on body fluid is demonstrated in three

能载气。也就是说,气必须依附于血,才不致于流散不收。临床上大出血病人往往有气随血脱的表现,治疗时除补血止血外,还需要益气固脱以急救之。

2. 血生气

气与血,一阴一阳,具有互生互化的作用。元气的生成来源,有肾中所藏的先天之精气和脾胃运化的水谷之精气,而这两脏都需要血的滋养,使其功能正常,才能化生元气。通过血液运行,不断地给脏腑经络输送精微物质,脏腑经络之气的功能才能保持正常。因此,血生气主要是通过血对脏腑经络的营养作用来实现的。

二、气与津液的关系

气与津液的关系类似于气与血的关系。由于津液是血液的组成成分之一,所以在血脉中气与津液的关系和气与血的关系是一致的。同时,津液还广泛存在于人体所有的组织器官中,不限于血脉内,故气与津液在作用方式上还是与气血关系有些不同。

(一)气对津液的作用

气对津液的作用,主要表

aspects: qi producing body fluid, qi promoting the flow of body fluid and qi controlling body fluid.

1. Qi producing body fluid

Body fluid comes from the water and nutrients of food transformed by the spleen and stomach. The spleen and stomach play an important role in the production of body fluid. If spleen-qi and stomach-qi are sufficient and if the digesting and absorbing functions are normal, the transformation and production of body fluid will be sufficient; if spleen-qi and stomach-qi are deficient and if the digesting and absorbing functions are abnormal, the transformation and production of body fluid will be reduced.

2. Qi promoting the flow of body fluid

The flow of body fluid, including the distribution and excretion, depends on the propelling function of qi. At the early stage body fluid is transported by spleen-qi to the heart and the lung; heart-qi propels body fluid and blood to flow; lung-qi disperses the fluid in the skin and viscera on the one hand, and descends the fluid to the kidney and the bladder on the other; the kidney and the bladder, through qi-transformation, transports the lucid part of the fluid to the heart and the lung on the one hand, and descends the turbid part of the fluid to transform it into urine to be discharged out of the body on the other. Since the flow and metabolism of body fluid all depend on the propelling and transforming functions of qi, the state of qi and the activity of qi directly affect the flow and metabolism of body fluid. If qi deficiency or qi stagnation occurs, the fluid will accumulate and turn into phlegm and edema. That is why it is said in TCM that "normal flow of qi ensures normal flow of water and stagnation of qi leads to stagnation of water."

现在气生津液、气行津液、气摄津液三个方面。

1. 气生津液

津液生成于脾胃,是从饮食物中吸收水分和营养而形成的。在生成津液的过程中,脾胃之气起着决定性作用。脾胃之气充足,消化吸收功能正常,津液的化生就充盛;若脾胃之气衰,消化吸收功能减弱,津液化生必然会减少。

2. 气行津液

津液的运行,包括津液的输布和排泄两方面,而这两方面的生理过程都必须依靠气的推动作用才能完成。津液最初由脾气进行转运,上输于心肺;心气推动津液与血液一起运行;肺主通调水道,肺气一方面将水液宣发于皮肤腠理,布散于五脏六腑,另一方面将水液肃降于肾与膀胱;肾与膀胱通过气化作用,将水液之清蒸腾向上,复归于心肺,将水液之浊推动下行,形成小便排出体外。由于津液的整个运行代谢过程完全依赖于气的推动、气化作用,所以气的充足与否,气机是否调畅,都会影响津液的运行代谢。若发生气虚或气滞等情形,就会导致津液停聚,形成痰饮、水肿之类病变,故中医学有

3. Qi controlling body fluid

Under the propelling and transforming action of qi, the metabolism of the body is demonstrated in two ways: opening and closing. Opening means to excrete the remaining part of fluid out of the body and closing means to keep certain amount of water needed in the body. The way that qi keeps body fluid in the body is called "qi controlling body fluid". The ways to excrete water from the body include urination and sweating. If qi fails to control body fluid due to deficiency, it will lead to abnormal urination and sweating, such as poliguria, incontinence of urine, enuresis and polyhidrosis, etc.

3.4.2.2　The effect of body fluid on qi

The effect of body fluid on qi is demonstrated in two ways: carrying qi and producing qi.

1. Body fluid carrying qi

Body fluid is the carrier of qi and qi must attach itself to body fluid in order to flow to the whole body. This theory can be understood from two angles. On the one hand, blood produced by body fluid in the vessels can carry the nutrient qi; on the other hand, body fluid flowing in other tissues and organs can carry the defensive qi. If great quantity of body fluid is lost, qi will be exhausted accordingly. This state is called "loss of body fluid followed by exhaustion of qi". In severe cases, it will become "loss of body fluid followed by loss of qi".

2. Body fluid producing qi

Body fluid, just like blood, can produce qi. On the one hand, body fluid inside the vessels transforms into blood to nourish the viscera so as to maintain sufficiency of qi in these viscera and the body. On the other hand,

"气行则水行，气滞则水滞"的说法。

3. 气摄津液

在气的推动和气化作用下，津液的代谢表现为开、合两种方式。开，即将剩余水液排泄出去；合，即将人体需要的水液保留在体内。气对水液的这种保留作用，就是"气摄津液"。人体排泄水液的途径主要是尿与汗。如果气虚不能固摄津液，可导致尿与汗的异常排出，如小便多、小便失禁、遗尿、多汗等。

（二）津液对气的作用

津液对气的作用，主要表现在津液载气和津液生气两个方面。

1. 津液载气

津液也是气的载体，气必须依附于津液而流布于全身。这种作用包括两个方面：脉内之津液化生血液，能运载营气；脉外之津液流行贯注于各组织器官，能运载卫气。如果津液大量流失，气也将随之耗散，这称为"气随津泄"，严重者可导致"气随液脱"。

2. 津液生气

津液能化生气，与血生气的机理是基本一致的。一方面，脉内的津液化生血液，与血液共同滋养脏腑形体，保证

body fluid outside the vessels nourishes the muscles and orifices to maintain their normal functions. At the same time body fluid outside the vessels keeps a constant communication with body fluid inside the vessels and supplements each other. If body fluid becomes deficient, its function to nourish and moisten will be weakened, leading to decline of visceral qi.

3.4.3　The relationship between blood and body fluid

Both blood and body fluid are liquid substances and function to nourish and moisten the viscera and the body. Compared with qi, both blood and body fluid pertain to yin. Physiologically blood and body fluid depend on and transform into each other. Pathologically, blood and body fluid affect each other.

Blood is made up of body fluid and the nutrient qi. After the transformation by the spleen and stomach, body fluid is transported first to the vessels and then flows with blood to the whole body. Part of body fluid extravasates from the vessels and flows outside the vessels to moisten and nourish the viscera and the body. At the same time part of body fluid flowing outside the vessels enters the vessels again to participate in the production of blood. In fact, body fluid inside and outside the vessels frequently transforms and supplements each other. Normally there is a dynamic balance maintained between them. Under pathological condition, if great quantity of body fluid is consumed or if great amount of body fluid comes out of the vessels, it will lead to insufficiency of blood inside the vessels. On the contrary, if too much body fluid outside the vessels enters the vessels because of massive hemorrhage, it will lead to insufficiency of body fluid. As a result, a morbid state of scanty fluid and dryness of blood is

其气的持续充足。另一方面,脉外的津液能滋养肌肤孔窍,以维持其正常的功能,并与脉内的津液相互流通补充。若津液亏虚,滋养濡润功能减弱,脏腑之气也会虚衰。

三、血与津液的关系

血与津液均为液态物质,都有营养和滋润作用,与气相对而言,两者都属阴。血与津液在生理上具有非常密切的相互依存、相互转化的关系,故在病理上也常相互影响。

血液是由津液和营气两部分所组成,故津液在脉内是血液的一个组成部分。津液最初通过脾胃的运化等功能产生后,首先进入血脉,随血液流布于全身,然后一部分津液从脉内渗出脉外,成为脉外之津液。脉外之津液直接滋润、营养脏腑形体,同时也有一部分津液回渗于脉内,参与血液的生成。实际上,脉内的津液与脉外的津液经常处于相互渗透、相互转化、相互补充的过程中,正常情况下两者之间维持着一种动态的平衡关系。在病理情况下,如果津液大量耗损,脉内的津液过多地渗出脉外,会导致血脉空

caused due to insufficiency of body fluid and blood.

Sweat, transformed from body fluid, is closely related to blood. Blood deficiency, usually followed by insufficiency of body fluid, cannot be treated simply by diaphoresis because profuse sweating consumes body fluid and further aggravates the deficiency of blood. On the other hand, profuse sweating and scanty body fluid, often accompanied by insufficiency of blood, cannot be simply treated by blood-breaking therapy because excessive bleeding exhausts the blood and further aggravates the scanty state of body fluid. That is why it is said in *Lingshu* that "the patients with massive bleeding cannot be treated by diaphoresis while the patients with profuse sweating should not be treated by bloodletting therapy."

Blood and body fluid not only depend on and transform into each other, but also share the same origin. That is to say that both of them come from the food nutrients. Such a relationship between blood and body fluid is generalized as "body fluid and blood sharing the same origin" in TCM.

虚;反之,如果失血过多,脉外的津液将过多地渗入脉内,从而引起津液不足。其结果,津液与血液皆不足,就形成津枯血燥的病变。

汗液源于津液,与血液有密切的关系。凡血虚之人,津液也不充裕,不宜再用发汗疗法,出汗多则津液耗损,将会加重血虚。凡多汗津亏之人,血液也显不足,不宜再用破血疗法,出血多则血脉空虚,将会加重津亏。故《灵枢·营卫生会》说:"夺血者无汗,夺汗者无血。"

血与津液之间不但存在着相互依存、相互转化的关系,而且它们的生成来源也相同,都是源于水谷精微。中医学把血与津液之间的这种同源互化关系,概括为"津血同源"。

4 The meridians and collaterals

第四章 经络

The meridians and collaterals are important components of the body. They are linear in form and subdivide into several levels of branches which are interconnected with each other and form into a network. The main function of the meridians and collaterals is to transport qi and blood, connect the viscera with other organs and combine the body into an organic whole.

The meridians are the main trunks in the system of the meridians and collaterals while the collaterals are the branches of the meridians. The collaterals stem from the meridians and fork into different levels of smaller and finer ones.

经络是人体结构的重要组成部分。经络呈线状,反复分支并相互联络,整体上构成网状结构。经络的作用主要是通行气血,沟通脏腑器官,把人体联系成一个有机的整体。

经络是经脉和络脉的总称。经脉是经络系统的主干部分,络脉是经络系统的分支部分。络脉从经脉主干上分出,并不断反复分支,越分越细,以至形成网状遍布全身。

4.1 The content of the theory of meridians and collaterals

第一节 经络学说的内容

The system of meridians and collaterals is described in the following figure.

经络系统包括经脉和络脉两部分,其主要组成如下图:

Three yin meridians of hand
- the lung meridian of hand-taiyin
- the pericardium meridian of hand-jueyin
- the heart meridian of hand-shaoyin

Three yang meridians of hand
- the large intestine meridian of hand-yangming
- the triple energizer meridian of hand-shaoyang
- the small intestine meridian of hand-taiyang

Three yin meridians of foot
- the spleen meridian of foot-taiyin
- the liver meridian of foot-jueyin
- the kidney meridian of foot-shaoyin

Three yang meridians of foot
- the stomach meridian of foot-yangming
- the gallbladder meridian of foot-shaoyang
- the bladder meridian of foot-taiyang

Twelve meridians

Appendix
- the twelve branches of the meridians
- the twelve tendons
- the twelve skin divisions

Meridians

Eight extraordinary vessels
- the thoroughfare vessel
- the conception vessel
- the governor vessel
- the belt vessel
- the yin-heel vessel
- the yang-heel vessel
- the yin-link vessel
- the yang-link vessel

System of Meridians and Collaterals

Collaterals
- the fifteen divergent collaterals
- the floating collaterals
- the minute collaterals

十二经脉

手三阴经
- 手太阴肺经
- 手厥阴心包经
- 手少阴心经

手三阳经
- 手阳明大肠经
- 手少阳三焦经
- 手太阳小肠经

足三阴经
- 足太阴脾经
- 足厥阴肝经
- 足少阴肾经

足三阳经
- 足阳明胃经
- 足少阳胆经
- 足太阳膀胱经

附
- 十二经别
- 十二经筋
- 十二皮部

经脉

奇经八脉
- 冲脉
- 任脉
- 督脉
- 带脉
- 阴跷脉
- 阳跷脉
- 阴维脉
- 阳维脉

经络系统

络脉
- 十五别络
- 浮络
- 孙络

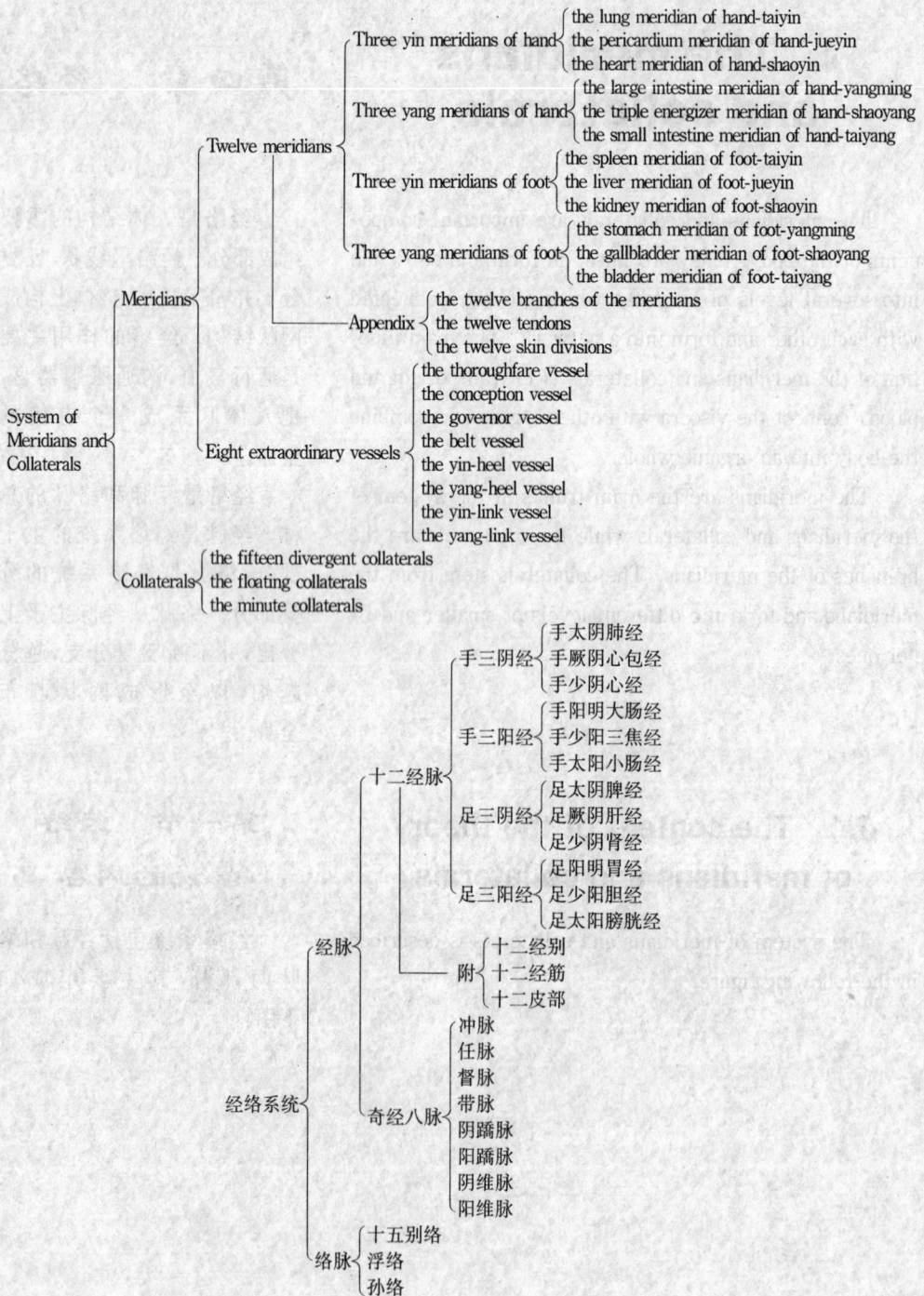

Fig. 4 - 1　The system of meridians and collaterals
图 4 - 1　经络系统

This section is devoted to the introduction of the twelve regular meridians and the eight extraordinary vessels. The running routes of the meridians and other concerned content are described in detail in the fascicle of *Chinese Acupuncture and Moxibustion*.

4.1.1 The twelve meridians

4.1.1.1 The names of the twelve meridians

The names of the twelve meridians are the lung meridian of hand-taiyin, the pericardium meridian of hand-jueyin, the heart meridian of hand-shaoyin, the large intestine meridian of hand-yangming, the triple energizer meridian of hand-shaoyang, the small intestine meridian of hand-taiyang, the spleen meridian of foot-taiyin, the liver meridian of foot-jueyin, the kidney meridian of foot-shaoyin, the stomach meridian of foot-yangming, the gall-bladder meridian of foot-shaoyang and the bladder meridian of foot-taiyang.

The names of the twelve meridians contain three parts: ① whether the part that certain meridian runs along the four limbs is the hand or foot; ② whether a certain meridian pertains to yin or yang; ③ whether a certain meridian belongs to a zang-organ or a fu-organ. Take the lung meridian of hand-taiyin for example. It runs on the hand, pertains to taiyin and belongs to the lung.

There are two ways to abbreviate the names of the twelve meridians. One is to omit hand or foot and yin or yang. The other is to omit the names of the zang-organs and fu-organs. For example, the lung meridian of hand-taiyin can be abbreviated into "the lung meridian" or "hand-taiyin meridian". Compared with the eight extraordinary vessels, the twelve meridians is also called "the twelve regular meridians".

本节主要介绍有关十二经脉和奇经八脉的基础知识,关于经脉的具体循行路线及其他有关内容,请参阅《中国针灸》分册。

一、十二经脉

(一) 名称

十二经脉的名称是:手太阴肺经;手厥阴心包经;手少阴心经;手阳明大肠经;手少阳三焦经;手太阳小肠经;足太阴脾经;足厥阴肝经;足少阴肾经;足阳明胃经;足少阳胆经;足太阳膀胱经。

十二经脉的名称包括三个部分的含义:① 指出某一经脉在四肢循行的部位是手还是足。② 指出某一经脉的阴阳属性。③ 指出某一经脉所隶属的脏腑。如手太阴肺经循行于手,属太阴经,隶属于肺。

十二经脉名称有两种简称法。一是略去手、足及其阴阳属性,只取其脏腑名称。二是略去脏腑名称,只取其手、足及其阴阳属性名称。如手太阴肺经可简称"肺经"、"手太阴经"等。相对于奇经八脉,十二经脉也称为"十二

The twelve meridians can be divided into four groups. The hand-taiyin meridian, the hand-jueyin meridian and the hand-shaoyin meridian are collectively called "three yin meridians of the hand"; the hand-yangming meridian, the hand-shaoyang meridian and the hand-taiyang meridian are collectively called "three yang meridians of the hand"; foot-taiyin meridian, foot-jueyin meridian and foot-shaoyin meridian are collectively called "three yin meridians of the foot"; foot-yangming meridian, foot-shaoyang meridian and foot-taiyang meridian are collectively called "three yang meridians of the foot".

4.1.1.2 The flowing and infusing order of the twelve meridians

The main function of the twelve meridians is to transport qi and blood. Qi and blood flowing in the meridians follow certain directions. For example, qi and blood in the lung meridian start to flow from the lung, emerging the surface of the body from the lateral side of the chest and moving downward to the tip of the thumb along the medial side of the upper limbs. When qi and blood flow to the end along a certain meridian, they enter another meridian and continue their flow. Such a continuous flow of qi and blood in the meridians is called "flowing and infusing".

Qi and blood in the twelve meridians follow a certain order to flow and infuse. When they have flown and infused for one cycle in the twelve meridians, they return to the original meridian and start another cycle of flowing and infusing. The flowing and infusing order is demonstrated in the following figure：

正经"。

十二经脉也可分为四组：手太阴经、手厥阴经、手少阴经合称"手三阴经"，手阳明经、手少阳经、手太阳经合称"手三阳经"，足太阴经、足厥阴经、足少阴经合称"足三阴经"，足阳明经、足少阳经、足太阳经合称"足三阳经"。

（二）流注次序

十二经脉的基本功能之一是通行气血。气血在十二经脉中运行有一定的方向性，如手太阴肺经的气血是从肺发出，从胸部外侧出于体表，沿上肢内侧前缘向下运行至拇指端。气血沿某一经脉运行至其终端，就传注于另一经脉继续运行，这种气血在经脉之间相互传注的现象，称为"流注"。

十二经脉气血按一定次序流注，运行于十二经脉一周，又回到原来的经脉，这样周而复始，循环不息。其流注次序如下图 4-2：

| The lung meridian of hand-taiyin | → | The large intestine meridian of hand-yangming | → | The stomach meridian of foot-yangming | → | The spleen meridian of foot-taiyin |

The flowing diagram (Fig. 4-2) reads as follows:

The lung meridian of hand-taiyin → The large intestine meridian of hand-yangming → The stomach meridian of foot-yangming → The spleen meridian of foot-taiyin

The liver meridian of foot-jueyin ↑   ↓ The heart meridian of hand-shaoyin

The gallbladder meridian of foot-shaoyang   The small intestine meridian of hand-taiyang

The triple energizer meridian of hand-shaoyang ← The pericardium meridian of hand-jueyin ← The kidney meridian of foot-shaoyin ← The bladder meridian of foot-taiyang

手太阴肺经 → 手阳明大肠经 → 足阳明胃经 → 足太阴脾经

足厥阴肝经   手少阴心经

足少阳胆经   手太阳小肠经

手少阳三焦经 ← 手厥阴心包经 ← 足少阴肾经 ← 足太阳膀胱经

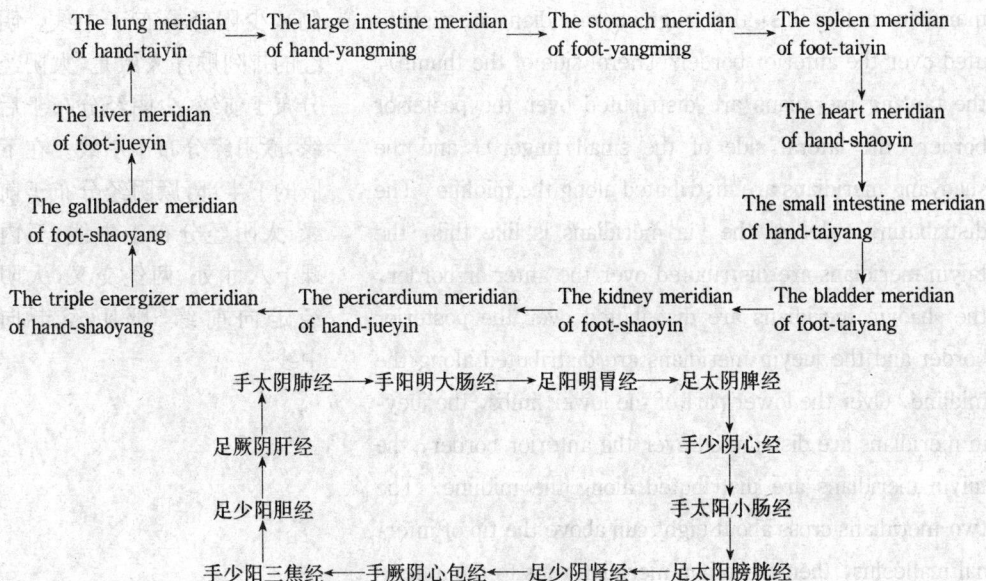

Fig. 4 - 2   The flowing and infusing order of the twelve meridians
图 4 - 2   十二经脉流注次序

4.1.1.3   The distribution of the twelve meridians

The distribution of the twelve meridians follows a certain rule. The rule varies according to the running routes of the meridians.

Head and face: The hand-yangming meridian and foot-yangming meridian run over the face and the forehead; the hand-shaoyang meridian and foot-shaoyang meridian run along the lateral sides of the head; the foot-taiyang meridian runs over the vertex and the nape; the hand-taiyang meridian runs over the cheeks.

The four limbs: The three yin meridians of the hand and the three yang meridians of the hand run along the upper limbs; the three yin meridians of the foot and the three yang meridians of the foot run along the lower limbs. The yin meridians run along the medial side of the four limbs while the yang meridians run along the lateral side of the four limbs. The distributing order of the yang

(三) 分布规律

十二经脉在体表的分布是有规律的。根据经脉所在部位的不同,其规律如下:

头面部:手阳明经、足阳明经行于面部、额部;手少阳经、足少阳经行于头部两侧;足太阳经行于头顶、后项;手太阳经行于面颊部。

四肢部:手三阴经、手三阳经行于上肢,足三阴经、足三阳经行于下肢。其中阴经行于四肢内侧面,阳经行于四肢外侧面。阳经的排列顺序是,阳明经分布于前缘(拇指侧),太阳经分布于后缘(小指

meridians is like this: the yangming meridians are distributed over the anterior border (lateral side of the thumb), the taiyang meridians are distributed over the posterior border (the lateral side of the small finger), and the shaoyang meridians are distributed along the midline. The distributing order of the yin meridians is like this: the taiyin meridians are distributed over the anterior border, the shaoyin meridians are distributed over the posterior border and the jueyin meridians are distributed along the midline. Over the lower part of the lower limbs, the jueyin meridians are distributed over the anterior border, the taiyin meridians are distributed along the midline. The two meridians cross about eight cun above the tip of internal malleolus, then the taiyin meridian runs to the anterior border and the jueyin meridian runs to the midline.

The trunk: The three yang meridians of the hand run over the scapula; among the three yang meridians of the foot, the yangming meridian runs over the front (the chest and abdomen), the taiyang meridian runs along the back and the shaoyang meridian runs along the side of the body; the three yin meridians of the hand all emerge from the armpit; the three yin meridians of the foot all run over the chest and abdomen. The meridians running on the chest and abdomen from the medial to the lateral are foot-shaoyin meridian, foot-yangming meridian, foot-taiyin meridian and foot-jueyin meridian respectively.

4.1.1.4　The external and internal relationships

The twelve meridians can be grouped into six pairs, each pair is internally and externally related to each other. The meridians in external and internal relationship with each other pertain to yin and yang respectively. The yin meridian is the internal and the yang meridian is the external. The meridians in external and internal relation-

侧），少阳经分布于中线。阴经的排列顺序大致是，太阴经分布于前缘，少阴经分布于后缘，厥阴经分布于中线。在下肢的下半部，厥阴经分布于前缘，太阴经分布于中线，至内踝上八寸处，两经交叉，太阴经走向前缘，厥阴经走向中线。

躯干部：手三阳经行于肩胛部；足三阳经则阳明经分布于前（胸、腹面），太阳经分布于后（背面），少阳经分布于侧面；手三阴经均从腋下走出；足三阴经均行于胸、腹面。循行于胸、腹面的经脉自内向外的顺序为足少阴经、足阳明经、足太阴经、足厥阴经。

（四）表里关系

十二经脉分为六对，每一对都是互为表里的。互为表里的经脉有阴阳之分，其阴经为里，阳经为表。表里两经在四肢末端相互交接。表里两经所隶属的脏腑也互为表里。

ship with each other are connected with each other at the
extremities of the four limbs. The viscera to which the
meridians in external and internal relationship with each
other pertain are also related to each other externally and
internally. In this way the meridians and the viscera in
external and internal relationship with each other respectively associate with each other. The yin meridian pertains to the zang-organ and connects the fu-organ with its
collaterals while the yang meridian pertains to the fu-organ and connects the zang-organs with its collaterals.

The external and internal relationships among the
twelve meridians are demonstrated in the following table:

表里两经与互为表里的脏腑
形成相互属络关系,其阴经属
脏而络腑,阳经属腑而络脏。

十二经脉的表里相合关系如
下表:

Table 4 - 1 The external and internal relationships among the twelve meridians

External	Internal
The lung meridian of hand-taiyin	The large intestine meridian of hand-yangming
The pericardium meridian of hand-jueyin	The triple energizer meridian of hand-shaoyang
The heart meridian of hand-shaoyin	The small intestine meridian of hand-taiyang
The spleen meridian of foot-taiyin	The stomach meridian of foot-yangming
The liver meridian of foot-jueyin	The gallbladder meridian of foot-shaoyang
The kidney meridian of foot-shaoyin	The bladder meridian of foot-taiyang

表 4 - 1 十二经脉的表里相合关系

里	表
手太阴肺经	手阳明大肠经
手厥阴心包经	手少阳三焦经
手少阴心经	手太阳小肠经
足太阴脾经	足阳明胃经
足厥阴肝经	足少阳胆经
足少阴肾经	足太阳膀胱经

4.1.2 The eight extraordinary vessels

4.1.2.1 The nomenclature

The names of the eight extraordinary vessels are du-
mai (the governor vessel), renmai (the conception vessel), chongmai (the thoroughfare vessel), daimai (the

二、奇经八脉

(一) 名称

奇经八脉的名称是:督
脉;任脉;冲脉;带脉;阴蹻脉;
阳蹻脉;阴维脉;阳维脉。

belt vessel), yinqiao (the yin-heel vessel), yangqiao (the yang-heel vessel), yinwei (the yin-link vessel) and yang-wei (the yang-link vessel).

The eight extraordinary vessels are different from the twelve regular meridians. Compared with the twelve regular meridians, the eight extraordinary vessels are characterized by no regular distribution, no direct connection with the viscera and no internal and external relationship between each other.

4.1.2.2 The running features of the eight extraordinary vessels

The eight extraordinary vessels are different from the twelve regular meridians in running routes and functions.

1. The thoroughfare vessel, the conception vessel and the governor vessel are "three separate vessels that originate from the same source"

The thoroughfare vessel, the conception vessel and the governor vessel all start from the lower abdomen (the uterus for women) and run downward to the perineum where they begin to run in the different directions. The trunk of the governor vessel runs posteriorly from the perineum, penetrates the spine, moves upward to the forehead from the neck and midline of the head and then runs downward from the nose to the labial frenum. The branches of the governor vessel are connected with the kidney and the brain. The conception vessel runs forward from the perineum, moves upward from the pubic region, the abdomen, the midline on the chest, the throat and the mandible to the mouth where it runs around the lips and then upward in lines to the region below the eye socket

奇经八脉是不同于十二正经的另一类经脉,所以称为"奇经"。与十二正经相比,奇经八脉有如下特点:① 其分布不像十二经脉那样规则。② 与脏腑没有直接的属络关系。③ 相互之间没有表里关系。

(二)循行特点

奇经八脉在循行上有着与十二经脉完全不同的特点,这些特点使得奇经八脉具有特殊功能。

1. 冲、任、督三脉"一源而三歧"

冲脉、任脉、督脉三者皆起于小腹中(在女子即为女子胞),下行出于会阴,从此分道而行。督脉主干从会阴向后,贯脊柱上行,经项、头部正中线绕至前额,经鼻下行至上唇系带处;分支联系于肾、脑。任脉从会阴向前,经阴阜,沿腹部和胸部正中线上行,经咽喉上行至下颌部,环绕口唇,沿面颊分行至目眶下。冲脉主干从会阴至气街,与足少阴经并行,挟脐向上,散布于胸中,再上行环绕口唇,至目眶

from the cheeks. The trunk of the thoroughfare vessel runs from the perineum to qijie (pathway of qi) where it runs parallel to the foot-shaoyin meridian upward beside the navel, dispersing in the chest, moving upward around the lips and below the region of the eye socket. One of the branch of the thoroughfare vessel runs downward along the medial side of the thigh to the foot. The other branch stems from the abdomen, is connected with the governor vessel from the posterior region and runs upward in the spine.

下;其分支之一从气街沿大腿内侧下行至足,另一分支从小腹中向后与督脉相通,上行于脊柱内。

The governor vessel, known as "the sea of the yang meridians", governs all the yang meridians in the body. The conception vessel, known as "the sea of the yin meridians", governs all the yin meridians in the body. The thoroughfare vessel, known as "the sea of blood" and "the sea of the twelve meridians", is the place where all qi and blood in the body converge on the one hand and regulates qi and blood in the twelve meridians on the other. Since all these three vessels start from the uterus in women, they are closely related to the physiological activities of women.

督脉能总督一身之阳经,故称其为"阳脉之海"。任脉能总任一身之阴经,故称其为"阴脉之海"。冲脉为全身气血会聚之所,能调节十二经气血,故称其为"血海"、"十二经之海"等。在女子,由于冲、任、督三脉皆起于女子胞,所以它们都与女子的特殊生理活动有关。

2. The belt vessel runs transversely around the body and controls all the other meridians and vessels

The belt vessel is the only one that runs transversely around the body. It starts from the hypochondria, runs obliquely downward to the lower abdomen and then transversely around the body like a belt. That is why it can control qi and blood in the other meridians and vessels.

2. 带脉横行,约束诸经

带脉是经脉系统中唯一横行的经脉,它起于季胁,斜向前下至少腹,然后绕身一周,状如束带,所以带脉有约束诸经气血的作用。

3. The link vessels and heel vessels contact with qi and blood in the twelve meridians

The yin-link vessel starts from the medial side of the shank, runs upward along the medial side of the lower limbs and, across the abdomen, the chest and the throat,

3. 维脉、蹻脉联络十二经气血

阴维脉起于小腿内侧,沿下肢内侧上行,经腹、胸至咽喉,与任脉相会;阳维脉起于

connects with the conception vessel; the yang-link vessel starts from below the external ankle, runs upward along the lateral side of the lower limb and, across the lateral side of the head and the nape, connects with the governor vessel. These two vessels run across the twelve meridians and connect with the twelve meridians. The yin-link vessel is connected with all the yin meridians while the yang-link vessel is connected with all the yang meridians. The yin-heel vessel starts from below the internal ankle and the yang-heel vessel starts from below the external ankle. They run upward along the medial side and lateral side of the lower limbs respectively to the inner canthus of the eyes where they converge with each other and combine with the hand-taiyang and the foot-taiyang meridians. So these two vessels are mainly responsible for the movement of the eyes and the lower limbs.

Appendix: The twelve branches of the meridians, the twelve tendons, the twelve skin divisions, the fifteen divergent collaterals, the floating collaterals and the minute collaterals

The twelve branches of the meridians:

They stem from the twelve regular meridians, also pertaining to the twelve regular meridians. They all stem from the twelve regular meridians on the four limbs, then entering the cavity of the body and the viscera, eventually emerging from the surface of the body, running upward to the head where the yin branches converge with the branches of the yang meridians that are in external and internal relationships with the meridians from which they stem, finally returning to the yang meridians they pertain to.

The twelve tendons:

They refer to the muscular system that are connected

外踝下,沿下肢外侧上行,至头侧及项后与督脉会合。此二经穿行于十二经脉之间,起联络沟通作用。阴维脉联络所有阴经,阳维脉联络所有阳经。阴跷脉起于内踝下,阳跷脉起于外踝下,分别沿下肢内侧和外侧上行,至目内眦,二经相合,并合于手、足太阳经,故此二经主管目与下肢的运动。

附:十二经别、十二经筋、十二皮部、十五别络、浮络、孙络

(一)十二经别

十二经别是从十二经脉别出的经脉,也属于正经。它们都是从十二经脉的四肢部分别出,然后进入体腔脏腑深部,再浅出体表而上行头面,阴经的经别合入相表里的阳经的经别,最后回到所属的阳经。

(二)十二经筋

十二经筋,指十二经所联

with the twelve meridians.

The twelve skin divisions：

They refer to the twelve skin areas divided according to the twelve meridians.

The fifteen divergent collaterals：

The fifteen collaterals include twelve collaterals of the twelve meridians (one for each of the twelve meridians respectively), the collateral of the governor vessel, the collateral of the conception vessel and the major collateral of the spleen.

The floating collaterals：

They refer to the superficial collaterals.

The minute collaterals：

They refer to the smallest collaterals in the collateral system, similizing as "grandson-collateral" in TCM.

属的筋肉系统的部分。

（三）十二皮部

十二皮部，指体表皮肤按十二经脉划分的十二个区域。

（四）十五别络

十五别络，由十二经脉、督脉、任脉各分出一支络脉，再加上脾之大络组成。

（五）浮络

浮络，指浅行于体表部位的络脉。

（六）孙络

孙络，指络脉系统中最细小的络脉。

4.2   The basic functions of the meridians and collaterals

There are two basic functions of the meridians and collaterals. One is to connect the external with the internal as well as to connect the viscera with other organs. The other is to transport qi, blood, yin and yang to nourish the viscera and the body. In physiology, pathology and treatment, the meridians and the collaterals are responsible for the transmission and conduction of physiological and pathological information as well as the regulation of the physiological functions of the body.

4.2.1   To connect the external with the internal as well as to connect the viscera with other organs

The body is an organic whole. It is the meridians and

第二节   经络的基本功能

经络的基本功能有二，一是沟通表里上下，联络脏腑器官，二是通行气血阴阳，濡养脏腑形体。在这两个基本功能的基础上，经络在生理、病理和治疗上具有感应传导、调节功能平衡的作用。

一、沟通表里上下，联络脏腑器官

人体是一个有机的整体，

collaterals that connect the viscera, the body, the five sensory organs and the nine orifices together. The meridians internally pertain to the viscera and externally connect the limbs. Since the meridians are composed of various collaterals of different levels, they have formulated the whole body into a network. There are three basic ways with which the meridians to connect all parts of the body together.

4.2.1.1　The relationships between the viscera, the body, the sensory organs and the orifices

The connection between the external and the internal as well as the viscera and other organs is mainly accomplished by the twelve meridians. On the one hand the twelve meridians and their branches accomplish such a connection by emerging from the external of the body and entering the internal of the body. On the other hand, they reinforce such a connection with the twelve branches, twelve tendons and twelve skin divisions.

4.2.1.2　The relationships between the zang-organs and fu-organs

The twelve meridians has formed six pairs of external and internal relationships which enable the zang-organs and the fu-organs in external and internal relationships to connect with each other. The meridians stemming from the viscera associate with several internal organs during their running processes. As a result each zang-organ or fu-organ is connected with several meridians.

4.2.1.3　The relationships among the meridians

The twelve meridians are connected with each other, follow a certain running and infusing order and together form a large circulatory system. The twelve meridians and the eight extraordinary vessels have formulated a

而在脏腑、形体、五官九窍之间起联络作用的正是经络。经络内属于脏腑，外络于肢节，出入上下，联系极其广泛。由于经络可以反复分支，网络全身，所以经络四通八达，无所不至。经络的联络与沟通作用有以下三种基本方式。

（一）脏腑与形体官窍之间的联系

经络联系脏腑与形体官窍，主要通过十二经脉来进行。十二经脉一方面通过其本经及其分支出入于表里，另一方面又通过十二经别、十二经筋、十二皮部来加强这种联系。

（二）脏腑之间的联系

十二经脉构成六对表里相合关系，使相表里的脏腑之间具有相互属络关系。发源于脏腑的经脉在体内循行过程中还联系于多个其他脏腑，每一脏或腑都有数条经脉与之相联系。

（三）经络之间的联系

十二经脉的阴阳表里相接，有一定的流注次序，并形成一个大的循环系统。十二经脉与奇经八脉之间纵横交错，奇

crisscross network. The extensive association among the meridians and collaterals enables the body to become an organic whole.

经八脉之间又彼此相互联系。经络之间的广泛联系,使人体上下内外完全沟通起来,形成一个密不可分的有机整体。

4.2.2   To transport qi, blood, yin and yang to nourish the viscera and the body

All the viscera and other parts of the body depend on qi, blood, yin and yang to nourish and maintain their physiological functions. It is the meridians that transport qi, blood, yin and yang to the whole body. In fact, the meridians and collaterals are the passages of qi, blood, yin and yang. The purpose of the meridians to connect the viscera and the body is to transport qi, blood, yin and yang. With the extensive distribution of the meridians and collaterals, qi, blood, yin and yang in the body can flow freely to maintain a holistic balance of the body.

二、通行气血阴阳,濡养脏腑形体

人体所有脏腑形体,都需要气血阴阳的濡养,才能维持正常的生理功能。气血阴阳之所以能通达全身,有赖于经络的传注输送。经络实质上是气血阴阳的通道,经络在脏腑与形体之间联络与沟通的目的就在于通行气血阴阳。通过经络的广泛分布,人体气血阴阳上下内外相互交通贯注,维持着整体的协调与平衡。

Appendix: The functional characteristics of the eight extraordinary vessels

Apart from sharing the same functions with the twelve meridians, the eight extraordinary vessels still have three special functions. The first is to strengthen the connection of the twelve meridians. For example, the governor vessel accumulates qi and blood in all the yang meridians; the conception vessel accumulates qi and blood in all the yin meridians; the thoroughfare vessel accumulates qi and blood in the twelve meridians; the yang-link vessel connects all the yang meridians together; and the yin-link vessel connects all the yin meridians together. The second is to regulate qi and blood in the twelve meridians. When qi and blood in the twelve meridians are ex-

附: 奇经八脉的功能特点

奇经八脉除了也具有沟通表里上下、联络脏腑器官及通行气血阴阳、濡养脏腑形体的基本功能外,还具有自身的功能特点。奇经八脉有三个方面的功能特点:① 加强十二经脉之间的联系,如督脉会聚诸阳经气血,任脉会聚诸阴经气血,冲脉会聚十二经气血,阳维脉联络诸阳经,阴维脉联络诸阴经等。② 调节十二经气血。十二经气血有余

cessive, they then flow into the eight extraordinary vessels to store up. If qi and blood in the twelve meridians are insufficient, the eight extraordinary vessels will infuse some qi and blood stored in them into the twelve meridians. The third is to govern some of the special physiological activities of women. Since the thoroughfare, conception and governor vessels all start from the uterus, they are closely related to the menstruation, pregnancy and labor of women. Since the belt vessel runs transversely around the lower abdomen, it can protect fetus and controls leukorrhea.

4.3   The clinical application of the theory of meridians and collaterals

4.3.1   To explain pathogenesis and pathological transmission

4.3.1.1   To explain the pathogenesis

The occurrence of exogenous disease is usually caused by invasion of pathogenic factors which first attack the surface of the body, then invade the collaterals with scanty defensive qi, and gradually get into the internal part of the body. The occurrence of endogenous disease is caused either by insufficiency or imbalance of qi, blood, yin and yang. If qi, blood, yin and yang are insufficient, the meridians and collaterals will become empty; if qi, blood, yin and yang have lost balance, the meridian qi will be stagnated or in disorder, leading to the occurrence of disease.

4.3.1.2   To explain pathological transmission

Disease is usually transmitted along the meridians. The exogenous pathogenic factors are transmitted from

时,则流注于奇经八脉,蓄积以备用;十二经气血不足时,奇经八脉中蓄积的气血就溢出于十二经中,给予补充。③ 主持女子的特殊生理活动。冲、任、督三脉同起于女子胞,与女子月经和胎产均有密切关系;带脉横围于小腹,能固护胎儿,主司带下。

第三节　经络学说的临床应用

一、说明疾病发生与传变的机理

(一)说明疾病发生的机理

外感病的发生,是由于邪气的侵袭。外邪最初侵入人体,是从肌表开始,首先侵入卫气空虚的络脉,然后逐步向里传变。内伤病的发生,或由于气血阴阳的不足,或由于气血阴阳的失调。若气血阴阳不足,则经络空虚;若气血阴阳失调,则经气阻滞或逆乱,都能导致疾病发生。

(二)说明疾病传变的机理

疾病的传变常常以经络为途径。外邪由表入里,从络

the external to the internal, from the collaterals to the meridians, and from the meridians to the viscera. Thus the pathological changes of the viscera can be transmitted by the meridians. For example, disease of the zang-organs can be transmitted to the fu-organs and the disease of fu-organs can be transmitted to the zang-organs by the meridians in external and internal relationship with each other. On the other hand, the diseases of the five zang-organs can be transmitted among them because of the multiple relationships among the meridians and collaterals. For example, the liver disease can be transmitted to the lung and the stomach; the kidney disease can be transmitted to the heart and the lung; etc. Besides, disease of the internal organs can be transmitted to the surface of the body, leading to pathological changes of the related constituents, organs and orifices. For example, angina pectoris may lead to tenderness on medial side of the upper limb along which the heart meridian runs; the disease caused by stomach-fire may cause swelling pain of the gums through which the stomach meridian runs; up-flaming of liver-fire may cause ocular disease, etc.

4.3.2   To guide the diagnosis and treatment of disease

4.3.2.1   To guide the diagnosis of disease

Since the meridians run along certain routes and pertain to certain viscera, there is a special relationship between different parts of the body and the internal organs. Clinically the relationship between the pathological location or the disease and the meridians can be used to decide which meridian and viscus are involved so as to make an accurate diagnosis. For example, the liver meridian distributes over the hypochondrium, so hypochondriac pain indicates liver disease; the lung meridian emerges from

脉传入经脉,从经脉再传入脏腑。脏腑的病变,可以通过经络相互传变,如脏病可以传腑,腑病可以传脏,是通过表里经的相互属络关系进行传变。五脏之间也可以通过经络的多种相互联系而传变,如肝病传肺、胃,肾病传心、肺等。内脏病变也可以通过经络传出体表,出现相关形体官窍的病变,如真心痛可在上肢内侧手少阴心经经过的部位有痛感,胃火病人可在阳明经所经过的牙龈出现肿痛,肝火上炎可见目赤等。

二、指导疾病的诊断和治疗

(一)指导疾病的诊断

由于经络有一定的循行部位和所属脏腑,因此人体各部与内脏之间存在着特定的联系。临床上可以根据病变或证候所在的部位与经络的关系,判断疾病所属的经络与脏腑,从而作出诊断,如肝经布于胁,胁痛可以诊断为肝病;肺经出于缺盆,缺盆中痛

the supraclavicular fossa, pain in the supraclavicular fossa indicates lung disease. Take headache for another example. It usually appears in different regions. Pain in the forehead is related to the yangming meridian; pain in both sides of the head is usually related to the shaoyang meridian; and pain in the nape is often related to the taiyang meridian. Besides, some diseases show special reaction points on certain acupoints. If tenderness appears on these reaction points, it is very helpful for diagnosis. For example, intestinal abscess will lead to tenderness on Lanwei (EX-LE7), gallbladder disease will bring on tenderness on Yanglingquan (GB 34).

4.3.2.2 To guide the treatment of disease

The theory of the meridians and collaterals is extensively used in clinical treatment, especially in acupuncture and moxibustion, massage and drug treatment.

The treatment of disease by acupuncture, moxibustion and massage is usually done by needling or massaging the acupoints proximal or distal to the affected part on the meridians to regulate the functional activities of the meridian qi and blood. To select acupoints, one has to differentiate the syndrome first with the theory of the meridians and collaterals to decide which meridian the disease is related to, and then select acupoints in the light of the running route and coverage of the meridian. Such a way to select acupoints is called "selection of acupoints along the meridians".

Drug treatment also has to be done according to the theory of meridians and collaterals because the meridians and collaterals can transport the effect of the drugs to the affected part. In the long course of clinical practice, TCM has developed the theory of "meridian tropism of drugs"

可以诊断为肺病。又如头痛往往出现在不同部位,若前额痛则与阳明经有关,两侧头痛多与少阳经有关,后项头痛则与太阳经有关。此外,某些疾病在体表特定经穴有特殊反应点,该反应点出现压痛时往往是诊断的重要依据,如肠痛在足阳明经的阑尾穴有压痛,胆病在足少阳经的阳陵泉有压痛等。

(二)指导疾病的治疗

经络学说被广泛用于临床各科的治疗,特别是对针灸、按摩和药物治疗,具有重要指导意义。

针灸疗法与按摩疗法,主要是对于某一经或某一脏腑的病变,在其病变的邻近部位或经络循行的远隔部位上取穴,通过针灸或按摩,以调整经络气血的功能活动,从而达到治疗的目的。而穴位的选取,首先必须按经络学说来进行辨证,断定疾病属于何经后,再根据经络的循行分布路线和联系范围来选定,这就是"循经取穴"。

药物治疗也是以经络为渠道,通过经络的传导转输,才能使药到病所,发挥其治疗作用。中医学通过长期的临床实践经验的总结,创立了

which holds that each drug can enter one or more meridians. With the guidance of this theory, clinically drugs are selected, based on syndrome differentiation, according to their state of "meridian tropism" to treat disease so as to improve the therapeutic effect. Again take headache for example. If it is related to the taiyang meridian, Qianghuo (*Rhizoma seu Radix Notopterygii*) should be used; if it is related to the yangming meridian, Baizhi (*Radix Angelicae Dahuricae*) should be used; if it is related to the shaoyang meridian, Chaihu (*Radix Bupleuri*) should be used, because these drugs enter to these meridians respectively. In the formulation of a prescription, one or two drugs that enter a certain meridian can be added in order to guide the other drugs, which normally do not enter that meridian, to work on that meridian. The drug that leads other drugs to work on a certain meridian or organ is called "guiding drug".

"药物归经"的理论。"药物归经"理论认为,不同的药物将以不同的经络为通路,到达不同的脏腑器官。每一种药物可以归入一经或数经。这样,临床治疗时就可以在辨证的基础上,有目的地选择能直达病所的药物,从而提高治疗效果,如治头痛,属太阳经的可用羌活,属阳明经的可用白芷,属少阳经的可用柴胡,这是因为这些药物能归入相应的经络。此外,处方时也可以在众多不具有直达病所作用的一般药物中加入一两味能归入某一经络的药物,以引导其他药物到达病所,这些起引导作用的药物被称为"引经药"。

5 Causes of disease

第五章 病因

Causes of disease refer to various pathogenic factors, the differentiation of which decides the differentiation of syndromes, the cogniton of disease and the selection of correct therapeutic methods. In fact, the treatment of disease in TCM is causal treatment and the differentiation of syndromes, to a large degree, is causal differentiation of syndromes, known as "differentiation of syndromes to find causes", "analysis of symptoms to find the causes" and " analysis of causes to decide treatment".

病因,即致病因素,指各种能使人发生疾病的原因。病因理论在中医学中的地位极其重要,因为它关系到整个辨证论治过程。中医学认为,只有正确辨认疾病的原因,才能认识疾病的本质,才有可能制订正确的治疗方案。中医治病实质上是一种病因治疗,而辨证在很大程度上就是辨病因,所以有"辨证求因"、"审症求因"、"审因论治"等说法。

The pathogenic factors in TCM can be divided into four categories: ① exogenous pathogenic factors including six climatic factors and pestilence. ② endogenous pathogenic factors including seven emotions, improper diet and overstrain, etc. ③ secondary pathogenic factors including phlegm, retention of fluid and blood stasis. ④ other pathogenic factors including various traumatic injuries, injuries due to physical and chemical factors and injuries caused by insects and animals. This chapter is mainly devoted to the discussion of the six abnormal climatic factors, seven emotions, improper diet, overwork and over-rest, phlegm, retention of fluid and blood stasis, etc.

病因可分为四类: ① 外感病因,包括六淫、疫疠。② 内伤病因,包括七情、饮食失宜、劳逸过度等。③ 继发病因,包括痰饮、瘀血。④ 其他病因,包括各种外伤、理化因素致伤、虫兽所伤等。本书重点介绍外感六淫、内伤七情、饮食失宜、劳逸过度、痰饮、瘀血等内容。

5.1 The six climatic factors

第一节 外感六淫

The six climatic factors are pathogenic wind, pathogenic cold, pathogenic summer-heat, pathogenic dampness,

六淫,即风、寒、暑、湿、燥、热(火)六种外感病邪的

pathogenic dryness and pathogenic heat (fire).

Wind, cold, summer-heat, dampness, dryness and heat (fire) are six kinds of natural climatic factors known as "six qi". Human beings living in the natural world constantly contact with these natural factors. Under normal condition, the human body can adapt to the changes of climate which are indispensable to the existence of human beings. If the harmonious relationship between human beings and nature is broken, the body is unable to adapt itself to the changes of the climate, leading to the occurrence of disease. Under such a condition, these six natural climatic factors become pathogenic factors.

The six climatic factors are either abnormal changes of the climate or normal factors of the climate. When the climate suddenly changes, many people cannot adapt themselves to such a violent change and fall ill. Only those with very strong constitution can avoid being attacked. However sometimes under normal condition, some people can be attacked by the climatic factors and fall ill because of weak constitution that makes them unable to adapt to the normal changes of the climate.

The six climatic factors are characterized by the following features in causing disease:

(1) The cause of disease by the six climatic factors is usually related to seasonal changes and living conditions

总称。

风、寒、暑、湿、燥、热（火），本是六种正常的自然气候因素,合称为"六气"。人生存在自然环境中,不可避免地要与自然界各种气候变化"打交道"。正常情况下,人体对各种自然气候的变化具有充分的适应能力,自然气候有序的变化也是人类生存不可缺少的条件。如果人与自然环境相适应的协调关系被打破,不能适应自然气候的变化,就会导致疾病。此时,六气相对于人体就成为致病的因素,中医学把这类致病因素叫做"六淫"。

六淫可以是气候的反常变化,也可以是正常的气候因素。当气候发生反常变化时,人群中多数人不能适应,所以会有较多的人感受外邪而生病,只有那些体质特别强健的人才可以避免。但是在正常的气候条件下,也会有一部分人感受外邪而生病,是因为这部分人体质较弱,或因为某种原因降低了他们对正常环境的适应能力,于是就容易感受外邪而发病。

六淫致病,一般具有以下几个特点。

（1）六淫致病多与季节气候、居住环境有关。因为风、

because the occurrence of wind, cold, summer-heat, dampness, dryness and heat (fire) is specifically related to the four seasons. For example, spring is prone to wind, summer is prone to summer-heat (fire), late summer is prone to dampness, autumn is prone to dryness and winter is prone to cold. The living environment can be regarded as a small environment with its own climatic states. For example, long-term living in damp area is subject to attack by pathogenic dampness and working in the area with high temperature is subject to attack by pathogenic dryness and heat.

(2) The six climatic factors may singly or collectively attack people. For example, pathogenic wind may combine with cold, dampness, dryness and heat to attack people and lead to wind-cold syndrome, wind-dampness syndrome, wind-dryness syndrome and wind-heat syndrome.

(3) The nature of the diseases caused by the six climatic factors may be the same as or different from that of the six climatic factors. For example, invasion of pathogenic cold may deepen internally to transform into heat and accumulation of pathogenic dampness also may transform into heat. Sometimes the nature of the disease caused by various pathogenic factors may vary due to the difference in constitution, which is called "secondary transformation". For example, frequent abundance of yang or frequent deficiency of yin may transform into heat after the invasion of exogenous pathogenic factors; frequent abundance of yin or frequent deficiency of yang may transform into cold after invasion of exogenous pathogenic factors; frequent abundance of dampness or deficiency of the spleen may lead to transformation of dampness, etc.

(4) The six climatic factors usually invade people from the skin into the muscles or from the mouth and nose

寒、暑、湿、燥、热(火)的出现与季节有某种特殊联系,所以春季易感受风邪,夏季易感受暑、热(火),长夏易感受湿邪,秋季易感受燥邪,冬季易感受寒邪。居住环境可视为小环境,也有相应的小气候。如久居湿地容易感受湿邪,在高温环境下工作容易感受燥热邪气等。

(2) 六淫邪气可单独侵袭人体,也可以相互兼挟侵入人体而使人发病。如风邪可兼寒、湿、燥、热等邪,而形成风寒、风湿、风燥、风热等证。

(3) 六淫所致疾病的性质可以与其原始性质一致,也可以因个体的体质因素及其反应性的差异而发生转化。如感受寒邪,可以入里化热,湿邪蕴积日久也可以化热。感受各种邪气,还可以因其体质不同而表现为不同性质的疾病,中医学把这种现象叫做"从化"。如素体阳盛或阴虚者,感受外邪后易从热化;素体阴盛或阳虚者,感受外邪后易从寒化;素体湿盛或脾虚者,感受外邪后易从湿化等。

(4) 六淫邪气往往从外感受而发病,或从皮肤侵入肌

into the lung and the defensive qi. That is why external syndromes tend to appear at the early stage of disease caused by the six climatic factors and gradually transmit to the internal.

Besides, clinically there are some diseases due to dysfunction of the viscera that appear similar to the pathological changes caused by pathogenic wind, pathogenic cold, pathogenic dampness, pathogenic dryness and pathogenic heat (fire), known as "five endogenous pathogenic factors", such as endogenous wind, endogenous cold, endogenous dampness, endogenous dryness and endogenous heat (fire) which are not directly caused by, but can result from, the six exogenous climatic factors. For example, attack by exogenous pathogenic wind can stir the endogenous pathogenic wind and exogenous pathogenic dampness can induce endogenous pathogenic dampness.

5.1.1 Wind

Wind is the main climatic factor in spring. That is why wind tends to cause disease in spring. But in other seasons wind also can cause disease.

Wind is characterized by the following features:

1. Wind tends to float

Wind is a pathogenic factor of yang nature, characterized by floating and dispersion because of lightness. That is why wind attacks the upper part (the head and face) and skin first when it invades the body. So the disease caused by wind mainly involves the surface of the body, the head and the face with the manifestations of headache, running nose, sweating and aversion to cold, etc.

2. Wind tends to move

Wind is mobile and the disease caused by it is also

表,或从口鼻侵入肺卫。因此,外感六淫早期多先出现表证,然后逐步向里传变。

此外,临床上还有某些并非感受六淫外邪,而是由脏腑功能失调所致的类似于风、寒、湿、燥、热(火)的病理变化,中医学称为"内生五邪"、"内生五气"等,如内风、内寒、内湿、内燥、内热(火)之类。内生五邪(内生五气)虽然不是由外感六淫所致,但常可因外感六淫邪气而引发,如外感风邪可引动内风,外感湿邪可引动内湿等。

一、风

风为春季的主气,故风邪致病多见于春季,但在其他季节也可感受风邪。

风邪的性质及致病特点如下:

1. 风性浮越

浮,即上浮;越,指外越。风为阳邪,具有轻扬、开泄的特性,轻扬则易上浮,开泄则易外越,故风邪侵袭人体,常先侵袭人体上部(头面)及肌表。因此,风邪致病主要表现为肌表及头面部症状,如头痛、流鼻涕、汗出、恶风等。

2. 风性善动

风气具有运动不息的特

migration (such as migratory pain of limbs in wind-bi syndrome), tremor of the limbs (such as convulsion, spasm due to some special pathogenic factors of wind) and dizziness (such as subjective feeling of shaking or faintness or like sitting in a boat or car). Dizziness is usually caused by dysfunction of the viscera complicated by liver-wind. Exogenous pathogenic wind is often the factor that induces endogenous wind.

3. Wind tends to change

Wind tends to change. So the disease caused by wind is often characterized by sudden onset, immediate transmission and change as well as fast healing. For example, rubella is marked by quick fluctuation of cutaneous pruritus without a fixed location.

4. Wind tends to be complicated by other pathogenic factors

Since it is easier for wind to attack the body, other factors in the six exogenous factors often attach themselves to wind when they invade the body, frequently leading to exogenous wind-cold syndrome, exogenous wind-heat syndrome, exogenous wind-dampness syndrome and exogenous wind-dryness syndrome. That is why TCM holds that "wind is the leading one among the six exogenous pathogenic factors", "all diseases are caused by wind" and "wind is the leading cause of all diseaes".

5.1.2   Cold

Cold is the dominant climatic factor in winter. So

性,故风邪致病也具有善动的特征。风性善动有以下几种表现形式:① 病位游移,行无定处。如"风痹"可见肢节游走性疼痛,痛无定处。② 肢体振颤,运动异常。如各种抽搐、痉挛,中医学称为"风气内动",是因某些特殊风邪所致。③ 眩晕。表现为自觉身体动摇,或天旋地转,或如坐车船之中。眩晕症一般是由脏腑功能失调并挟"肝风"所致,而外感风邪具有引动内风的作用。

3. 风性多变

风气具有变幻无常的特性,故风邪致病往往变化多端,来去迅速。如风邪致病往往发病迅速,传变快,痊愈也快;"风疹"病见皮肤瘙痒此起彼伏,发无定处等等。

4. 风易兼邪

风邪最易侵犯人体,故六淫中其他邪气往往依附于风而来,从而出现外感风寒、风热、风湿、风燥等。因此,中医学认为风是其他邪气侵犯人体的先导,故有"风为六淫之首"、"风为百病之始"、"风为百病之长"等说法。

二、寒

寒为冬季的主气,故寒邪

cold diseases, though also encountered in other seasons, are usually seen in winter. The invasion of cold into the body is frequently due to cold weather and lack of cold control measures. Sometimes it is due to drench, walking in water and exposure to wind in sweating.

The invasion of wind is either superficial or internal. The former refers to external cold syndrome caused by cold when it attacks the surface of the body and stagnates the defensive qi while the latter refers to internal cold syndrome caused by cold when it directly attacks the internal of the body and impairs the visceral yang-qi.

The following is a brief description of the nature of pathogenic cold and its characteristics in causing diseases.

1. Cold tends to impair yang

Cold pertains to yin and tends to impair yang. When cold attacks the surface of the body, it will impair yang in the superficies; when it attacks the internal of the body, it will impair the visceral yang. If yang-qi is impaired and cannot warm and transform qi, it will lead to cold syndrome due to functional decline. If cold impairs the superficies, the defensive qi will be stagnated, leading to aversion to cold and anhidrosis; if cold directly invades the spleen and the stomach, the spleen-yang will be impaired, leading to cold pain in the stomach and abdomen, vomiting and diarrhea; if cold directly attacks shaoyin, it will impair heart-yang and the kidney-yang, leading to aversion to cold, lying with the knees drawn up, dispiritedness, cold hands and feet, diarrhea with undigested food, profuse and clear urine, thin and indistinct pulse.

2. Cold tends to coagulate

Qi, blood and body fluid in the body flow continuously inside the body because they are constantly warmed and propelled by yang-qi. If the pathogenic cold obstructs

致病多见于冬季,但在其他季节也可感受寒邪。感受寒邪往往与气候寒冷及人们防寒保暖不够有关,淋雨、涉水、汗出当风等因素也可感受寒邪。

由于感寒途径不同,所感寒邪轻重不一,故寒邪致病有伤寒、中寒两种情形。若寒邪伤于肌表,郁遏卫阳,出现表寒证的,称为"伤寒";寒邪直中于里,伤及脏腑阳气,出现里寒证的,则为"中寒"。

寒邪的性质及致病特点如下。

1. 寒易伤阳

寒为阴邪,故易损伤阳气。寒邪袭表,则伤表阳;寒邪伤里,则损脏腑之阳。阳气受损,失其正常的温煦、气化作用,可出现功能减退的寒证。如寒邪损伤肌表,卫阳被遏,则见恶寒、无汗;寒邪直中脾胃,脾阳受损,可见脘腹冷痛、呕吐、腹泻;寒邪直中少阴,伤及心肾之阳,可见畏寒蜷卧、精神委靡、手足厥冷、下利清谷、小便清长、脉微细等症。

2. 寒性凝滞

凝滞,即凝结、阻滞不通之义。人身之气血津液之所以能运行不息,通畅无阻,全

yang-qi, then qi, blood and body fluid cannot flow freely and will coagulate in the vessels, bringing on pain. If cold attacks the viscera, the visceral qi and blood will be stagnated, causing abdominal pain; if cold attacks the muscles and joints, qi and blood in the muscles and joints will coagulate, resulting in pain in the muscles and joints.

3. Cold tends to contract

Cold pertains to yin and tends to restrain the activity of qi, leading to contracture of muscles, tendons and vessels. If cold attacks the superficies, the muscular interstices will be stagnated, the muscles will be contracted and the defensive qi cannot disperse, leading to aversion to cold, anhidrosis and papules; if cold invades the limbs and joints, the tendons and vessels will become contracted, bringing on somatic pain, headache and spasm of the limbs.

5.1.3　Summer-heat

Summer-heat is transformed from heat and fire in summer. Summer-heat pertains to yang and usually appears after summer solstice and before autumn solstice. The attack by summer-heat is either due to hot weather or due to low adaptability of the body to the environment.

Summer-heat is characterized by the following features:

1. Summer-heat is hot

Summer-heat pertains to yang and is hot in nature. So the disease caused by summer-heat is usually marked by a series of yang symptoms such as high fever, dysphoria, reddish complexion, thirst with preference for cold

赖一身阳气的温煦推动。若遇寒邪郁遏阳气,则气血津液运行受阻,凝结于经脉,使经脉阻滞不通,于是发生疼痛。寒在脏腑,脏腑中气血凝结而经脉不通,则心腹中疼痛;寒在肌肉关节,肌肉关节中气血凝结而经脉不通,则肌肉关节疼痛。

3. 寒性收引

收引,即收缩牵引之义。寒为阴邪,易使气机收敛,导致肌肤收缩,筋脉牵引。若寒袭肌表,使腠理闭塞,肌肤收缩,卫阳不得宣泄,则见恶寒无汗,皮肤粟起;若寒客肢节,使筋脉牵引,血脉挛缩,可见头身疼痛,肢体拘急不伸。

三、暑

暑为夏季的主气,为火热所化。暑邪属阳邪,具有明显的季节性,主要出现在夏至以后、立秋之前。感受暑邪既与气候炎热有关,也与人体对环境的适应能力下降有密切关系。

暑邪的性质及致病特点如下。

1. 暑性炎热

暑属阳邪,其性炎热,故暑邪伤人,多出现一系列阳热症状,如高热、心烦、面赤、口渴喜冷饮、脉象洪大等。

drink and full and large pulse, etc.

2. Summer-heat tends to disperse

Summer-heat pertains to yang and tends to disperse and elevate. Summer-heat disturbs the mind when it elevates, leading to dysphoria and dizziness or even sudden coma and unconsciousness in severe cases. Summer-heat induces sweating and consumes body fluid when it disperses, leading to thirst with preference for drinking water and reddish and scanty urine. If there is profuse sweating, qi will get lost, eventually bringing on shortness of breath and lassitude due to qi deficiency.

3. Summer-heat is often complicated by dampness

In the hot season, heat fumigates dampness. That is why dampness is exuberant in summer and often mixes up with heat to attack people. Thus disease caused by summer-heat-dampness is often, apart from fever and extreme thirst, characterized by lassitude of the four limbs, chest oppression, vomiting and unsmooth loose stool, etc.

5.1.4　Dampness

Dampness is predominant in late summer but also can be encountered in other seasons. Since it is hot in late summer, dampness permeates everywhere due to fumigation and frequently causes disease. Sometimes drench or living in damp area also results in disease of dampness.

The following is a brief description about the nature and characteristics of dampness in causing disease:

1. Dampness is heavy and turbid

Dampness pertains to yin, so it is heavy. The attack by dampness will lead to such symptoms as heaviness of

2. 暑性升散

暑为阳邪,故易上升、发散。暑邪上升,则干扰神明,使人心烦、头昏,严重者突然昏迷,不省人事。暑邪发散,则汗出过多,耗伤津液,可出现口渴喜饮,尿赤短少;汗出过多则气随津泄,导致气虚,出现气短、乏力等症。

3. 暑多挟湿

暑热季节,热蒸湿动,故湿气也盛。人在暑湿之中,二者容易相兼伤人。故夏季感受暑邪者,多挟有湿邪。暑湿致病,除有发热、烦渴等暑热症状外,常兼见四肢困倦、胸闷呕恶、大便溏泄而不爽等湿阻症状。

四、湿

湿为长夏的主气,但在其他季节特定环境下也能感受湿邪。长夏气候炎热,氤氲薰蒸,则湿气弥漫,人多易感受湿邪而致病。若淋雨涉水,或居处潮湿,也能感受湿邪。

湿邪的性质及致病特点如下。

1. 湿性重浊

重,即沉重;浊,指秽浊。湿为阴邪,故有沉重的特性。

the body, or heaviness of the four limbs, or heaviness of the head like being bound, or heaviness and lassitude of the whole body. Dampness is similar to water and it often mixes up with water. That is why it is turbid. Invasion of dampness into the body often brings on the symptoms of turbid secreta and excreta, dirty complexion, excessive secretion of gum in the eyes, loose stool, mucous and bloody dysentery, turbid urine, leukorrhea and oozing eczema.

2. Dampness tends to block qi

Dampness moves slowly because it is heavy. So it tends to retain in the viscera and meridians, inhibits the flow of qi and disturbs the activity of qi, frequently leading to chest oppression and fullness, scanty and unsmooth urination and inhibited defecation. On the other hand, dampness pertains to yin and tends to impair yang-qi. Thus prolonged blockage of qi by dampness will prevent yang-qi from flowing, often causing exuberance of dampness and decline of yang. Since dampness pertains to earth in the five elements and is related to the spleen, it tends to impair the spleen, bringing on encumbrance of the spleen by dampness and stagnation of qi in the middle energizer. If dampness impairs yang, it will inactivate spleen-yang and further accumulate water and dampness, leading to diarrhea, scanty urine, edema and ascites.

3. Dampness is sticky and stagnant

These characteristics of dampness usually affect people in two ways. One is that the disease caused by dampness is not brisk. For example, the secreta and excreta are too sticky to be excreted. The second is that the disease caused by dampness is obstinate and recurring with long duration, such as damp-bi syndrome (damp-blockage syndrome), eczema and damp-warm syndrome.

感受湿邪,病人会有身体沉重的感觉,或四肢沉重,或头重如裹,或全身困重而乏力。湿类于水,水邪互结则秽浊不洁。感受湿邪,常见排泄物、分泌物秽浊不清,出现面垢眵多、大便溏泄、下痢粘液脓血、小便混浊、妇女白带过多、湿疹浸淫流水等症。

2. 湿易阻气

由于湿性沉重,运行迟缓,故易留滞于脏腑经络,阻遏气的运行,使气机升降失常,常出现胸闷脘痞、小便短涩、大便不爽等症。又由于湿为阴邪,易伤阳气,故湿邪阻气日久,阳气不得运行,往往形成湿盛阳微的局面。因湿气属土而内通于脾,故湿邪最易伤脾,而致湿邪困脾,气壅中焦;若湿盛伤阳,则脾阳不振,运化无权,更使水湿停聚,发为腹泻、尿少、水肿、腹水等病症。

3. 湿性粘滞

粘,即粘腻;滞,即停滞。湿邪具有粘腻停滞的性质,主要表现在两方面:一是指湿邪所致病证多粘滞而不爽,如排泄物及分泌物多粘腻涩滞而排出不畅;二是指湿邪为病往往胶着难化,缠绵难愈,病程较长或反复发作,如湿痹、湿

疹、湿温等病即具有这种
特征。

4. Dampness tends to move downward

Dampness is similar to water, so it tends to move downward. Firstly, it impairs the lower part when it attacks the body. That is why *Huangdi Neijing* says that "when dampness attack the body, it first impairs the lower part of the body". Secondly, the disease caused by dampness usually involves the lower part of the body. For example, edema often mostly involves the lower limbs; stranguria, leukorrhagia and dysentery all occur in the lower part of the body. Thirdly, the disease caused by dampness usually is transmitted from the upper to the lower. For example, damp-warm disease is usually transmitted from the upper energizer to middle energizer and lower energizer; stranguria, leukorrhagia and dysentery may be caused by downward migration of dampness.

4. 湿性趋下

湿类于水,故其性趋下。
湿性趋下有三个方面的含义:
① 湿邪伤人,先伤人体下部,
故《黄帝内经》有"伤于湿者,
下先受之"的理论。② 湿邪为
病多见下部症状,如水肿多以
下肢较为明显,淋浊、带下、泄
痢等湿邪所致病证都表现在
下部。③ 湿邪致病的传变特
征是由上向下,如湿温病有从
上焦依次传至中焦、下焦的规
律,淋浊、带下、泄痢等症也可
由湿邪下注所引起。

5.1.5 Dryness

Dryness is predominant in autumn. So disease caused by dryness mostly appears in autumn. In late summer dampness permeates. But in autumn dampness disappears and the weather becomes cool and dry. Dryness can be divided into warm-dryness and cool-dryness due to difference in weather. The disease occurring at the early stage of autumn is a kind of warm-dryness because there is still some remaining summer-heat; the disease occurring at the late stage of autumn is a kind of cool-dryness syndrome because the weather is already cold in late autumn.

The following is a brief description of the nature and characteristics of dryness in causing disease:

1. Dryness is xerotic and unsmooth

Dryness is usually caused by insufficiency of body fluid. So the attack by dryness tends to consume body fluid and

五、燥

燥为秋季的主气,故感受
燥邪多见于秋季。长夏湿气
弥漫,入秋湿气一去,天气忽
然清肃,故易生燥邪。感受燥
邪,因气候寒温不同而有温
燥、凉燥之分。初秋有夏热之
余气,燥与温热结合而侵犯人
体,则成温燥;深秋有近冬之
寒气,燥与寒气相合而侵犯人
体,则表现为凉燥。

燥邪的性质及致病特点
如下。

1. 燥性干涩

燥多由津液匮乏所致,因
其津液不足,失于流利,故表

lead to dryness of the mouth and nose, dry throat, dry skin or even rhagas, scanty urine and retention of dry feces.

2. Dryness tends to impair the lung

Dryness is prevailing in autumn and is associated with the lung. So dryness tends to impair the lung when it invades the body. If it impairs the lung, the lung-fluid will be consumed and the function of the lung to depurate and descend will be affected, leading to dry cough with scanty phlegm, or sticky sputum difficult to expectorate, or blood sputum, dyspnea and chest pain.

5.1.6　Heat (fire)

Heat (fire) is the predominant climatic factor in summer. So disease due to pathogenic heat (fire) usually occurs in summer. However it can also be encountered in other seasons. Since there are two ways to describe the order of pathogenic factors in *Huangdi Neijing*, namely "wind, cold, summer-heat, dampness, dryness and heat" and "wind, cold, summer-heat, dampness, dryness and fire", so "fire" and "heat" are often mentioned in the same breath. If we make a comparison between the fire and the heat, we can say that the heat is the manifestation of the fire and the fire is the nature of the heat. They are, to a certain degree, different from each other but intrinsically related to each other.

The following is a brief description of the nature and the characteristics of heat (fire) in causing disease:

1. Heat (fire) tends to flame up

Heat (fire) pertains to yang and tends to flame up. So the disease caused by the pathogenic heat (fire) is marked by high fever, aversion to heat, extreme thirst,

现为干涩。感受燥邪,最易耗伤人体的津液,造成阴津亏虚的病变,可见口鼻干燥、咽干、皮肤干涩甚则皲裂、小便短少、大便干结等症。

2. 燥易伤肺

燥生于秋,秋气通于肺,故燥邪易于伤肺。若肺为燥邪所伤,则肺津受损,影响肺的宣发肃降功能,可出现干咳少痰,或痰液胶黏难咯,或痰中带血,以及喘息胸痛等症。

六、热(火)

热(火)为夏季的主气,故感受热(火)邪以夏季为多,但在其他季节也能感受热(火)邪。因《黄帝内经》有"风寒暑湿燥热"和"风寒暑湿燥火"两种提法,所以历来把"热"与"火"相提并论。以热与火相比较,则热为火之表现,火为热之本性,两者有区别也有本质联系。由于它们的性质和致病特点相同,所以一般不加以严格区分。

热(火)邪的性质及致病特点如下。

1. 热(火)性炎热

热(火)为阳邪,其性炎热,易升腾上炎,故热(火)邪伤人,多见高热、恶热、烦渴、

sweating and full pulse. When the pathogenic heat (fire) attacks the body, it may disturb the mind, leading to dysphoria, insomnia, mania, coma and delirium, etc. Since the pathogenic heat is responsible for irritability and rapid movement, the disease caused by it is characterized by acute onset and rapid transmission.

2. Heat (fire) tends to consume qi and impair body fluid

Heat (fire) pertains to yang and tends to consume yin-fluid. If there is superabundant heat, it will drive body fluid out of the body in the form of sweat. So the disease caused by the pathogenic heat, apart from the manifestations of heat, is often accompanied by thirst with preference for drinking water, dry throat and tongue, dark and scanty urine and retention of dry feces due to consumption and impairment of body fluid.

Huangdi Neijing says that "strong fire consumes qi". The pathogenic heat (fire) is strong fire, so it consumes the healthy qi. Besides, profuse sweating due to exuberance of heat also impairs the healthy qi. So at the late stage of febrile disease healthy qi is still deficient though the pathogenic factors have already been eliminated.

3. Heat (fire) tends to produce wind and disturb blood

When heat (fire) invades the body, it usually scorches the liver meridian, consumes body fluid and deprives the tendons of moisture and nourishment, leading to occurrence of liver-wind with the manifestations of high fever, epistaxis, coma, delirium, convulsion of the four limbs, staring straight upward, stiff neck and opisthotonus.

Blood coagulates with cold and moves fast with heat.

汗出、脉洪数等症,并可上扰神明,出现心烦失眠、狂躁妄动、神昏谵语等症。由于阳热之气主躁动而急速,故感受热(火)邪往往发病急,传变快。

2. 热(火)易耗气伤津

热(火)为阳邪,阳盛则阴病,故易伤阴津。热盛之时,迫津外泄,出汗较多,则使阴津消灼,故热(火)邪致病除热象外,往往伴有口渴喜饮、咽干舌燥、小便短赤、大便秘结等津液耗伤之症。

《黄帝内经》有"壮火食气"的理论。壮火,即阳热亢盛之实火;食,消耗的意思。感受热(火)邪,便是壮火,故能消耗人体正气。同时热盛汗出过多,气随津泄,也能耗伤人体正气。所以热病后期,邪气虽去,而正气往往不足,需要一个逐渐恢复的过程。

3. 热(火)易生风动血

热(火)邪侵袭人体,往往燔灼肝经,劫耗阴液,使筋脉失其滋养濡润,而致肝风内动,称为"热极生风",表现为高热、神昏谵语、四肢抽搐、目睛上视、颈项强直、角弓反张等。

血液得寒则凝,得热则

But if the heat is excessive, it will drive blood to flow very fast or scorch the vessels or even compel blood to flow out of the vessels, leading to various hemorrhage, such as hematemesis, hematochezia, hematuria, eruptions, profuse menorrhea and sudden profuse uterine bleeding.

4. Heat (fire) tends to cause swelling and ulceration

When heat (fire) invades blood phase and accumulates in local area, it will putrefy blood and muscles, causing abscess, furuncle and ulceration. These kinds of problems are marked by redness, swelling, heat and pain which are the manifestations of heat (fire). Heat (fire) responsible for abscess, furuncle and ulceration is called heat (fire) toxin. That is why it is said in TCM that "abscess and furuncle are caused by fire-toxin".

Appendix: Pestilence and five endogenous pathogenic factors

Pestilence

Pestilence is a kind of strong infectious pathogenic factor, quite similar to the pathogenic heat (fire) in the six pathogenic climatic factors in nature, but more serious than the pathogenic heat in toxicity. The diseases caused by pestilence are marked by acute onset, severe pathological condition, similar symptoms, strong infection and easiness to spread. Historical records show that diseases caused by pestilence often spread the disease far and wide with high mortality.

行。但热势过盛,血行加速,或灼伤脉络,可致血热沸腾,甚则迫血妄行,而致各种出血,如吐血、衄血、便血、尿血、皮肤发斑及妇女月经过多、崩漏等病症。

4. 热(火)易致肿疡

热(火)邪入于血分,聚于局部,可腐蚀血肉而发为痈肿疮疡。凡痈肿疮疡之证,多有红、肿、热、痛的特征,即是感受热(火)邪的表现。痈肿疮疡之热(火)邪,一般称为热(火)毒,故中医学有"痈疽原是火毒生"的说法。

附:疫疠、内生五邪

疫疠

疫疠,是一类具有强烈传染性的病邪,又有"疫气"、"疠气"、"毒气"等多种名称。一般来说,疫疠病邪的性质与六淫中的热(火)邪颇同,故也具有热(火)邪的性质和致病特征。但是疫疠病邪具有比一般热(火)邪毒性更强的特点,主要表现在感受疫疠病邪后的发病情形更为严重。疫疠病邪具有发病急骤、病情重笃、症状相似及传染性强、易于流行等特点。从以往的记载来看,疫疠之邪可导致疾病

The commonly encountered diseases caused by pestilence are facial erysipelas, mumps, pestilent dysentery, diphtheria, scarlet fever, smallpox, cholera and plague.

Five endogenous pathogenic factors

The so-called five endogenous pathogenic factors are endogenous wind, endogenous cold, endogenous dampness, endogenous dryness and endogenous heat (fire). Though they are called wind, cold, dampness, dryness and heat (fire), they are actually pathogenic factors due to dysfunction of the viscera. That is why the word "endogenous" is used to modify their names.

1. Endogenous wind

Endogenous wind is produced by the liver, so it is usually called "liver-wind" and "internal disturbance of liver-wind". There are four factors responsible for the occurrence of endogenous wind. The first is extreme heat producing wind, referring to the disease marked by convulsion due to exuberant heat that scorches liver-yin and deprives the tendons of nourishment; the second is transformation of liver-yang into wind, referring to the disease marked by dizziness and infantile convulsion resulting from hyperactivity of yang transforming into wind and disturbing the upper orifices; the third is yin-deficiency stirring wind, referring to the disease marked by infantile convulsion and convulsion resulting from declination of liver-yin and inability of yang to hide that lead to failure of the yin-fluid to nourish the tendons; the fourth is blood-deficiency stirring wind, referring to the disease marked by muscular peristalsis and tremor resulting from failure of the deficient blood to nourish the liver and the tendons.

大规模流行,而且患病死亡率高。

常见的疫疬所致的疾病有大头瘟(面部丹毒)、虾蟆瘟(流行性腮腺炎)、疫痢(中毒性痢疾)、白喉、烂喉丹痧、天花、霍乱、鼠疫等。

内生五邪

内生五邪,即内风、内寒、内湿、内燥、内热(火),也称"内生五气"。内生五邪虽有风、寒、湿、燥、热(火)等名称,但它们皆由脏腑功能失常所产生,故皆冠以"内"字。

1. 内风

内风皆生于肝,故也称"肝风"、"肝风内动"。其形成原因有:① 热极生风:因热邪炽盛,灼伤肝阴,筋脉失养,而致动风,出现以抽搐为特征的病变。② 肝阳化风:因阳亢化风,上扰清窍,出现眩晕、惊厥等症。③ 阴虚风动:由肝阴虚竭,阳不潜藏,阴液不能滋养其筋,又被阳亢化风所扰,从而发生惊厥、抽搐等症。④ 血虚风动:由肝血亏虚,血不养肝,筋失濡养,而致风动,表现为肌肉蠕动、震颤等。

2. Endogenous cold

The occurrence of endogenous cold is due to the deficiency of yang. The deficiency-cold of the viscera can be caused by either the deficiency of the kidney-yang or the spleen-yang or heart-yang. Since the kidney-yang is the source of yang-qi in the whole body, the deficiency of the kidney-yang is the predominant factor responsible for the occurrence of endogenous cold.

3. Endogenous dampness

Endogenous dampness results from the spleen. Usually failure of water to transform due to dysfunction of the spleen may produce the endogenous dampness which encumbers the spleen and affects the transporting and transforming functions of the spleen or accumulates into phlegm and retention of fluid, further resulting in other diseases.

4. Endogenous dryness

Endogenous dryness results from insufficiency of body fluid and is related to yin-deficiency. Since body fluid and blood can transform into each other, the deficiency of blood also causes dryness. The manifestations of endogenous dryness are often related to the intestines, the stomach, the lung and other orifices, such as dry nose, dry throat, dry eyes, scanty urine and retention of dry feces, etc.

5. Endogenous heat (fire)

The causes of endogenous heat (fire) are various, such as exogenous wind, exogenous cold, exogenous dampness and exogenous dryness that all can transform into heat; mental upset and extreme changes of emotions that often turn into fire; predomination of yang and deficiency of yin that usually produce the endogenous fire and heat; and excessive qi that frequently leads to fire, etc.

2. 内寒

内寒生于阳虚。或肾阳虚，或脾阳虚，或心阳虚，都可引起相应的脏腑虚寒。由于肾阳为一身阳气之根本，故肾阳虚是形成内寒的首要因素。

3. 内湿

内湿生于脾。凡脾虚失于健运，水湿不化，即能生湿。湿邪既生，乃困阻于脾，妨碍脾的运化功能；或聚湿成痰、成饮，进一步发展变化成其他病变。

4. 内燥

内燥皆由津液不足所致，与阴虚相关联。由于津血同源互化，故血虚也能生燥。内燥主要表现在肠胃、肺及有关的孔窍，因失于滋润而致鼻干、咽燥、两目干涩、小便短少、大便干结等。

5. 内热(火)

内热形成原因众多。外感风、寒、湿、燥，皆可化热；情志不遂，五志皆可郁而化火；阴阳不调，阳盛及阴虚皆可有火热内生；气有余便是火，等等。

5.2 Internal impairment due to seven emotions

The seven emotions refer to joy, anger, anxiety, contemplation, grief, fear and terror which are different responses of the body to the environmental stimuli and are normal psychological activities. Normally the seven emotions will not cause disease, but sudden, violent or prolonged emotional stimuli, beyond the range of physiological activities, will cause disorder of qi activity and disharmony of visceral yin, yang, qi and blood which consequently lead to disease. Since the seven emotions are endogenous and directly affect visceral qi and blood, the internal disorder caused is called "internal impairment due to seven emotions".

The seven emotions are the physiological responses of visceral qi, blood, yin and yang. Different visceral qi, blood, yin and yang differ from each other in moving styles, leading to different emotional responses. In *Huangdi Neijing*, the seven emotions are matched with the five viscera: the heart governs joy, the liver governs anger, the spleen governs contemplation, the lung governs grief, and the kidney governs fear. Terror and anxiety are also closely related to the activity of qi in the five zang-organs.

The attribution of the seven emotions to the five zang-organs is not absolute. On the one hand, the same viscus may produce different emotional responses because of different pathophysiological states. For example, excess of liver-qi causes anger while deficiency of liver-qi brings on fear; excess of heart-qi brings on joy while deficiency of heart-qi leads to grief; etc. On the other hand,

第二节　内伤七情

七情,是喜、怒、忧、思、悲、恐、惊七种情志变化的总称。七情是人体对外界事物的不同反应,属正常的心理活动方式,一般不会致病。只有突然、强烈或长期持久的情志刺激,超过了正常的生理活动范围,导致人体气机紊乱,脏腑阴阳气血失调,才会导致疾病的发生。因七情生于内,直接影响脏腑气血,是导致内伤病的主要因素之一,所以称为"内伤七情"。

七情,是脏腑气血阴阳的运动变化在心理上的反映,不同脏腑的气血阴阳运动变化形式不同,故出现的情绪反应也不同。《黄帝内经》把七情与五脏一一相配合,建立了五脏主五志的理论,即心主喜、肝主怒、脾主思、肺主悲、肾主恐。惊和忧也与五脏气机运动密切相关。

七情虽分属五脏,但也不是绝对的。其一,同一内脏的不同生理病理状态,可有不同的情绪反应。如肝气实则表现为怒,肝气虚则表现为恐;心气实则表现为喜,心气虚则表现为悲,等等。其二,所有

the seven emotions are exclusively dominated by the heart. In fact all the emotional activities are controlled by the heart and all the emotional responses are the manifestations of heart-spirit.

The following is a brief generalization of the effect of the seven emotions on the activity of qi:

Excessive joy relaxes the activity of qi; excessive anger drives qi to move upwards; excessive contemplation stagnates qi; excessive grief exhausts qi; fear drives qi to move downwards; excessive terror disturbs qi; and excessive anxiety depresses qi.

The following is a brief description of the characteristics of the seven emotions in causing disease.

5.2.1　Directly impairing the internal organs

Since the seven emotions are endogenous, they can directly impair the internal organs. For example, excessive joy impairs the heart, excessive anger impairs the liver, excessive contemplation impairs the spleen, excessive grief impairs the lung and excessive fear impairs the kidney, etc. The relationships among the five zang-organs are complicated, so the impairment of one viscus by the seven emotions may involve several zang-organs and fu-organs. For example, depression and rage impair the liver. But the adverse flow of liver-qi often attacks the spleen and the stomach, leading to imbalance between the liver and the spleen as well as disharmony between the liver and the stomach. Since the heart is the supreme dominator of the mental activities, the impairment caused by the seven emotions is closely related to the heart. Clinically the seven emotions often impair the heart, the liver and the spleen.

5.2.2　Disordering the activity of qi

When the seven emotions impair the internal organs,

情志活动实际上都必须通过心才能体现出来,一切情绪反应实质上仍是心神的表现,因此七情最终要归心所主管。

七情对气机的作用是:

喜则气缓;怒则气上;思则气结;悲则气消;恐则气下;惊则气乱;忧则气郁。

七情致病有以下特点。

一、直接伤及内脏

七情生于内,故直接伤及内脏。如喜伤心,怒伤肝,思伤脾,悲伤肺,恐伤肾等。由于内脏之间存在着多种复杂的关系,所以七情损伤某一内脏时,其病理反应会波及多个脏腑。如郁怒伤肝,肝气横逆,又常犯脾胃,出现肝脾不调、肝胃不和等证。同时,由于心为精神活动的最高主宰,故七情所伤都与心有密切关系。从临床来看,七情所伤以心、肝、脾三脏为多见。

二、导致气机紊乱

七情损伤内脏,主要是影

they mainly affect the activity of visceral qi, leading to disorder of the activity of qi and, in turn, bringing on the disorder of blood circulation because the blood flows together with qi. Prolonged emotional upset may transform into fire known as "transformation of five emotions into fire", resulting in disharmony between yin and yang because fire consumes yin.

5.2.2.1 Excessive joy relaxing the activity of qi

"Relax" here also means "slack". Joy is controlled by the heart. Normally joy can harmonize qi and blood, smooth the activity of the nutrient qi and defensive qi as well as ease the mind. If it becomes excessive, it may slack heart-qi, derange the mind and lead to inability to concentrate and even mania.

5.2.2.2 Excessive anger driving qi to move upwards

Anger is controlled by the liver. Excessive anger drives liver-qi, together with the blood, moving adversely upwards and leading to dizziness, distending headache, reddish complexion and redness of the eyes or hematemesis, or even sudden syncope. Under excessive anger, liver-qi may flow adversely and attack the spleen and stomach, causing anorexia, chest oppression and belching or even diarrhea.

5.2.2.3 Excessive anxiety inhibiting qi

Anxiety is related to the liver and the lung. Excessive anxiety may impair the lung and the liver. Anxiety usually inhibits qi and leads to depression of lung-qi or stagnation of liver-qi. The depression of lung-qi causes chest oppression and unsmooth breath; stagnation of liver-qi leads to hypochondriac distension and fullness or pain, unhappiness and reduced appetite.

响脏腑气机，导致气机紊乱。血随气行，气机紊乱则血行失常。情志不调，日久不解则化火，称为"五志化火"。火邪伤阴，则导致阴阳失调。

（一）喜则气缓

缓有"缓和"与"涣散"双重含义。喜为心之志，正常情况下，喜能使气血和缓，营卫通利，心情舒畅；若大喜过度则导致心气涣散，神不守舍，出现精神不集中，甚则失神狂乱等症状。

（二）怒则气上

怒为肝之志，大怒使肝气横逆上冲，血随气逆，并走于上，可出现头昏胀痛、面红目赤，或呕血等症，甚至突然昏厥。大怒而肝气横逆，犯脾乘胃，则令脾胃受制，使人不欲饮食，脘闷嗳气，或见大便泄泻。

（三）忧则气郁

忧与肺、肝均有关，忧愁过度，可伤及肺、肝。忧则气郁，可导致肺气抑郁或肝气郁结。肺气抑郁则使人心胸满闷，呼吸不畅；肝气郁结可致胁肋胀满或疼痛，心中不快，饮食减少等。

5.2.2.4 Excessive contemplation stagnating qi

Contemplation is controlled by the spleen. So excessive contemplation will stagnate spleen-qi and affect transportation and transformation, leading to gastric and abdominal distension and fullness, anorexia and loose stool, etc. Prolonged indulgence in contemplation consumes yin-blood and deprives the heart-spirit of nourishment, often bringing on palpitation, amnesia, insomnia and dreaminess, etc.

5.2.2.5 Excessive grief exhausting qi

Grief is dominated by the lung, so excessive grief exhausts lung-qi. Usually excessive grief affects the normal functions of the lung to depurate, descend, disperse and distribute, leading to failure of the nutrient qi and the defensive qi to distribute and consumption of the pectoral qi. So excessive grief often impairs the lung, leading to dizziness, lassitude and dispiritedness, etc.

5.2.2.6 Excessive terror driving qi to move downwards

Terror is dominated by the kidney. So sudden terror drives qi to move downwards, leading to incontinence of urine and feces due to failure of kidney-qi to fixate or weakness and atrophy of the bones and seminal emission due to failure of the kidney to store essence. Prolonged state of terror may lead to various diseases due to failure of qi to elevate, decline of the visceral functions and inability of healthy qi to defend the superficies.

5.2.2.7 Excessive fear disturbing qi

Fear and terror are all caused by similar external stimuli, but they are different in the responses of visceral qi activity. Terror, dominated by the kidney, drives qi to move downwards; fear, originating from the heart, disturbs the activity of qi. So when frightened, the main

（四）思则气结

思为脾之志,思虑过度则导致脾气郁结,运化功能障碍,从而出现脘腹胀满、食欲不振、大便溏薄等症。久思不解,阴血暗耗,心神失养,则出现心悸、健忘、失眠、多梦等症。

（五）悲则气消

悲为肺之志,过悲可使肺气消减。凡悲哀至极,肺气过于敛肃,宣发输布失职,营卫不能布散,胸中大气(宗气)于是耗损。故悲哀伤肺者,常见头昏、乏力、精神不振等症。

（六）恐则气下

恐为肾之志,大恐则令肾气过度下沉,固摄无权,气泄于下,导致二便失禁;或精失所藏,而致骨酸痿厥、遗精等症。恐惧日久不解,气机不能升发,脏腑功能减退,正气不能卫外,也易感受各种外邪而发病。

（七）惊则气乱

惊与恐可由相似的外界刺激因素所引起,但二者在脏腑气机上的反应有明显区别。恐生于肾,导致气机下行;惊生于心,引起气机紊乱。因此,人受

responses are disorder of heart-qi, derangement of the mind, indecision and bewilderment. Disorder of the activity of qi damages the harmony between qi and blood and weakens the defensive qi, leading to invasion of pathogenic factors into the body and occurrence of disease.

5.2.3 Causing or aggravating certain diseases

Emotional factors can cause certain diseases. For example, people with frequent superabundance of liver-yang tend to flare into violent rage which brings on violent hyperactivity of liver-yang, leading to sudden dizziness and syncope or unconsciousness, paralysis and distorted face. Besides, certain diseases may become aggravated or worsened because of abnormal changes of emotions. For example, the heart disease can be caused and quickly worsened by sudden terror.

5.3 Improper diet

Diet is indispensable to human existence and is the main route for human being to obtain nutrient substances from the natural world. However, the intake of food has to follow certain rules. If the diet is improper, it may impair the body and become pathogenic factors.

Improper diet includes three aspects: starvation and overeating, unhygienic food and food partiality.

5.3.1 Starvation and overeating

Starvation refers to two different things: prolonged

惊吓之时,主要反应为心气紊乱,神无所主,虑无所定,不知所措。由于气机紊乱,于是气血不调,卫外不固,邪气便能乘虚而入,导致疾病的发生。

三、引发或加重某些疾病

情志因素可引发某些疾病。如素体肝阳偏亢者,若遇事恼怒,肝阳暴张,可突发眩晕、昏厥,或昏仆不语,半身不遂,口眼歪斜等。某些疾病过程中,可因异常的情绪波动而使病情加重,或迅速恶化,如心脏病患者,可因突然受惊恐刺激而骤然发病,并迅速恶化。

第三节 饮食失宜

饮食是人类生存的必要条件,是人体从外界获得营养物质的主要方式。然而,饮食的摄取,应当遵循满足人体对营养素需求的正常进食规律,才能有益于健康。如果饮食失宜,反而会对人体造成伤害,而成为一种致病因素。

饮食失宜包括饥饱失度、饮食不洁、饮食偏嗜三个方面的内容。

一、饥饱失度

饥饱失度包括过饥和过

lack of food and protracted insufficient intake of food.

Prolonged lack of food cannot provide the body with enough nutrient substance, leading to insufficient production of qi and blood and sudden decline of the visceral functions with the manifestations of dizziness and lassitude of the four limbs or even death in severe cases. Protracted insufficient intake of food will lead to malnutrition, deficiency of qi and blood, weakness of the body , susceptibility to invasion of pathogenic factors and various diseases.

Overeating means two different things: crapulence and protracted excessive intake of food. Crapulence impairs the spleen and stomach because the food taken is beyond the normal functions of the spleen and stomach to digest, transport and transform, leading to gastric and abdominal distension and fullness, eructation with fetid and acid odor, anorexia, vomiting and diarrhea, etc. In severe cases the intestinal and gastric vessels and collaterals will be impaired, causing abdominal pain or hemorrhoid bleeding, etc. Protracted excessive intake of food will bring on supernutrition, delayed transformation of qi and failure of the nutrients of food and water to transform into qi and blood. Instead, the nutrients of food and water turn into phlegm and accumulate in the body to hinder the flow of qi and blood, leading to obesity, dizziness, palpitation and chest oppression; or transforming dampness into heat to invade the vessels and causing abscess, carbuncle, sores and ulcers, etc.

5.3.2 Unhygienic food

If food contains unhygienic elements, it will cause diseases. Usually unhygienic food can cause gastrointestinal

饱两个方面。

过饥有连续饥饿和长期摄食不足两种情况。在连续饥饿状态下，由于无法从饮食中获取充足的营养，气血生化乏源，脏腑功能骤然减退，会出现头昏目眩、四肢无力等症状，严重时可危及生命。长期摄食不足，营养不良，人体气血得不到足够的补充而逐渐亏虚，不但身体日渐衰弱，还容易感受其他邪气而继发多种疾病。

过饱有暴饮暴食和长期摄入过量两种情况。暴饮暴食，超过脾胃的承受能力，饮食不能正常地腐熟和运化，阻滞于中，反使脾胃受伤，出现脘腹胀满、嗳腐泛酸、厌食、吐泻等症，严重者可伤损肠胃脉络，引起腹痛或痔疮出血等症。长期摄入过量，营养过剩，气化不及，水谷精微不化气血，反变生痰饮而停聚于体内，阻碍气血运行，出现形体肥胖、头昏目眩、心悸胸闷等症；或酿湿蕴热，侵淫血脉，变生痈疽疔疮等。

二、饮食不洁

饮食中混有不洁之物，食之可使人致病。一般不洁之

disorders, such as abdominal pain, vomiting and diarrhea. If food is contaminated with parasitic ovum, it will cause various parasitic diseases. Putrid food is poisonous and can cause acute abdominal pain, vomiting and diarrhea if it is taken.

Unhygienic water is also a pathogenic factor. The natural source of water in a industrialized society is often contaminated with various poisonous or harmful elements. Drinking such water can also lead to various acute or chronic diseases due to water poisoning.

5.3.3   Food partiality

Normally people should take a variety of food in proper proportions in order to ensure a balanced nutrition. Protracted food partiality leads to insufficient intake of certain substances and excessive intake of other substances which will cause imbalance of visceral qi, blood, yin and yang.

There are two different cases in food partiality: partiality to cold or hot food and partiality to the five flavors.

1. Partiality to cold or hot food

Food is either cold and cool or warm and hot in property. It can be cooked or uncooked. Partiality to cold and cool food or excessive intake of uncooked and cold food will impair yang-qi in the spleen and the stomach, leading to endogenous cold-dampness and causing abdominal pain and diarrhea. Partiality to warm and dry food or excessive intake of hot food accumulates heat in the stomach and the intestines, leading to thirst, abdominal fullness, distension and pain, constipation or hemorrhoids, etc.

物主要引起腹痛、吐泻等胃肠道病症;若饮食中混有寄生虫卵,可引起各种寄生虫病;若食物已腐败变质,则有毒,食之可发生中毒症状,出现剧烈腹痛、吐泻等。

饮水不洁,也是重要致病因素之一。工业社会中的自然水源往往因受污染而混有多种有毒或有害物质,饮用这种水也会导致多种急性或慢性中毒性疾病。

三、饮食偏嗜

正常人的饮食应多品种均匀搭配,以保证营养的全面性。如果听任嗜好,长期偏食,就会形成某些营养物质摄入不足而另一些营养物质摄入过量,导致脏腑气血阴阳失调。

饮食偏嗜表现在两个方面,一是偏寒偏热,一是五味偏嗜。

1. 偏寒偏热

饮食物也有寒凉、温热之性,又有生冷、炙热之别,若偏好寒凉饮食,或过食生冷,可损伤脾胃阳气,导致寒湿内生,发生腹痛、泄泻等症;若偏喜温燥之物,或多食炙热,可使胃肠积热,出现口渴、腹满胀痛、便秘,或酿成痔疮等。

2. Partiality to the flavors

The five flavors are attributed to the five zang-organs respectively: the sour flavor enters the liver, the bitter flavor enters the heart, the sweet flavor enters the spleen, the acrid flavor enters the lung and the salty flavor enters the kidney. If the five flavors are not evenly contained in the food, the relationships among the five zang-organs will be broken. For example, partiality to the sour flavor strengthens liver-qi and weakens spleen-qi because predominant liver-qi will over restrict spleen-qi. Partiality to salty flavor consolidates kidney-qi and inhibits heart-qi because water restricts fire, leading to stagnation of the vessels. Partiality to the sweet flavor invigorates spleen-qi and restricts kidney-qi, making it difficult for the essence to produce marrow and transform blood, resulting in osteodynia, loss of hair and early senility. Partiality to bitter flavor makes heart-qi hyperactive and lung-qi hypoactive, leading to retention of food nutrients in the middle energizer and malnutrition of the skin and hair. Partiality to the acrid flavor makes lung-qi hyperactive and liver-qi hypoactive, leading to spasm or flaccidity of the tendons and vessels due to failure of the blood to nourish the tendons.

2. 五味偏嗜

五味与五脏各有归属，即酸味入肝，苦味入心，甘味入脾，辛味入肺，咸味入肾。若饮食中五味不均匀，五脏之间的关系就会失衡。如偏食酸味，肝气偏强，脾气就会因受肝气制约太过而日益衰竭；偏食咸味，肾气过强，水旺克火，心气受抑，血脉就会凝滞；偏食甘味，脾气偏盛，肾气受制，精不生髓、化血，于是骨痛、发落而早衰；偏食苦味，心气太盛，肺金受邪，宣发输布失职，水谷精微郁滞于中焦，皮毛却得不到滋养；偏食辛味，肺气偏盛，肝气受制，血不养筋，则筋脉拘急或弛缓无力，等等。

5.4　Overwork and over-rest

Work and rest are two activities indispensable to human existence. Normal work is helpful for the flow of qi and blood and strengthening the body. Necessary rest can eliminate fatigue and restore strength and vitality. Overwork and over-rest all lead to disease.

第四节　劳逸过度

劳，即劳动，包括各种劳作和运动。逸，指休息和静养。劳和逸都是人类生活的需要，两者不可缺一。正常的劳作和运动，有助于流通气血，增强体质；必要的休息和静养，可以消除疲劳，恢复体力和精神。如果过度劳累，或过度安逸，都会使人致病。

5.4.1 Overwork

Overwork covers three aspects: overstrain, over-work with the mind and excessive sexual activity.

Overstrain refers to protracted physical hard work, such as over physical work and over sports activity. Protracted physical hard work consumes great amount of qi and blood and causes disease if the energy and vitality are not supplemented and restored in time. Other activities, such as protracted standing, prolonged walking and speaking for a long time, also lead to overstrain.

Overwork with the mind refers to excessive contemplation that consumes heart-blood and causes asthenia disease. Overwork with the mind not only consumes heart-blood, but also impairs the spleen. So the symptoms caused by overwork with the mind are usually palpitation, amnesia, insomnia and dreaminess due to malnutrition of heart-spirit, often complicated by anorexia, abdominal distension and loose stool due to dysfunction of the spleen.

Normal sexual activity is helpful for the flow of qi and blood and the regulation of yin and yang. However, excessive sexual activity consumes kidney-essence, weakens qi and blood and malnourishes the five zang-organs, leading to early senility with the symptoms of aching and weakness of the waist and knees, dizziness and tinnitus, dispiritedness, or impotence, seminal emission and premature ejaculation due to kidney deficiency.

5.4.2 Over-rest

Over-rest means lack of enough activity. Protracted lack of enough activity will lead to slow movement of qi and blood, hypofuncton of the viscera, poor appetite, fatigue, dispiritedness, weakness of the four limbs or obesity, intolerance to work, palpitation, asthma and sweating

一、过劳

过劳,包括劳力过度、劳神过度和房劳过度三个方面。

劳力过度,指长时间过度用力,如体力劳动过度、运动过度等,气血消耗太过,得不到及时补充和恢复,从而积劳成疾。诸如久立、久行、言语过久等所致损伤,也属劳力过度。

劳神过度,指用心思虑太过,耗伤心血,导致虚损性疾病。凡劳神太过,不仅心血耗伤,而且思虑则伤脾,故一方面表现为心神失养的心悸、健忘、失眠、多梦,同时多兼有脾不健运的纳呆、腹胀、便溏等症。

房劳过度,即房事过度。夫妇间正常的房事,可以通行气血,调和阴阳。但房事太多,肾精耗损过度,气血也随之衰弱,五脏失养,导致早衰,出现腰膝酸软、眩晕耳鸣、精神委靡,或阳痿、遗精、早泄等肾亏之症。

二、过逸

过逸,主要指运动太少。长期过度安逸,缺少锻炼,气血运行迟缓,脏腑功能减退,使人食少乏力,精神不振,肢体软弱,或发胖臃肿,不耐劳

when moving. Prolonged lack of activity will give rise to the production of phlegm, dampness and blood stasis inside the body and invasion of pathogenic wind, cold and dampness from the outside, eventually binging on various diseases.

动,动则心悸、气喘及汗出等。日久痰湿、瘀血生于内,风寒湿邪袭于外,可继发多种疾病。

5.5　Diseases caused by phlegm, rheum and blood stasis

Phlegm and blood stasis are pathological substances produced during the course of disease due to certain pathogenic factors. They may directly or indirectly affect the viscera and the body, leading to secondary disease. So phlegm and blood stasis are both pathological substances and pathogenic factors. Since they have resulted from primary disease, they are called secondary pathogenic factors.

5.5.1　Phlegm and rheum

5.5.1.1　The basic concept of phlegm and rheum

Phlegm is a pathological substance caused by disturbance of body fluid. Generally speaking, the thick part is called phlegm while the thin part is called rheum.

Phlegm is either substantial or insubstantial. Substantial phlegm is visible, palpable and audible, such as sputum, scrofula and nodules in the skin and muscles and borborygmus. Insubstantial phlegm is invisible, unpalpable and inaudible. But there are pathological manifestations of phlegm. Substantial phlegm is identical with insubstantial phlegm in nature. When accumulating, it is

第五节　痰饮、瘀血致病

痰饮和瘀血是人体受某种致病因素作用后在疾病过程中所形成的病理产物。这些病理产物形成之后,又能直接或间接作用于人体脏腑或形体,导致继发性疾病。所以,痰饮、瘀血既是病理产物,又是致病因素。因其继发于原发疾病之后,故称其为继发病因。

一、痰饮

(一)痰饮的基本概念

痰饮是人体津液代谢障碍所形成的病理产物。一般以较稠浊的称为痰,较清稀的称为饮。

痰饮分为有形之痰饮和无形之痰饮。有形之痰饮是指视之可见、触之可及、闻之有声的实质性痰饮,如咯吐所出之痰液,皮肤肌肉间形成的瘰疬、痰核及腹中有辘辘水声等。无形之痰饮是指视之不

substantial; when dispersing, it is insubstantial.

Jingui Yaolüe (*Synopsis of Golden Chamber*) classifies rheum into four categories according to their location, namely phlegmatic rheum in the abdomen, suspending rheum in the chest and diaphragm, sustaining rheum in the rib-sides and overflowing rheum in the skin and muscles.

Phlegm, rheum, water and dampness are all pathological substances caused by disturbance of body fluid. But they are different from each other. The one that spreads and appears substantial is dampness; the one that accumulates and appears substantial is rheum; the one that is thin and clear is water; the rheum that is condensed is phlegm. That is to say that all of them result from disturbance of body fluid and can transform into each other.

5.5.1.2 The formation of phlegm and rheum

Phlegm and rheum are caused by disturbance of body fluid involving the spleen, the lung, the kidney, the liver and triple energizer. Various pathogenic factors, including the six abnormal climatic factors, internal impairment due to seven emotions, improper diet, overwork and over-rest, can impair the viscera and affect qi-transformation, leading to disturbance of body fluid and the production of phlegm and rheum due to the accumulation of body fluid.

The spleen governs the transportation and transformation of water and dampness, the lung regulates the water passage, the kidney governs water, the liver promotes

见、触之无物、闻之无声的非实质性痰饮,虽无形质可见,却有因痰饮所致的病理表现。有形之痰饮与无形之痰饮本质是相同的,差别在于聚之则有形,散之则无形。

《金匮要略》把饮分为四类,即痰饮、悬饮、溢饮、支饮。这是根据饮邪所在部位不同而规定的名称。如饮停于腹中名"痰饮",饮悬于胸膈名"悬饮",饮支撑两胁名"支饮",饮溢于肌肤名"溢饮"。

痰、饮、水、湿四者都是津液代谢障碍所形成的病理产物,但相互之间有一定区别。其弥漫无形者为湿气,停聚有形者为水饮;饮之更清稀者为水,饮之煎炼而成者为痰。也就是说,四者皆源于津液代谢障碍,并可互相转化。

(二)痰饮的形成

痰饮皆由津液代谢障碍所致,涉及到脾、肺、肾、肝、三焦等多个脏腑。各种致病因素,如外感六淫、内伤七情、饮食失宜、劳逸失当等,都可损伤脏腑,使其气化功能失常,津液代谢障碍,停聚而成痰饮。

因脾主运化水湿,肺主通调水道,肾主水,肝主疏泄能促进津液代谢,三焦为水道,

the metabolism of body fluid and the triple energizer serves as the water passage. The disorder of any of these organs will lead to retention of body fluid and accumulate dampness into phlegm and rheum which then affect the viscera and impair their functions, leading to repeated production of phlegm and rheum. For example, accumulation of phlegm and dampness in the lung causes cough and asthma which are clinically attributed to the deficiency of the spleen. That is why the ancient people believed that "the spleen is the source of phlegm and the lung is the container of phlegm".

The production of phlegm and rheum is also related to cold and heat which are either exogenous or endogenous due to disharmony of visceral yin and yang. If there is cold in the viscera, the activity of qi-transformation will be slowed down and the transformation of body fluid will be difficult, giving rise to the production of phlegm and rheum, especially rheum. If there is heat in the viscera, it will scorch or coagulate body fluid into phlegm. If there is heat in the viscera, it scorches body fluid into either rheum or phlegm, frequently condensing into phlegm. If there is cold in the lung, it will retain rheum in the lung and cause frothy and thin sputum, known as "retention of cold rheum in the lung". If there is heat in the lung, it will block phlegm in the lung and cause yellowish, thick and purulent sputum, known as "accumulation of phlegm-heat in the lung".

5.5.1.3　The characteristics of phlegm and rheum in causing diseases

1. Hindering the flow of qi and blood

Phlegm and rheum can flow with qi to anywhere. If phlegm and rheum flow in the meridians, they tend to block the meridians and hinder the flow of qi and blood,

若脾失健运,或肺失通调,或肾不主水,或肝失疏泄,或三焦气化失常,使水湿不化,津液停聚,皆可聚湿而成痰饮。痰饮形成以后,又可在脏腑之间相互影响,进而使多个脏腑气化失常,导致痰饮的反复形成。如痰湿蕴肺而致咳嗽、气喘,临床多责之于脾虚,故古人有"脾为生痰之源,肺为贮痰之器"的说法。

痰饮的形成还与寒热因素有关。寒热可由外感而得,也可由脏腑阴阳失调所致。脏腑有寒,则气化迟滞,津液不化,形成痰饮,而以饮为多;脏腑有热,则煎熬津液,津液或沸腾为饮,或凝结为痰,而以痰为多。如肺寒可致饮停于肺,咳吐清稀泡沫痰液,称为"寒饮伏肺";肺热可致痰阻于肺,咳吐黄稠脓痰,称为"痰热蕴肺"等。

(三) 痰饮致病的特点

痰饮致病有以下特点。
1. 阻碍经脉气血运行
痰饮随气流行,无所不至。若痰饮流注于经络,易使经络阻滞,气血运行不畅,出现肢体

leading to numbness and inflexibility of the limbs, or even paralysis. If accumulating in local areas, they frequently cause scrofula, subcutaneous nodules and cold abscess.

2. Hindering the ascent and descent of qi

Phlegm and rheum result from water and dampness. Retention of phlegm and rheum in the viscera tends to hinder the activity of qi and prevent visceral qi from ascending and descending. Take the lung for example. The normal function of lung-qi is to depurate and descend. Retention of phlegm and rheum in the lung will lead to chest oppression, cough and dyspnea, etc. Take the stomach for another example. The normal function of the stomach-qi is to descend. Retention of phlegm and rheum in the stomach will cause nausea and vomiting, etc.

3. Frequently confusing the mind

If phlegm disturbs the upper and blends lucid yang, it will lead to dizziness; if phlegm confuses the mind or phlegm-fire disturbs the heart, it will cause chest oppression, palpitation, unconsciousness and delirium or mania, etc.

4. Complicated symptoms and constant change

Since phlegm and rheum are caused by various factors, involve many parts of the body and flow to anywhere with qi, the diseases caused by them are various, involving many viscera and tissues and marked by complicated symptoms and constant change. Clinically the diseases caused by phlegm and rheum may involve the five zang-organs and six fu-organs, the body, the sensory organs, the orifices, the four limbs and the skeleton. The symptoms are chest oppression, cough, asthma, expectoration, nausea, vomiting, palpitation, dizziness, mania, numbness of the limbs, arthralgia or swelling of joints, subcutaneous swelling or suppuration, edema, ascites and diarrhea, etc. Generally speaking, obstinate disease and disease

麻木、屈伸不利,甚至半身不遂等。若结聚于局部,可形成瘰疬痰核、阴疽流注等。

2. 阻滞脏腑气机升降

痰饮为水湿所聚,若停滞于脏腑,易于阻遏气机,使脏腑气机升降失常。如肺以肃降为顺,若痰饮停肺,肺失宣肃,可出现胸闷、咳嗽、喘促等症;胃以降为和,痰饮停胃,胃失和降,则出现恶心呕吐等症。

3. 易于蒙蔽神明

痰浊上扰,蒙蔽清阳,可致头昏目眩;痰迷心窍,或痰火扰心,心神被蒙,可致胸闷心悸、神昏谵妄,或引起癫狂惊痫等。

4. 症状复杂,变化多端

由于痰饮形成的原因多,痰饮关联部位广,并且能随气升降,上下内外无所不至,故痰饮所致疾病种类多,影响脏腑组织也多,症状极为复杂,且变化多端。从临床表现来看,五脏六腑、形体官窍、四肢百骸,皆可因痰饮而致病,其症状表现如胸闷、咳嗽、气喘、咯痰、恶心、呕吐、心悸、眩晕、癫狂、肢体麻木、关节疼痛或肿胀、皮下肿块或溃破流脓,以及水肿、腹水、泄泻等。凡

without evident cause are all related to phlegm and rheum. That is why it was believed in ancient times that "strange diseases are mostly caused by phlegm" and "many diseases are exclusively caused by phlegm".

Since phlegm and rheum can ascend and descend with qi, the disease caused by them is usually marked by constant change and recurrence. Take epilepsy for example. It attacks when phlegm ascends with qi and stops when phlegm descends with qi.

5.5.2　Blood stasis

5.5.2.1　The basic concept of blood stasis

Blood stasis is a kind of pathological substance caused by disturbance of blood circulation. Normally the blood is propelled by heart-qi to flow in the vessels. If blood circulation is stagnated or slowed down by certain factors, it will lead to retention of blood in the vessels or viscera or overflow of blood out of the vessels, causing blood stasis.

Blood stasis is substantial pathological substance, such as clot in the blood, subcutaneous purpura or lump in the body. Sometimes blood stasis is insubstantial, referring to certain symptoms related to blood stasis, such as various kinds of pain, palpitation and mania, etc.

Blood stasis and blood stagnation are two different concepts. The former is a kind of pathological substance while the latter is a pathological process. The former is the result of the latter while the latter inevitably leads to the former.

5.5.2.2　The formation of blood stasis

There are various factors responsible for blood sta-

种种疑难杂病、不明原因疾病,都可能与痰饮有关,所以古人有"怪病多痰"、"百病多由痰作祟"的说法。

由于痰饮可以随气升降,故其病证往往容易变化,呈反复发作性。如癫痫病,痰随气升则病发,痰随气降则病止,反复多次。

二、瘀血

(一)瘀血的基本概念

瘀血,是由血液运行障碍所产生的一种病理产物。正常血液由心气推动着在血脉中不停地运行,若因某种原因导致血液停滞,或血行迟缓,阻滞于经脉或脏腑,或离经之血存积体内,皆称为瘀血。

瘀血作为一种病理产物,可以是有形的,如出血中带有瘀血块,或皮下出现紫斑,或体内形成肿块等;也可以是无形的,只是出现一些与瘀血有关的症状,如多种疼痛、心悸、狂躁等。

瘀血与血瘀的概念不同,瘀血是一种病理产物,而血瘀则是一个病理过程。血瘀的过程可以产生瘀血,瘀血必然是血瘀病理过程的产物。

(二)瘀血的形成

瘀血形成的原因很多。

sis. It may be caused by six exogenous climatic factors. For example, cold stagnates and tends to block blood vessels. It may be caused by seven emotions. For example, anxiety binds qi and tends to slow down blood circulation. It may be caused by consumptive disease and overstrain. The following is a brief description of the causes of blood stasis:

1. Qi stagnation

Blood circulates with qi. If qi stagnates, it will inevitably lead to blood stasis. Blood stasis results from inhibited blood circulation caused by hindrance of qi activity due to exogenous cold and dampness or agglomeration of qi due to excessive anxiety or failure of liver-qi to disperse or unsmooth flow of qi due to internal blockage of phlegm. For example, protracted stagnation of liver-qi and blood vessels will bring on mass with the manifestations of hypochondriac pain and palpable lumps.

2. Qi deficiency

Qi is the commander of blood. Deficiency of qi makes it difficult for qi to propel the blood, eventually causing blood stasis. Various factors are responsible for qi deficiency and blood stasis, such as hypofunction of the viscera, consumptive disease, overstrain, improper diet, protracted disease or puerperium. Patients with protracted disease usually suffer from deficiency of qi and unsmooth blood circulation. General treatment is often ineffective. The proper treatment should focus on supplementing qi to promote blood circulation.

3. Blood-cold

Blood flows with warmth and coagulates with cold. Blood-cold usually slows down blood circulation and causes blood stasis. Various factors are responsible for blood-cold and blood stasis, such as invasion of exogenous cold in the vessels, damage of yang-qi due to predominant dampness,

有外感六淫所致者,如寒性凝滞,可使血脉瘀滞;有内伤七情所致者,如忧思气结,可使血行迟缓;也有虚损、劳伤等因素所致者。归纳起来,瘀血的形成机理有以下几个方面。

1. 气滞

血随气行,气滞则血瘀,可导致瘀血。外感寒、湿阴邪,阻碍气机运行;或忧思气结,肝气失疏;或痰浊内阻,气机不畅等,皆可使血行受阻而形成瘀血。如肝气郁滞,血脉瘀滞,日久则形成癥积,出现胁下疼痛,可触及坚硬肿块等。

2. 气虚

气为血帅,气虚则推动无力,血行迟缓,而形成瘀血。凡脏腑功能减退,或虚损劳伤,或饮食失调,或久病,或产后,皆可导致气虚,而形成瘀血。如久病之人,往往气虚,血行不畅,所以一般治疗不易收效,必须补气以行血,待气血畅旺,方能祛邪外出,促使疾病痊愈。

3. 血寒

血液得温则行,得寒则凝。若血中有寒,则血行迟缓,从而形成瘀血。外感寒邪侵淫血脉;或湿盛日久损伤阳气;或命门火衰,元阳不足;或

decline of fire in the life gate, insufficiency of primordial yang and stagnation of cold in the vessels due to excessive intake of cold food. Invasion of cold in the uterus will stagnate uterine vessels, leading to lower abdominal pain during menstruation, purplish menses or menses with blood clot, or delayed menstruation or amenorrhea, etc.

4. Blood-heat

Blood flows with warmth. But there is excessive heat, it will drive the blood to overflow and cause blood stasis. If heat is mingled with the blood, it will consume body fluid and condense the blood into stasis. Take taiyang syndrome of blood accumulation in *Shanghan Lun* for example. It is caused by blood and heat mingled in the lower abdomen with the symptoms of acute abdominal agglomeration and mania. So this syndrome should be treated by Taohe Chengji Decoction for activating blood to resolve stasis and promoting defecation to eliminate stasis and heat.

5. Traumatic injury

Apart from damaging the tendons, bones and muscles, traumatic injury also impairs the vessels and causes blood stasis. That is why traumatic injury is often accompanied by local hematoma which is a sign of blood stasis. If traumatic injury drives blood to flow out of the vessels and accumulate in the body, it will also cause blood stasis.

6. Hemorrhage

Blood cannot flow with qi if it flows out of the vessels. If the blood that flows out of the vessels is not eliminated and accumulates in local areas, it becomes blood stasis. There are various factors responsible for hemorrhage, such as qi deficiency, failure of the spleen to command blood, failure of the liver to store blood, abnormal flow of blood due to heat, disturbance of blood due to fire transforming from the five emotions and traumatic injury, etc.

过食寒凉,血脉寒滞等,皆可使血寒而致瘀血。如女子寒阻胞宫,血脉瘀滞,可见经行少腹疼痛,经色紫黑或挟有瘀血块,或经期延后,或经闭不来等,都与瘀血有关。

4. 血热

血液得温则行,但温热太过,则血热妄行,造成离经之血积存体内,而形成瘀血;或血与热结,阴津耗伤,血液凝结而成瘀血。如《伤寒论》所述太阳蓄血证,即是血热互结于少腹,而致少腹急结,神志错乱如狂,故用桃核承气汤活血化瘀,通下瘀热。

5. 外伤

外伤除了能损伤筋骨肌肉外,也可损伤血脉,形成瘀血,故外伤患者一般都有局部血肿,是瘀血的特征表现。若外伤出血,血液离经而积存于体内,也形成瘀血。

6. 出血

血液离经,便不能再随气运行。离经之血若未能排出体外,停积于局部,就成为瘀血。导致出血的原因很多,如气虚出血、脾不统血、肝不藏血、血热妄行、五志化火动血、外伤出血等。

5.5.2.3 The characteristics of blood stasis in causing diseases

The manifestations of diseases caused by blood stasis are various. The following are the common ones.

1. Pain

It is marked by stabbing, fixed and unpapable pain that turns worse at night. If it is caused by blood stasis due to protracted disease and deficiency of qi and blood, the pain is vague and lingering.

2. Lump

Protracted blood stasis gradually develops into lumps which appear hard and fixed. If the lumps are subcutaneous, the skin usually turns cyanotic. If the lumps are in the viscera, hard mass will be caused.

3. Hemorrhage

Hemorrhage can lead to blood stasis. If blood stasis is retained in the vessels, the impairment caused is very hard to heal and tends to bring on repeated hemorrhage. In this case blood stasis becomes the cause of hemorrhage which can only be stopped by activating blood to resolve stasis to repair the injured vessels. Hemorrhage caused by blood stasis often appears cyanotic and accompanied by blood clot.

4. Cyanosis

The patient with blood stasis is characterized by cyanotic complexion, lips and nails.

5. Tongue variations

The tongue is cyanotic or has ecchymosis and petechia.

6. Pulse variations

The pulse is thin, unsmooth, deep and taut, or knotted or slow regular intermittent.

Besides, there are still some other commonly

（三）瘀血致病的特点

瘀血致病的表现很多,归纳起来主要有以下共同特点。

1. 导致疼痛

主要表现为刺痛,痛处固定不移,拒按,夜间痛甚。若因久病、气血虚衰而致瘀血疼痛,可表现为隐痛绵绵。

2. 形成肿块

瘀血日久,凝结不化,逐渐形成肿块。瘀血所致肿块,质地坚硬,固定不移。肿块在体表,可见皮色青紫;肿块在内脏,则形成癥积,坚硬如石。

3. 引起出血

出血可导致瘀血,瘀血阻于损伤的血络,则其损伤不能愈合,可导致反复出血。此时瘀血成了出血的原因,必须活血化瘀,使损伤的血络得到修复,出血才可治愈。瘀血所致出血,其血色紫暗,常伴有血块。

4. 出现紫绀

瘀血患者可见面色、口唇、爪甲呈青紫色。

5. 舌质变化

舌质可呈紫暗色,或出现瘀点、瘀斑。

6. 脉象变化

脉象细、涩、沉、弦,或出现结、代脉。

此外,面色黧黑、肌肤甲

encountered symptoms, such as blackish complexion, squamous and dry skin, purpura on the skin, amnesia and mania, etc.

Apart from the points mentioned above, clinically blood stasis is diagnosed with the consideration of the following points.

(1) If there are traumatic injury, hemorrhage and history of menstruation, pregnancy and labor, the patient tends to have internal retention of blood stasis.

(2) If the treatment is ineffective before the application of the therapy for activating blood to resolve stasis, the patient must have insubstantial blood stasis though there are no signs of blood stasis.

(3) Protracted disease involving the collaterals often causes blood stasis. If it is lingering, blood stasis has to be taken into consideration.

The above three points are the supplementary methods for diagnosing blood stasis.

错、皮肤紫癜、善忘狂躁等也是瘀血的常见症状。

临床上判断是否有瘀血存在,除了根据上述瘀血的致病特点外,还可从以下几点加以分析:① 发病有外伤、出血、经胎产史者,多有瘀血内积。② 虽无瘀血特征,但未用活血化瘀法前屡治无效者,可能是一种无形的瘀血证。③ 久病入络,多有瘀血,若久治不愈,应考虑瘀血的存在。此三点可作为判断瘀血证的辅助方法。

6 Pathogenesis

Pathogenesis studies how pathogenic factors affect the human body and cause disease as well as how disease develops and changes.

6.1 Causes of disease

Disease means the damage of health. TCM believes that the healthy state implies the balance of yin and yang, the manifestation of which is high coordination and unity between the viscera, the meridians, qi, blood and body fluid as well as the body and the external environment. If such a state of high coordination and unity is broken by various pathogenic factors, disease will be caused. The occurrence of disease is actually concerned with pathogenic factors and healthy qi (body resistance). Besides, constitution is also an important factor responsible for the occurrence of disease.

第六章　病机

病机,指疾病发生、发展与变化的机理。疾病发生的机理,即发病机理,研究致病因素作用于人体而引起疾病的机理;疾病发展变化的机理,简称病变机理,研究疾病形成的内在本质及其传变的机理。

第一节　发病机理

发病机理,也称"发病机制"、"发病原理"。

人体在发病前应当是健康的,疾病就是对健康的否定。中医发病学认为,所谓健康状态,其本质即是阴阳平衡,表现为人体各脏腑、经络、气血津液之间,以及人体与环境之间的高度协调与统一。如果在各种致病因素的作用下,这种高度的协调与统一状态被破坏,就会发生疾病。疾病的发生,实际上关系到邪气(病因)与正气(抗病能力)两个基本方面,不同的体质对发病也有重要影响。

6.1.1　Occurrence of disease and the relationship between pathogenic factors and the healthy qi

The occurrence of disease is a very complicated process of mutual struggle between pathogenic factors and the healthy qi.

6.1.1.1　Deficiency of healthy qi and invasion of pathogenic factors: two important aspects of the occurrence of disease

The healthy qi, one kind of qi that constitutes the body and maintains life activities, exists in all the internal organs and meridians and ensures their normal functions. When pathogenic factors attack the body, healthy qi fights against pathogenic factors and protects the body. That is why it is literally called "righteous qi" in TCM.

Only when healthy qi is superabundant can it fight against pathogenic factors. The state of healthy qi is decided by the congenital kidney-qi and the acquired gastro-splenic qi. Since essence, blood, body fluid, yin and yang can transform into each other, they directly influence the state of the healthy qi. If healthy qi is insufficient, the body resistance will be weakened, giving rise to the invasion of pathogenic factors.

一、邪正与发病

疾病的发生是一个极其复杂的过程,但其本质在于邪气与正气的相互斗争,邪正斗争贯穿于疾病过程的始终。

(一)正虚、邪侵是发病的两个重要因素

疾病的发生必须具备两个条件,一是正气不足,二是邪气侵袭。

正气,是相对于邪气而言的,实际上它就是构成人体和维持人体生命活动的基本物质之一的"气",它广泛存在于人体脏腑经络之中,一般情况下发挥着维持脏腑经络正常功能的作用。当邪气侵袭人体时,这种"气"又担负着抗御邪气、保卫人体的作用,故也称其为"正气"。

正气必须保持充盛,才能抗御邪气的侵袭。正气的充盛与否,取决于气的生成,即先天肾气和后天脾胃之气是否强盛。由于气与精、血、津液、阴、阳之间存在着相互化生的关系,所以这些物质的充足与否也直接影响着正气的盛衰。如果正气不足,人体抵抗邪气的能力下降,邪气即易

Pathogenic factors, the factors that directly disturb the normal physiological functions of the body, include six abnormal climatic factors, pestilence, abnormal changes of the seven emotions, improper diet, overwork, over-rest, phlegm, rheum and blood stasis, etc.

The occurrence of disease results from invasion of pathogenic factors into the body and struggle between pathogenic factors and the healthy qi. The invasion of pathogenic factors into the body is exclusively caused by insufficiency of the healthy qi. Since pathogenic factors can only attack the body when healthy qi is deficient, they are called "deficient pathogenic factors". The combination of "deficient pathogenic factors" with the deficiency of healthy qi is prerequisite to the occurrence of disease, which is described in *Huangdi Neijing* as "when two conditions of deficiency combine with each other, pathogenic factors begin to attack the body".

6.1.1.2 The effect of healthy qi and pathogenic factors on the occurrence of disease

Insufficiency of healthy qi and invasion of pathogenic factors are two important elements in causing disease. However, their role in causing disease is different. TCM believes that insufficiency of healthy qi is the intrinsic cause of disease while invasion of pathogenic factors is an important condition for the occurrence of disease.

1. Insufficiency of healthy qi: the intrinsic cause of disease

TCM pays great attention to the role of healthy qi in causing disease. It believes that normal visceral functions, superabundance of healthy qi, exuberance of qi and blood, and compactness of the defensive qi will prevent pathogenic factors from invading the body. That is why

于侵袭人体而导致发病。

邪气是直接干扰人体正常生理功能的因素,包括六淫、疫疠、七情致病、饮食所伤、劳逸失当、痰饮、瘀血等。

疾病的发生,是邪气侵入人体,与正气相互斗争的结果。邪气之所以能侵入人体,与人体正气的不足有密切关系。由于邪气只有在正气虚弱时才能侵袭人体,故中医学把这种邪气称为"虚邪"。虚邪与人体正气之虚相合,是疾病产生的两个必要条件,所以《黄帝内经》有"两虚相得,乃客其形"的理论。

(二)正气与邪气在发病过程中的不同作用

虽然正气不足与邪气侵袭是发病的两个重要因素,但邪气与正气在发病过程中所起的作用是不同的。中医学认为,正气不足是发病的内在根据,邪气侵袭是发病的重要条件。

1. 正气不足是发病的内在根据

中医发病学非常重视人体正气的作用,认为若内脏功能正常,正气旺盛,气血充盈,卫外固密,病邪难以侵入,疾病就无从发生。所以,《黄帝

Huangdi Neijing says that "with sufficient healthy qi inside the body, pathogenic factors will have no way to invade the body". Only when healthy qi becomes deficient and the defensive qi is weakened can pathogenic factors invade the body, leading to disorder of yin and yang in the body, disturbance of the visceral functions and occurrence of disease. That is why *Huangdi Neijing* says that "if pathogenic factors invade the body, qi in the body must be deficient." Obviously TCM emphasizes the role of healthy qi in causing disease.

Insufficiency of healthy qi is responsible for invasion of pathogenic factors into the body. However, insufficiency of healthy qi manifests in different ways, including general insufficiency and local insufficiency as well as constant insufficiency and temporary insufficiency. General insufficiency usually leads to general disease or transmission of pathogenic factors from local region to other areas. Local insufficiency leads to local disease that will not be transmitted to other areas. Constant insufficiency is usually marked by weak constitution that gives rise to frequent invasion of pathogenic factors and frequent occurrence of disease. Temporary insufficiency is usually due to fatigue, hunger, mental impairment, sexual intercourse, menstruation and labor, though the constitution is usually strong.

Pathological changes may vary due to different degrees of insufficiency of healthy qi and invasion of pathogenic factors. Generally speaking, pathological changes are serious if insufficiency of healthy qi is severe and

内经》有"正气存内,邪不可干"的论述。只有在人体正气相对虚弱,卫外不固,抗邪无力的情况下,邪气方能乘虚而入,使人体阴阳失调,脏腑功能紊乱,从而导致发病。故《黄帝内经》又说:"邪之所凑,其气必虚。"这可以看出,中医学强调正气在发病中的主导地位。

正气不足导致邪气侵袭有不同情况,既有整体正气不足者,也有局部正气虚弱者;既有一贯正气不足者,也有暂时正气虚弱者。整体正气不足者,感邪后易导致全身性疾病;或邪气先侵犯局部,然后向其他部位传变,病变范围容易扩展。局部正气虚弱者,邪气主要侵犯虚弱之处而形成局部性病变,一般不易向别处传变。一贯正气不足者,体质较弱,邪气侵入机会多,发病机会也多。暂时正气虚弱者,平时体质尚好,若遇疲劳、饥饿、精神创伤、房事后、妇女经期、分娩等情形,即可出现一时性正气虚弱。此时若养护得法,可免受邪气侵袭;稍有不慎,邪气就会乘虚而入。

正气不足程度不同,所感邪气轻重不一,感邪后引起的病理反应强弱也不一。一般地说,正气虚弱较甚者,感邪

pathological changes are mild if insufficiency of healthy qi is light. The state of pathological changes is related to the struggle between healthy qi and pathogenic factors. If insufficiency of healthy qi is severe, it will be weak in fighting against pathogenic factors, leading to deficiency syndrome or syndrome of deficiency mingled with excess. If insufficiency of healthy qi is not very serious, it will be strong enough to fight against pathogenic factors, usually leading to excess syndrome due to severe struggle between healthy qi and pathogenic factors.

2. Invasion of pathogenic factors: an important condition for the occurrence of disease

Apart from emphasizing the role of healthy qi in causing disease, TCM also pays great attention to the role of pathogenic factors. Generally speaking, people with insufficient healthy qi only have clinical symptoms when they have been attacked by pathogenic factors. Pathogenic factors may dominate the occurrence of disease under certain conditions, such as high temperature, high-pressure electric current, chemical poison, wound caused by gun and bite by poisonous snake, etc. Take pestilence for example. It is also an important element in causing disease, usually leading to widely spreading disease. These pathogenic factors are usually hard to avoid, even for those with superabundance of healthy qi. That is why TCM advocates the idea of "avoiding poisonous factors" in cultivating health.

The pathological changes are related to the nature of

较重;正气虚弱不甚者,感邪也较轻。感邪引起的病理反应强弱,与邪正斗争的激烈程度有关。凡正气不足较严重者,抗邪无力,其病理反应往往较弱,多形成虚证或虚实错杂证;正气不足不甚严重者,由于正气尚能奋起抗邪,邪正相争激烈,其病理反应也较强,多形成实证。

2. 邪气侵袭是发病的重要条件

中医学虽重视正气,强调正气在发病中的主导地位,但并不排斥邪气在发病中的重要作用。一般正气不足之人,在未感受邪气之时,可无疾病表现,只有当邪气侵袭之后,邪气与正气相争,才会表现出明显的疾病症状。也就是说,邪气侵袭是疾病发生的一个重要条件。在某些特殊情况下,邪气也可以在发病中起主导作用,如高温、高压电流、化学毒剂、枪弹杀伤、毒蛇咬伤等,即使是正气强盛之人,也不免被伤害而致病。又如疫病病邪,常常成为疾病发生的决定因素,因而导致疾病的大流行。因此,在注意保护和增强正气的同时,古代中医养生学也提出了"避其毒气"的预防思想。

邪气作为发病的重要条

pathogenic factors, the severity of the attack and the regions being attacked.

(1) The nature of pathogenic factors and the occurrence of disease: Pathogenic factors of different nature may lead to different diseases. For example, attack by pathogenic wind leads to wind syndrome, attack by pathogenic cold leads to cold syndrome, attack by pathogenic dampness leads to dampness syndrome and attack by pathogenic heat leads to heat syndrome. Pestilence is more serious than six abnormal climatic factors and often causes infectious disease marked by quick spreading, acute onset and severity of morbid condition.

(2) The severity of the attack of pathogenic factors and the occurrence of disease: Generally speaking, light attack causes mild disease because the struggle between healthy qi and pathogenic factors is mild; serious attack causes serious disease because the struggle between healthy qi and pathogenic factors is serious. Take wind attack for example. It may lead to cold attack and wind attack due to different degree of the attack. If the attack is severe, it causes cold attack; if the attack is mild, it causes wind attack.

(3) The region being attacked and the occurrence of disease: Invasion of pathogenic factors into different regions may cause different diseases. For example, invasion of pathogenic cold into the muscles and meridians may cause headache and pain of the four limbs; invasion of pathogenic cold into the lung may cause cough and asthma; and invasion of pathogenic cold into the stomach may cause stomachache and vomiting.

件还表现在,感邪后所导致的病理变化与邪气的性质、感邪轻重以及邪气作用的部位有关。

(1) 邪气性质对发病的影响:不同性质的邪气,可导致不同性质的疾病。如感受六淫邪气,各有不同的病证表现,感受风邪则形成风证,感受寒邪则形成寒证,感受湿邪则形成湿证,感受热邪则形成热证等等。疫疠之邪比一般六淫邪气毒性更强,所以疫疠致病往往传染性强,容易流行,且发病急骤,病情重笃。

(2) 感邪轻重对发病的影响:感邪后发病的轻重,既与正气的强弱有关,也与感邪的轻重有关。一般来说,感邪轻者,其邪正相争较缓和,故发病较轻;感邪重者,其邪正相争也激烈,故发病较重。如同属风邪袭人,因感邪轻重不一,其病则有伤寒和伤风之不同。感邪重而深者形成伤寒,感邪轻而浅者形成伤风。

(3) 邪气作用部位对发病的影响:邪气侵入人体的部位不同,所形成的病证反应也不同。如寒邪客于肌表经脉,则头身四肢疼痛;寒邪袭肺,则咳嗽、气喘;寒邪犯胃,则脘痛、呕吐等。

6.1.2   Constitution and disease

Constitution is closely related to pathogenesis. That is why TCM pays great attention to constitutional factors.

6.1.2.1   The definition of constitution

Constitution is formed before birth and can be improved after birth. It is stable and also changeable.

Theoretically, constitution is the manifestation of the functional state of the internal organs, demonstrating the condition of qi, blood, yin and yang in the body. The body resistance in fighting against pathogenic factors is the specific manifestation of constitution in pathogenesis.

Temperament, a concept related to constitution, is a special response of constitution in psychology. Different constitution pairs with different temperament and vice versa.

6.1.2.2   The formation of constitution

Congenital essence is the base of constitution and decides the state of constitution. If constitution is different, its susceptibility to invasion of pathogenic factors is also different. Many hereditary or familial diseases all are related to the constitution of parents and their illness. Besides, the maternal nursing and care during pregnancy exerts great effect on the constitution of fetus.

二、体质与发病

体质与发病的关系非常密切,所以中医学历来重视人的体质因素。

(一)体质的定义

体质,指人的身体素质,它在先天基础上形成,在后天因素作用下也可逐渐改变,因而它既是相对稳定的,又是可变的。

从中医学理论上讲,体质的本质是人的脏腑器官的功能状态的表现,它反映了人体气血阴阳的盛衰状况。抗邪能力的强弱,是体质因素在发病中的表现。

与体质相关联的一个概念是"气质"。气质实际上是体质在心理上的一种特殊反应。不同的体质往往有与之相对应的气质表现,每一种气质类型,实质上都是以某种体质为其基础的。

(二)体质的形成

体质形成的基础秉承于父母的先天精气,中医将此称之为"禀赋"。凡禀赋强者体质也强壮,禀赋弱者体质也虚弱。体质强弱不等,对邪气的易感性差异就很大。许多遗传性或家族性疾病都与父母的身体素质及其患病情况有关。同时,母体怀孕期间的养护对

After birth, the base of constitution is fixed and usually unchangeable. In this sense, the congenital base of constitution influences the whole life of a person. However, the living state after birth also influences constitution. TCM holds that the cultivation of health after birth can accumulate essence to improve constitution, making strong constitution stronger and weak constitution better. On the contrary, lack of proper cultivation of health after birth may make strong constitution weaker and weak constitution worse or fatal. Of course the change of constitution is a slow process.

Specific immunity obtained from illness or vaccination is an important way to develop a certain kind of special constitution.

6.1.2.3 The classification of constitution

Constitution varies from person to person and the study of such a variation is helpful for expounding pathogenesis.

Constitution is generally classified into two categories: strong constitution and weak constitution. For thor-

胎儿体质的形成也有重要影响,所以中医学历来重视养胎。

婴儿出生后,其先天的体质基础已经形成,一般是不易改变的。从这个意义上讲,先天的体质基础可以影响人的一生。但是,后天的生活状况无疑会影响已经形成的体质。中医学认为,后天的诸多养生方法可以"积精全神",更充分地发挥先天的体质优势,或弥补先天的体质不足,从而达到增强体质的目的。这样,先天体质强者可以更强,先天体质弱者可以由弱转强。反之,若不注意养生,先天体质强者会由强变弱或过早衰竭,先天体质弱者则更促其多病甚或夭折。当然,体质的改变是一个缓慢渐进的过程。

因感受某种病邪或经预防接种后可获得对某种疾病的特异免疫力,这是后天通过获得性方式形成某种特异体质的重要形式。

(三)体质的分类

中医体质学说认为,人类体质是有差异性的。对这种差异性进行研究,就形成了关于体质的分类理论。体质的分类对进一步阐明发病学原理具有重要意义。

一般情况下,人们常把体质划分为强、弱两类。为了更

oughly explaining the pathogenesis of various diseases, there are different ways to divide constitution in TCM, generally including classification according to yin and yang theory, classification according to five elements theory, classification according to the viscera, classification according to qi, blood and body fluid, and synthetic classification. These ways to classify constitution are complicated, the following is a brief introduction to some commonly encountered types of constitution.

详细地阐述各种不同性质的疾病发生的原理,中医体质学提出了更具体的体质分类法。

从文献记载看,体质的分类方法很多,归纳起来大致有以下几种:① 阴阳分类法。② 五行分类法。③ 脏腑分类法。④ 气血津液分类法。⑤ 综合分类法。由于各种分类方法内容繁杂,且相互交叉重复,故本书不一一列出,特选择临床常用的几种体质类型加以介绍。

1. Constitution with superabundant yang

Superabundance of yang produces heat. So this type of constitution is marked by reddish complexion, sonorous voice, warm hands and feet, dry stool, slightly yellowish urine, tolerance to cold and intolerance to heat as well as slightly rapid pulse. This kind of syndrome can be further divided into specific types according to location of heat in different viscera, such as up-flaming of heart-fire, hyperactivity of liver-yang and exuberant fire in the heart and the liver, etc.

1. 阳盛质

阳盛质,指阳气偏盛的体质。阳盛则热,可表现为面色偏红,语声高亢,手足温暖,大便偏干,小便稍黄,耐寒不耐热,脉略数等。根据所在脏腑不同,可分为心火上炎、肝阳上亢、心肝火旺等类型。

2. Constitution with superabundant yin

Superabundant yin produces cold. So this type of constitution is marked by bluish complexion, low voice, cold hands and feet, soft stool, clear urine, tolerance to heat and intolerance to cold as well as slightly slow pulse, etc. This kind of syndrome can be further divided into specific types according to location of cold in different viscera, such as retention of cold in the lung, stagnation of cold in the liver meridian and accumulation of cold in the spleen and stomach, etc.

2. 阴盛质

阴盛质,指阴气偏盛的体质。阴盛则寒,可表现为面色偏青,语声低沉,手足不温,大便偏软,小便常清,耐热不耐寒,脉略迟等。根据所在脏腑不同,可分为寒邪伏肺、寒凝肝脉、寒积脾胃等类型。

3. Constitution with deficiency of yang

Deficiency of yang generates cold. So this type of constitution is marked by whitish complexion, cold feet and hands, spontaneous sweating, impotence, diarrhea, profuse clear urine and deep-slow pulse. This kind of syndrome can be further divided into specific types according to location of cold in different viscera, such as insufficiency of heart-yang, insufficiency of spleen-yang, insufficiency of kidney-yang (decline of fire in life-gate), etc.

4. Constitution with deficiency of yin

Deficiency of yin means insufficiency of yin-essence and deficiency of yin generates heat. So this type of constitution is marked by reddish cheeks, emaciation, feverish sensation in the soles and palms, dysphoria, insomnia, night sweating, seminal emission, dry stool, scanty brownish urine and thin-rapid pulse, etc. This kind of syndrome can be further divided into specific types according to location of heat in different viscera, such as insufficiency of heart-yin, insufficiency of liver-yin, insufficiency of lung-yin, insufficiency of spleen-yin and insufficiency of kidney-yin, etc.

5. Constitution with deficiency of qi

Deficiency of qi means insufficiency of the primordial qi and deficiency of qi leads to hypofunction of the viscera. So this type of constitution is marked by sallow complexion, dispiritedness, lassitude, low voice, poor appetite and weak pulse, etc. This kind of syndrome can be further divided into specific types according to the viscera involved, such as insufficiency of heart-qi, insufficiency of lung-qi, insufficiency of spleen-qi and insufficiency of kidney-qi, etc.

6. Constitution with deficiency of blood

Blood deficiency leads to malnutrition of the viscera. So this type of constitution is marked by pale complexion,

3. 阳虚质

阳虚质,指阳气不足的体质。阳虚则寒,可表现为面色偏白,畏寒,手足逆冷,自汗,阳痿,大便泄泻,小便清长,脉沉迟等。根据所在脏腑不同,可分为心阳不足、脾阳不足、肾阳不足(命门火衰)等类型。

4. 阴虚质

阴虚质,指阴精不足体质。阴虚则热,可表现为颧红,消瘦,手足心热,心烦少寐,盗汗,遗精,大便干结、小便短赤,脉细数等。根据所在脏腑不同,可分为心阴不足、肝阴不足、肺阴不足、脾阴不足、肾阴不足等类型。

5. 气虚质

气虚质,指元气不足体质。气虚则脏腑功能减退,可表现为面色萎黄,精神委靡,倦怠乏力,语声低微,食欲不振,脉虚弱无力等。根据所在脏腑不同,可分为心气不足、肺气不足、脾气不足、肾气不足等类型。

6. 血虚质

血虚质,指血液不足体质。血虚则脏腑失于濡养,可

dizziness, numbness of limbs, weakness of limbs, pale lips and nails, insomnia, dreaminess, scanty light-colored menses, light-colored tongue and thin-weak pulse, etc. This kind of syndrome can be further divided into specific types according to the viscera involved, such as insufficiency of heart-blood and insufficiency of liver-blood, etc.

7. Constitution with exuberant dampness

Exuberant dampness is caused by metabolic disturbance of body fluid due to prolonged living in humid areas and inhibited transformation of qi. The usual symptoms are obesity, dizziness, chest oppression, profuse phlegm, frequent nausea, poor appetite, mucous stool, profuse menorrhea, thick- greasy tongue coating and taut-slippery pulse, etc. This kind syndrome can be further divided into specific types according to the viscera involved, such as accumulation of phlegm-dampness in the lung, phlegm-dampness encumbering the spleen, phlegm-turbidity disturbing the heart and phlegm blocking the meridians, etc.

8. Constitution with blood stasis

Constitution with blood stasis means that internal retention of blood stasis due to unsmooth circulation of blood. The usual symptoms are grayish complexion, heaviness or pain of the head and limbs, or mass in the body, irregular menstruation or dysmenorrhea or purplish menses with blood clot, purplish tongue or tongue with petechia, thin and unsmooth pulse, etc. This kind of syndrome can be further divided into specific types according to the viscera involved, such as blockage of the liver collaterals, blockage of the heart meridian and blockage of the uterus, etc.

The types of constitution sometimes are mingled with each other, such as constitution with superabundant yin

表现为面色淡白,头昏眼花,肢体发麻,四肢无力,口唇及爪甲淡白,少寐多梦,妇女月经量少、色淡,舌质淡,脉细弱等。根据所在脏腑不同,可分为心血不足、肝血不足等类型。

7. 痰湿质

痰湿质,指津液代谢障碍,水湿停聚而痰湿久居的体质。痰湿久居,气化不利,可表现为形体肥胖,眩晕,胸闷,痰多,常恶心,纳食少,大便常挟粘液,妇女带下量多,舌苔厚腻,脉弦滑等。根据所在脏腑不同,可分为痰湿蕴肺、痰湿困脾、痰浊扰心、痰阻经脉等类型。

8. 瘀血质

瘀血质,指血液运行失畅,凝滞血脉而瘀血久居的体质。瘀血久居,经脉不畅,可表现为面色晦暗,头身肢体重着或疼麻,体内或有癥积,妇女月经不调,或痛经、或经色紫黑有瘀血块,舌质紫暗,或有瘀点瘀斑,脉细涩等。根据所在脏腑不同,可分为肝络瘀阻、心脉瘀阻、瘀阻胞宫等类型。

以上各型体质可以相兼,如阴盛质可兼阳虚质,阳虚质

mingled with deficiency of yang, constitution with deficiency of yang mingled with deficiency of qi, constitution with exuberant dampness mingled with blood stasis, etc.

6.1.2.4　The influence of constitution on disease

Generally speaking, people with strong constitution infrequently contract disease because of superabundance of healthy qi; people with weak constitution frequently contract disease because of insufficiency of healthy qi. However, different types of constitution usually exert different effects on the occurrence of disease.

1. Different types of constitution and different levels of susceptibility to invasion of pathogenic factors

Different types of constitution are subject to invasion of different pathogenic factors. For example, people with superabundant yang and deficient yin are frequently attacked by wind and heat, but infrequently attacked by cold and dampness; people with superabundant yin and deficient yang are frequently attacked by cold and dampness, but infrequently attacked by wind and heat; people with insufficient body fluid and blood are frequently attacked by dryness, but infrequently attacked by dampness; people with exuberant phlegm and dampness are frequently attacked by dampness, but infrequently attacked by dryness.

2. Different types of constitution and the principle of pathogenesis

The location and nature of disease after the invasion of pathogenic factors are usually decided by the types of constitution. In people with frequent weak constitution, disease tends to transmit to the weak areas and develop into special pathological changes. For example, spleen

可兼气虚质,痰湿质可兼瘀血质等。

(四) 体质对发病的影响

一般说来,体质强者,正气充盛,邪气不易侵入,故较少发病;体质弱者,正气不足,易被邪气侵袭,故容易发病。然而,就具体的体质类型而言,它们对疾病的发生还有一些特殊的影响。

1. 不同体质类型对不同邪气的易感性不同

体质类型不同,对邪气的易感性也不同。如阳盛及阴虚体质的人,易感受风、热等阳邪,不易感受寒、湿等阴邪;阴盛及阳虚体质的人,易感受寒、湿等阴邪,不易感受风、热等阳邪;津血不足体质的人,易感受燥邪,不易感受湿邪;痰湿偏盛体质的人,易感受湿邪,不易感受燥邪等。

2. 不同体质类型感邪后的发病规律不同

邪气侵入人体后的发病部位及形成何种性质的疾病,受其体质类型的决定性影响。从发病部位来看,素体有虚弱之处,感邪后即易传向体虚部

deficiency tends to lead to direct invasion of pathogenic factors into the spleen meridian and bring on spleen disease; lung deficiency tends to lead to direct invasion of pathogenic factors into the lung meridian and bring on lung disease; liver deficiency tends to lead to direct invasion of pathogenic factors into the liver meridian and bring on liver disease; heart deficiency tends to lead to direct invasion of pathogenic factors into the heart meridian and bring on heart disease; kidney deficiency tends to lead to direct invasion of pathogenic factors into the kidney meridian and bring on kidney disease; superficial deficiency tends to lead to external lingering of pathogenic factors and bring on external syndrome; meridian deficiency tends to lead to transmission of pathogenic factors along the meridians and bring on disorder of the meridians, etc.

The types of constitution decide the nature of disease. For example, the constitution with superabundant yang tends to develop heat syndrome after being attacked by pathogenic heat and even by pathogenic wind, cold and dampness which will transfer into heat after invasion into the body; the constitution with deficiency of yin tends to develop cold syndrome after being attacked by pathogenic factors; the constitution with spleen deficiency tends to develop dampness syndrome after being attacked by pathogenic factors. Thus the invasion of pathogenic factors in the same environment will lead to diseases of different nature because of difference in constitution. Such a phenomenon in TCM is called "transformation according to constitution" or "transformation of nature of disease".

3. Different types of temperament and different levels of susceptibility to the invasion of pathogenic factors

Temperament is a special psychological reaction of constitution. Different types of temperament lead to

位而形成某种特殊病变。如脾虚者,邪气易传向脾而形成脾病;肺虚者,邪气易传向肺而形成肺病;肝虚者,邪气易传向肝而形成肝病;心虚者,邪气易传向心而形成心病;肾虚者,邪气易传向肾而形成肾病;表虚者,邪气易逗留于外而形成表证;经络虚者,邪气可传入经络而导致经络病变等。

体质类型还能决定感邪后形成病证的性质。如阳盛体质者,感受热邪后形成热证,风、寒、湿等邪气也将顺从其体质而化为热,形成热证;阳虚有寒者,感邪后易从寒化;脾虚有湿者,感邪后易从湿化等。因此,在同一环境中感受相同的邪气,不同体质者将形成不同性质的疾病。中医体质学把这种现象称为"从化"(也有人称之为"质化")。

3. 不同气质类型对不同邪气的易感性不同

气质是体质因素在精神心理方面的特殊反应形式,故

different levels of susceptibility to the invasion of pathogenic factors. This phenomenon is the same as that of different types of constitution leading to different levels of
susceptibility to the invasion of pathogenic factors. Generally speaking, the temperament with abundance of yang is
easy to be attacked by wind and heat and difficult to be attacked by cold and dampness; the temperament with
abundance of yin is easy to be attacked by cold and dampness and difficult to be attacked by wind and heat.

Huangdi Neijing also holds that braveness and ti-
midity also affect the occurrence of disease. After being
attacked by pathogenic factors, people with brave temperament are characterized by rapid flow of qi and blood, no
retention and quick elimination of pathogenic factors; people with timid temperament are marked by slow flow of qi
and blood and frequent retention of pathogenic factors,
leading to occurrence of disease.

6.2　Mechanism of pathological changes

Mechanism of pathological changes includes the nature of disease and its transmitting principles.

The occurrence of disease results from the struggle
between pathogenic factors and healthy qi which exists in
the whole course of disease. In the struggle between
pathogenic factors and healthy qi, various general or local
pathological changes will be caused if healthy qi is impaired, the balance between yin and yang is damaged, the
functions of meridians are in disorder and the flow of qi
and blood is disturbed. Though complicated, pathological

也属于体质的范畴。不同气
质类型对不同邪气的易感性
不同,这一点与上述"不同体
质类型对不同邪气的易感性
不同"是一致的。一般地说,
气质属阳刚者,易感受风、热
等阳邪,不易感受寒、湿等阴
邪;气质属阴柔者,易感受寒、
湿等阴邪,不易感受风、热等
阳邪。

《黄帝内经》还提出,人的
勇敢与怯懦也能影响发病。
人感受病邪之后,如果气质勇
敢者,其气血运行快疾,邪气
不得停滞,会很快被消除,人
体不易发病;若气质怯懦者,
其气血运行迟缓,邪气即易于
停留,从而导致发病。

第二节　病变机理

病变机理,是疾病发生以
后发展变化的机理,包括疾病
形成后的基本属性及其传变
的规律。

疾病的发生,是邪正斗争
的结果,整个疾病存在的过
程,始终贯穿着邪正斗争。在
邪正斗争过程中,如果正气受
到损伤,阴阳平衡被破坏,并
使脏腑、经络的功能失调,或
使气血津液运行紊乱,就会产
生全身或局部的多种多样的

changes generally can be classified into such categories as predomination and decline of pathogenic factors and healthy qi, imbalance of yin and yang as well as disorder of qi, blood and body fluid.

6.2.1   Predomination and decline of pathogenic factors and healthy qi

Predomination and decline of pathogenic factors and healthy qi refer to changes of pathogenic factors and healthy qi due to struggle between them. The result of predomination and decline of pathogenic factors and healthy qi affects the nature and transmission of disease.

6.2.1.1   Predomination and decline of pathogenic factors and healthy qi and the changes of deficiency and excess

The occurrence of disease is due to two factors, deficiency of healthy qi and attack of pathogenic factors. However, these two factors play different roles in a specific disease. Sometimes disease is caused by deficiency of healthy qi, and sometimes by attack of pathogenic factors, resulting in either deficiency syndrome or excess syndrome. *Huangdi Neijing* says: "Excess means predomination of pathogenic factors while deficiency means exhaustion of essence." That is to say that "excess" is related to pathogenic factors while "deficiency" is related to healthy qi.

病理变化。因此,尽管疾病的种类繁多,临床表现错综复杂、千变万化,每种疾病或症状都有各自的病变机理,但从总体来说,都离不开邪正盛衰、阴阳失调、气血津液失常等病机变化的一般规律。

一、邪正盛衰

邪正盛衰,是指在疾病过程中,人体正气和致病邪气之间由于相互斗争所发生的双方力量对比的盛衰变化。邪正盛衰变化的结果,一方面影响着病证性质的虚实变化,另一方面直接影响着疾病的转归。

(一)邪正盛衰与虚实变化

疾病的形成关系到两个方面的因素,一是正气不足,一是邪气侵袭。但是,这两方面的因素在每个具体疾病中的作用还是有所侧重的。有时正气不足是发病的主要因素,有时邪气侵袭是发病的主要因素,由此形成虚和实两种不同性质的病证。《黄帝内经》对虚和实有明确的定义,指出:"邪气盛则实,精气夺则虚。"也就是说,"实"是针对邪气而言的,"虚"是针对正气而

1. Excess syndrome

Excess syndrome is characterized by predomination of pathogenic factors and abundance or certain degree impairment of healthy qi. Violent struggle between pathogenic factors and healthy qi leads to a series of excess symptoms. That is why it is a syndrome of excess nature. Excess syndrome is often seen at the early and medium stages of diseases caused by six abnormal climatic factors or diseases caused by phlegm, rheum, blood stasis, retention of food and accumulation of dampness and water in the body. Clinically excess syndrome includes superabundance of phlegm, internal blockage of blood stasis, indigestion and abnormal flow of water and dampness as well as the manifestations of high fever, mania, sonorous voice and hoarse breath, unpalpable abdominal pain, constipation, anuria and powerful pulse, etc.

2. Deficiency syndrome

Deficiency syndrome is marked by deficiency of healthy qi. Though pathogenic factors are not totally eliminated, they are not strong enough to damage healthy qi. So the struggle between pathogenic factors and healthy qi is mild with symptoms of deficiency of healthy qi and hypofunction of the viscera. That is why this kind of syndrome is termed deficiency syndrome. Deficiency syndrome is often seen at the advanced stage of exogenous diseases. It usually results from non-restoration of healthy qi, or frequent weakness of the body, or exhaustion of essence due to serious disease, protracted disease and chronic disease, or damage of qi, blood and body fluid due to profuse sweating, violent vomiting and diarrhea and massive hemorrhage, etc. Clinically the manifestations of

言的。

1. 实证

实证,是以邪气盛为矛盾主要方面的一种病理反映。此时正气未虚,或虽有某种程度的耗损,但整体正气依然强盛,足以与邪气相争。由于邪正斗争剧烈,故疾病的反应非常明显,出现一派有余的症状,所以称为实证。实证常见于外感六淫致病的初期和中期,或由于痰饮、瘀血、食积、水湿等滞留于体内而引起的病证。如临床上见到的痰涎壅盛、瘀血内阻、食积不化、水湿泛滥等病变,以及壮热、狂躁、声高气粗、腹痛拒按、大小便不通、脉实有力等,都属于实证的表现。

2. 虚证

虚证,是以正气虚损为矛盾主要方面的一种病理反映。此时邪气已去,或虽然余邪未尽,但不会对正气造成大的伤害,邪正相争趋于缓和。由于邪正斗争不甚激烈,主要表现为一系列正气不足及脏腑功能减退的症状,所以称为虚证。虚证多见于外感病的后期,正气虚损未复,或素体虚弱,或由于大病、久病、慢性病等消耗精气,或因大汗、剧烈呕吐下利、大出血等耗伤人体气血津液所导致。凡临床见

deficiency syndrome include dispiritedness, sallow complexion, palpitation and shortness of breath, spontaneous
sweating, night sweating, or feverish sensation in the five
centers (palms, soles and chest), or aversion to cold and
cold limbs as well as weak pulse, etc.

3. Mixture of deficiency syndrome and excess syndrome

During the course of a disease, the predomination
and decline of pathogenic factors and healthy qi may lead
to either simple deficiency syndrome and excess syndrome
or mixture of deficiency syndrome and excess syndrome.
Mixture of deficiency syndrome and excess syndrome may
be caused by delayed or improper treatment of excess syndrome that leads to prolonged retention of pathogenic factors in the body and impairment of healthy qi, or by coag-
ulation of pathological substances like dampness, water
and blood stasis due to deficiency of healthy qi.

Mixture of deficiency syndrome and excess syndrome
is characterized by either deficiency complicated by excess
or excess complicated by deficiency. The former is
marked by domination of deficiency syndrome accompanied by excess of pathogenic factors, such as edema due to
inactivation of spleen-yang. The latter is marked by domination of excess syndrome accompanied by deficiency
manifestations, such as excess-heat consuming yin-fluid at
the medium stage of febrile diseases.

4. Mutual transformation between deficiency syndrome and excess syndrome

Deficiency syndrome and excess syndrome are not
fixed, they often transform into each other due to struggle
between pathogenic factors and healthy qi.

到神疲体倦、面色憔悴、心悸气短、自汗、盗汗，或五心烦热，或畏寒肢冷，脉虚无力等，都属于虚证的表现。

3. 虚证和实证的相互错杂

在疾病过程中，邪正的消长盛衰，不仅可以导致单纯的虚证和实证，也可以出现虚实相兼的病理变化，即虚实错杂证。若实证失治，或治疗不当，以致病邪久留，损伤了人体的正气；或因正气本虚，无力驱邪外出，而致水湿、痰饮、瘀血等病理产物凝结阻滞，都可以形成虚实错杂的病理变化。

虚实错杂有两种情形，一是虚中夹实，一是实中夹虚。虚中夹实是指疾病的病理变化以虚证为主，又兼实邪的病机。如脾阳不振又见水肿，即属虚中夹实。实中夹虚是指以实证为主，又夹正虚的病机。如外感热病热盛期，常见实热耗伤阴津，即属实中夹虚。

4. 虚证和实证的相互转化

虚证和实证形成之后，并不是一成不变的。由于邪正斗争中双方力量对比经常发生变化，因而虚证和实证之间

Such a mutual transformation is characterized by transformation either from excess into deficiency or from deficiency into excess. In excess syndrome, healthy qi is usually not deficient. However, delayed or improper treatment may prolong the course of duration, leading to impairment of healthy qi and the physiological functions of the viscera and resulting in transformation of excess into deficiency. In deficiency syndrome, there is no invasion of pathogenic factors. However, deficiency of healthy qi and hypofunction of the viscera may lead to abnormal flow of qi, blood and body fluid and bring on qi stagnation, blood stasis, phlegm and rheum as well as water and dampness, eventually resulting in deficiency complicated by excess. Though there is excess of pathogenic factors, healthy qi is still insufficient. Thus this morbid state is termed "excess caused by deficiency".

6.2.1.2　The relationship between the prognosis of disease and the state of pathogenic factors and healthy qi

In the course of struggle between pathogenic factors and healthy qi, healthy qi can eliminate pathogenic factors and pathogenic factors are also able to impair healthy qi. Thus the struggle between pathogenic factors and healthy qi is marked by constant variation of both sides. Such a variation decides the development of disease that manifests in two ways: recovery or death. If healthy qi becomes dominant, pathogenic factors will be reduced and disease will be improved and gradually cured; if pathogenic factors become dominant, healthy qi will be weakened and disease will become worsened or death will be caused.

也常发生相互转化。

虚证和实证相互转化有两种形式,一是由实转虚,一是因虚致实。实证正气本不虚,若由于误治、失治,使病情迁延日久,虽然邪气渐去,但人体的正气、脏腑的生理功能也受到损伤,其疾病的性质也就逐渐由实转虚。反之,原属虚证,并无邪气,若因正虚而脏腑功能减退,导致气、血、水等不能正常运行而出现了气滞、瘀血、痰饮、水湿等实邪停滞征象,就形成了夹实的病机。此时虽有实邪,但正气仍然不足,所以称其为"因虚致实"。因虚致实也可导致虚实错杂证。

(二)邪正盛衰与疾病转归

在邪正斗争过程中,正气有祛除邪气的能力,邪气也有损伤正气的作用。因此,邪正斗争的过程必然伴随着正气与邪气双方力量对比的不断变化,这种变化最终将决定疾病的转归。疾病的转归有两种基本形式,一是痊愈,一是死亡。这两种转归实际上是邪正斗争的不同结果:若正胜邪退,则疾病趋于好转和痊愈;若邪胜正衰,则疾病趋于恶化或死亡。

1. Domination of healthy qi and decline of pathogenic factors

Domination of healthy qi and decline of pathogenic factors are the necessary conditions for improvement and cure of disease. If healthy qi is sufficient, it will be powerful in resisting pathogenic factors and pathogenic factors will gradually be eliminated. If timely treatment is resorted to, pathogenic factors will be eliminated or reduced and healthy qi will be gradually restored. In both cases the functions of the viscera are improved, pathogenic factors are eliminated and eventually disease is cured.

The course of domination of healthy qi and decline of pathogenic factors may be long or short, depending on individual conditions. Generally speaking, the duration of exogenous disease and excess syndrome is short because pathogenic factors have not penetrated deep into the body and healthy qi is not seriously impaired. So exogenous disease and excess syndrome are easy to improve and cure. However, the duration of endogenous disease and deficiency syndrome is long because pathogenic factors have penetrated deep into the body and healthy qi is seriously impaired. So endogenous disease and deficiency syndrome are difficult to improve and cure. Usually correct and timely treatment can shorten the course of domination of healthy qi and decline of pathogenic factors. Incorrect and delayed treatment will certainly prolong the course of such a development.

2. Domination of pathogenic factors and decline of healthy qi

Domination of pathogenic factors and decline of healthy qi are the basic causes of aggravation of disease or death. Such a variation results either from frequent deficiency of healthy qi that fails to restrict the development of pathogenic factors, or from exuberance of pathogenic

1. 正胜邪退

正胜邪退,是疾病趋于好转和痊愈的必要条件。由于正气充盛,抗御病邪的能力不断增强,邪气将逐渐被清除;或因得到及时正确的治疗,邪气被祛除或削弱,正气的耗伤逐渐得到修复,最终脏腑功能完全恢复正常,邪气被完全祛除,疾病即告痊愈。

正胜邪退的过程长短不一,因人而异。一般外感病、实证、病程短者,邪气侵入不深,正气损伤不重,则好转快,痊愈也快。若属内伤病、虚证、病程长者,邪气侵入深,正气损伤重,则好转慢,痊愈也慢。如果治疗及时而恰当,正胜邪退的过程就会缩短,反之则会延长。

2. 邪胜正衰

邪胜正衰,是疾病趋于恶化或死亡的根本原因。由于人体正气本来不足,无力制止邪气的发展;或因邪气过于亢盛,超过了机体的抵御能力;

factors that go beyond the body resistance, or from wrong or delayed treatment that impairs healthy qi and strengthens pathogenic factors, resulting in declination of visceral functions and separation of yin and yang, and eventually leading to death.

In the course of the variation of healthy qi and pathogenic factors, if healthy qi is not strong enough to eliminate pathogenic factors and pathogenic factors are not strong enough to further develop, it will bring on such a condition in which healthy qi and pathogenic factors are at a stalemate or healthy qi is deficient and pathogenic factors are still lingering. In this case healthy qi is difficult to restore, disease may change from an acute one into a chronic one or become obstinate, or certain sequelae may be caused.

6.2.2　Imbalance between yin and yang

Imbalance between yin and yang is a summarization of all kinds of basic pathogenesis, including dysfunction of the viscera, disorder of the meridians and disharmony of qi and blood, etc.

Normally yin and yang in the body maintain a dynamic balance through the interactions of inter-opposition, inter-dependence, inter-restriction and inter-transformation. If such a dynamic balance is impaired by six exogenous abnormal climatic factors, endogenous impairment by abnormal changes of emotions, improper diet or overwork and over-rest, the normal relationships between the viscera, the meridians, qi and blood will be affected,

或因失治、误治损伤了正气，助长了邪气，使正气抗邪能力日益低下，机体的病理损害日趋严重，邪气越发鸱张，最终正气不支，脏腑功能衰竭，阴阳离决而死亡。

此外，在邪正消长盛衰的过程中，若正气不足以祛除邪气，邪气也不能进一步发展，出现邪正相持或正虚邪恋，正气难以完全恢复等情况，常可使许多疾病由急性过程转入慢性阶段，或留下某些后遗症，或经久不愈。

二、阴阳失调

阴阳失调，是指阴阳之间失去正常的协调平衡关系，从而出现的一种病机变化。阴阳失调是一种最基本的病机，是一切病机变化本质的最高概括。凡脏腑失常、经络失调、气血失和等，都是阴阳失调的表现形式。

正常情况下，人体的阴阳之间通过相互对立、互根、消长、转化等作用，维持着一种动态的协调平衡关系。若因外感六淫、内伤七情、饮食失宜、劳逸失当等因素，破坏了这种协调与平衡，就会导致阴阳失调。阴阳一旦失调，其脏

leading to various complicated pathological changes.

The main pathological changes caused by imbalance between yin and yang are predomination and decline of yin and yang, mutual impairment of yin and yang, mutual rejection of yin and yang, mutual transformation of yin and yang as well as loss of yin and yang.

6.2.2.1 Relative predomination and decline of yin and yang

Relative predomination and decline of yin and yang refer to the changes of yin and yang beyond the normal range due to various factors. Relative predomination and decline of yin and yang directly cause excess syndrome and deficiency syndrome. Relative predomination of yin and yang leads to excess syndrome while relative decline of yin and yang leads to deficiency syndrome. Predomination and decline of yin and yang also decide the nature of disease. Relative predomination of yang and deficiency of yin cause heat syndrome while domination of yin and deficiency of yang bring on cold syndromes.

1. Relative predomination of yin and yang

When yin or yang becomes predominant, it becomes a pathogenic factor and causes excess syndrome because "excess of pathogenic factors leads to excess syndrome". When yin becomes predominant, it will bring on cold syndromes; when yang becomes predominant, it will lead to heat syndromes.

（1）Relative predomination of yang: Relative predomination of yang refers to excess-heat syndrome marked by predomination of yang and non-deficiency of yin due to relative predomination of yang-qi and hyperactivity of body functions during the course of disease. It results either from imbalance between yin and yang, or from attack

腑、经络、气血津液等相互关系都会失调，从而出现多种多样错综复杂的病理变化。

阴阳失调主要表现为阴阳盛衰、阴阳互损、阴阳格拒、阴阳互转、阴阳亡失等病理变化。

（一）阴阳盛衰

阴阳盛衰，是由各种原因导致的阴或阳的消长变化超过了正常范围，所出现的偏盛和偏衰的病机变化。阴阳盛衰直接导致实证和虚证，阴阳偏盛则形成实证，阴阳偏衰则形成虚证。阴阳盛衰还决定了疾病性质的寒和热，阳盛、阴虚则形成热证，阴盛、阳虚则形成寒证。

1. 阴阳偏盛

阴或阳一旦偏盛，就成了邪气。"邪气盛则实"，所以阴偏盛或阳偏盛都形成实证。阴偏盛则形成实寒证，阳偏盛则形成实热证。

（1）阳偏盛：阳偏盛是由于人体阴阳平衡失调，表现为阳气偏盛、功能亢奋的一种病理状态，其病机特点多表现为阳盛而阴未虚的实热证。其形成的主要原因，常见于外感

of exogenous warm pathogenic factors, or from attack of pathogenic factors of yin nature that transforms into heat with yang, or from endogenous impairment due to abnormal changes of emotions and heat transformed from abnormal changes of emotions, or from heat transformed from qi stagnation, blood stasis, phlegm and retention of food that make yang-qi predominant. Predomination of yang leads to heat, so usual clinical manifestation is fever, accompanied by profuse sweating, thirst, reddish complexion, reddish tongue with yellowish coating, full and large or rapid pulse; or accompanied by pathogenic heat disturbing the interior with the symptoms of dysphoria, insomnia, mania, dry feces and scanty brownish urine, etc.

Predomination of yang impairs yin. So predomination of yang is usually characterized by consumption of yin-fluid. At the medium and advanced stages of disease, pathogenic yang gradually declines and the consumption of yin-fluid is more and more serious, eventually leading to yin-deficiency syndromes.

(2) Relative predomination of yin: Relative predomination of yin refers to excess-cold syndrome marked by relative predomination of yin-qi, decline of body functions and retention of pathological substances in the course of disease. It may result either from attack of pathogenic cold and dampness, or from excessive intake of cold and uncooked food that makes yin-qi in the body predominant. Predomination of yin generates cold and obstructs yang-qi, clinically leading to cold symptoms, such as chills, dispiritedness, pale complexion, anhidrosis, preference for hot water, cold limbs, loose stool, clear urine, whitish tongue coating, deep and slow pulse, etc.

温热阳邪,或感受阴邪从阳化热,或七情内伤、五志化火,或因气滞、血瘀、痰浊、食积等郁而化火,促使人体阳气偏亢而形成。阳盛则热,故临床表现以发热为主症,兼见多汗、口渴、面红、舌红苔黄、脉洪大或数;或火邪内扰,出现心烦、失眠、狂躁、大便干结、小便短赤等症。

由于阳盛则伤阴,所以阳偏盛者往往有阴津耗损的表现。病至中、后期,阳邪渐退,阴津耗损却日益显著,就会形成阴虚证。

(2) 阴偏盛:阴偏盛是由于人体阴阳平衡失调,表现为阴气偏盛、功能衰减及其病理性代谢产物滞留的一种病理状态,其病机特点多表现为阴盛而阳未虚的实寒证。其形成的主要原因,常见于感受寒湿阴邪,或过食生冷,致使人体阴气偏盛而形成。阴盛则寒,阳气被遏而不得舒展,也失去其温煦作用,故临床表现以发寒为主症,常见恶寒战栗、精神不振、面色苍白、无汗、喜热饮、四肢逆冷、大便稀、小便清、舌苔白、脉沉迟

Since predomination of yin leads to disorder of yang, relative predomination of yin obstructs or impairs yang. At the medium and advanced stages of disease, pathogenic yin gradually declines and yang-qi becomes more and more deficient, eventually bringing on yang-deficiency syndromes.

2. Relative decline of yin and yang

Normally both yin and yang pertain to healthy qi in the body. Once yin or yang declines, insufficiency of healthy qi will be caused. So both relative decline of yin and yang can lead to deficiency syndrome because "loss of essence causes deficiency". Usually relative decline of yin brings on deficiency-heat syndrome while relative decline of yang results in deficiency-cold syndrome.

(1) Relative decline of yang: Relative decline of yang results either from imbalance between yin and yang and excessive consumption of yang-qi, or from congenital weakness and insufficiency of fire in life-gate, or from improper postnatal care and impairment of yang-qi, or from impairment of yang-qi during the course of disease. Deficiency of yang-qi generates cold and clinically brings on deficiency-cold syndrome and decline or weakness of viscera functions, leading to the symptoms of aversion to cold, cold limbs, mental lassitude, poor appetite, loose stool, clear and profuse urine, and deep-slow-weak pulse, etc.

Yang-deficiency syndrome mainly involves the spleen and the kidney, mainly characterized by deficiency of kidney-yang. Since kidney-yang is the foundation of yang-qi in the other organs, deficiency of kidney-yang will make spleen-yang insufficient. Since the spleen is the acquired base of life, deficiency of spleen-yang weakens the functions of transportation and transformation, eventually

等症。

由于阴盛则阳病,所以阴偏盛往往有阳气受遏或损伤的表现。病至中、后期,阴邪渐退,阳气不足就越来越明显起来,从而形成阳虚证。

2. 阴阳偏衰

正常情况下,阴和阳都属于人体的正气。阴或阳一旦偏衰,就会形成正气不足的局面。"精气夺则虚",所以阴偏衰和阳偏衰都形成虚证。阴偏衰则形成虚热证,阳偏衰则形成虚寒证。

(1)阳偏衰:阳偏衰多由人体阴阳平衡失调,阳气消耗过度;或先天禀赋薄弱,命门火衰;或后天调养失当,损伤阳气;或因病阳气受损,使机体阳气不足而形成。阳虚则寒,故临床主要表现为虚寒证,脏腑功能减退或衰弱,出现畏寒怕冷、四肢不温、精神疲乏、食欲不振、大便溏泄、小便清长、脉沉迟无力等症。

阳虚证主要表现在脾、肾二脏,尤以肾阳虚为重点。因为肾阳为各脏腑阳气的根本,所以肾阳一虚,脾阳也显不足。脾为后天之本,所以脾阳不足则运化功能减弱,气血生化乏源,会使阳虚症情加重。

leading to insufficient production of blood and qi and aggravating the state of yang deficiency.

Deficiency of yang makes it difficult to restrict yin, leading to interior exuberance of yin-cold or retention of water-dampness or interior blockage of blood stasis which may further stagnate qi activity and bring on serious dysfunction of the viscera.

(2) Relative decline of yin: Relative decline of yin may result either from imbalance between yin and yang and excessive consumption of yin-essence, or from congenital weakness and insufficiency of yin-fluid, or from improper postnatal care and exhaustion of yin-fluid, or from insufficiency of yin-fluid in the course of disease. Deficiency of yin generates heat and clinically brings on deficiency-heat syndrome and various hyperactivities of viscera functions, leading to the symptoms of emaciation, low fever, feverish sensation in the five centers (palms, soles and chest), night sweating, dry mouth, dry feces, scanty urine, reddish tongue coating or no tongue coating, thin and rapid pulse, etc.

Deficiency of yin mainly involves the liver and the kidney, mainly marked by kidney-deficiency. Since kidney-yin is the foundation of yin in the other viscera, deficiency of kidney-yin makes liver-yin insufficient.

Deficiency of yin cannot restrict yang and brings on endogenous heat and fire with the symptoms of irascibility and insomnia, etc. Insufficiency of liver-yin makes liver-yang hyperactive. Hyperactivity of liver-yang transforms into fire that disturbs the upper orifices and leads to dizziness, headache or even apoplexy and syncope, etc.

6.2.2.2　Inter-consumption of yin and yang

Yin and yang depend on each other and insufficiency of any side will affect the other. Protracted deficiency of

由于阳虚则不能制阴,可导致阴寒内盛,或水湿停聚,或瘀血内阻,进一步阻滞气机,可以造成脏腑功能的严重障碍。

(2) 阴偏衰:阴偏衰多由人体阴阳平衡失调,阴精消耗过度;或先天禀赋薄弱,阴液亏虚;或后天调养失当,阴液耗竭;或因病阴液受损,使机体阴液不足而形成。阴虚则热,故临床主要表现为虚热证,脏腑功能相对亢奋,出现形体消瘦、低热、五心烦热、盗汗、口干、大便干结、小便短少、舌红苔少或无苔、脉细数等症。

阴虚证主要表现在肝、肾二脏,尤以肾阴虚为重点。因为肾阴为各脏腑之阴的根本,所以肾阴一虚,肝阴也显不足。

由于阴虚则不能制阳,可导致火热内生,出现烦躁易怒、失眠等症。肝阴不足,则肝阳易亢,阳亢化火,上扰清窍,则眩晕、头痛,甚至发生中风昏厥等危象。

(二) 阴阳互损

由于阴阳是互根的,所以阴或阳的任何一方不足,都可

yin will affect yang and cause deficiency of yang. Similarly, prolonged deficiency of yang will affect yin and cause deficiency of yin. Such an inter-consumption of yin and yang eventually results in deficiency syndrome of both yin and yang.

1. Deficiency of yin affecting yang

Deficiency of yin affecting yang means that consumption of yin-fluid involves yang-qi and makes yang-qi insufficient in production or exhausted, leading to a morbid state marked mainly by deficiency of yin with the manifestation of deficiency of both yin and yang.

2. Deficiency of yang affecting yin

Deficiency of yang affecting yin means that consumption of yang-qi involves yin-fluid and makes yin-fluid insufficient in production, leading to a morbid state marked mainly by deficiency of yang with the manifestation of deficiency of both yin and yang.

6.2.2.3　Inter-rejection of yin and yang

Inter-rejection of yin and yang, a special pathogenesis in imbalance between yin and yang, includes two aspects: predomination of yin rejecting yang and predomination of yang rejecting yin. The cause of such a pathological change lies in the fact that either yin or yang becomes predominant and drives the other side outside, leading to a complicated pathological condition marked by disagreement between the nature of disease and symptoms.

1. Predomination of yin rejecting yang

Predomination of yin rejecting yang refers to a pathological state in which predominant yin drives yang-qi outside, leading to a pathological change marked by true interior cold

影响另一方。阴虚日久，则累及阳气，导致阳气也虚；阳虚日久则累及阴分，导致阴精虚亏，这种阴阳之间虚损相互影响的病机过程，称为阴阳互损。阴阳互损的结果，最终导致阴阳两虚证。

1. 阴损及阳

阴损及阳，是指由于阴液亏损，累及阳气，使阳气生化不足或无所依附而耗散，从而在阴虚的基础上又导致了阳虚，形成了以阴虚为主的阴阳两虚的病理状态。

2. 阳损及阴

阳损及阴，是指由于阳气虚损，累及阴液，使阴液生化不足，从而在阳虚的基础上又导致了阴虚，形成了以阳虚为主的阴阳两虚的病理状态。

（三）阴阳格拒

阴阳格拒，是阴阳失调中比较特殊的一种病机，包括阴盛格阳和阳盛格阴两方面。形成阴阳格拒的机理，主要是由于某些原因引起阴或阳的一方偏盛至极而壅遏于内，将另一方排斥格拒于外，从而出现病证性质和症候表现不一致的复杂病理现象。

1. 阴盛格阳

阴盛格阳，是指体内阴寒过盛，将阳气格拒于外，出现内真寒外假热的一种病理变

and false exterior heat. The nature of this syndrome is cold, but the manifestations appear febrile because yang-qi is driven outside. Take deficiency of yang generating interior cold for example. If it develops to a stage marked by extreme predomination of yin-cold and external floating of yang, a pathological change of predominant yin rejecting yang will be caused, the manifestations of which include cold limbs, diarrhea with undigested food and indistinct pulse due to predominance of yin-cold as well as some pseudo-febrile signs such as fever in spite of desire for quilt in the body and reddish cheeks.

2. Predomination of yang rejecting yin

Predomination of yang rejecting yin refers to a pathological state in which predominant yang drives yin outside, leading to a cold-like pathological change. Since pathogenic heat has deepened into the body and cannot be dispersed outside, there is pseudo-cold symptoms though the syndrome is febrile in nature. Take exuberant interior heat in febrile disease for example. Since heat is superabundant, yin and yang are in disharmony and yin-qi is blocked and rejected. The manifestations include feverish sensation in the chest, dry mouth, and dry and red tongue as well as cold limbs and aversion to cold due to the fact that extreme change of yang appears like yin.

6.2.2.4 Inter-transformation of yin and yang

Inter-transformation of yin and yang means that yang-heat syndrome may change into yin-cold syndrome and yin-cold syndrome may turn into yang-heat syndrome in the course of a disease.

1. Transformation of yang into yin

The nature of the disease originally pertains to yang-heat. But when yang-heat develops to a certain degree, it will turn into yin-cold. For example, some febrile diseases

化。其病证性质虽然是寒,而被格拒于外的阳气却表现出热的假象。如阳虚而生内寒,若疾病发展至严重阶段,阴寒盛极,浮阳外越,就形成阴盛格阳的病理变化,其表现除有阴寒过盛之四肢厥逆、下利清谷、脉微欲绝等症外,又见身体反温(但欲盖衣被)、面颊泛红等假热之象。

2. 阳盛格阴

阳盛格阴,是指阳热盛极,格阴于外,反似寒证的一种病理变化。由于热邪深伏,不能外达,故外见假寒,其本质仍属热证。如温热病热盛于内,由于热势盛极,阴阳不相调和,阴气即受阻格,其表现除有心胸烦热、口干舌焦、舌红等症外,又有阳极似阴的四肢厥冷或微畏寒等症。

(四) 阴阳互转

阴阳互转,是指在疾病发展过程中,阳热证可逆转为阴寒证,阴寒证也可逆转为阳热证。

1. 由阳转阴

疾病的性质本属阳热,但阳热亢盛至一定程度时,可向阴寒方向转化。如某些热病

show a series of heat symptoms at the early stage, such as high fever, thirst, reddish tongue, yellowish tongue coating and rapid pulse, indicating that the syndrome is obviously of yang-heat. However, improper treatment or extreme exuberance of pathogenic factors may suddenly lead to such critical signs of yin-cold as low body temperature, cold limbs, cold profuse sweating and indistinct pulse. This shows that the nature of the disease has been changed. Such a change is quite different from true-heat and false-cold syndrome in yang syndrome appearing like yin syndrome.

2. Transformation of yin into yang

The nature of the disease originally pertains to yin-cold. But when yin-cold develops to a certain degree, it will turn into yang-heat. For example, attack of exogenous pathogenic cold leads to a series of wind-cold symptoms at the early stage, such as serious aversion to cold and light fever, headache, body pain, thin and whitish tongue coating, and floating-tense pulse, indicating wind-cold affecting the superficies. Eventually it develops into a yang-heat syndrome marked by high fever, sweating, thirst, reddish tongue, yellowish tongue coating and rapid pulse. This shows that yin syndrome has been transformed into yang syndrome and cold syndrome has been turned into heat syndrome. Such a change is quite different from true-cold and false-heat syndrome in yin syndrome appearing like yang syndrome.

6.2.2.5 Loss of yin and yang

Loss of yin and yang refers to a critical pathological state caused by sudden loss of great quantity of yin-fluid or yang-qi. Loss of yin or yang also pertains to relative predomination and relative decline of yin and yang, quite different from relative predomination and decline of yin or yang in the occurrence and severity of disease.

初期可见高热、口渴、舌红、苔黄、脉数等一派热象,显然属于阳热之证。由于治疗不当或邪毒太盛等原因,可突然出现体温下降、四肢厥逆、冷汗淋漓、脉微欲绝等阴寒危象。这是疾病性质的根本转变,与阳证似阴的真热假寒证有本质区别。

2. 由阴转阳

疾病的性质本属阴寒,但阴寒盛极至一定程度时,可向阳热方向转化。如外感寒邪,初期可见恶寒重发热轻、头身疼痛、苔薄白、脉浮紧等风寒束表之象,其后可发展为高热、汗出、口渴、舌红、苔黄、脉数等阳热之证。这就属于阴证转阳,寒证化热,与阴证似阳的真寒假热证完全不同。

(五) 阴阳亡失

阴阳亡失,包括亡阴和亡阳两个方面,是指机体的阴液或阳气突然大量地亡失,导致生命垂危的一种病理变化。亡阴和亡阳也属于阴阳偏衰的范畴,但它与一般阴阳偏衰在发病缓急和轻重程度上有较大差别。

1. Loss of yang

Loss of yang is usually caused by predomination of pathogenic factors and weakness of healthy qi to control pathogenic factors, frequent deficiency of yang and overstrain, wrong application of diaphoresis and profuse sweating that result in sudden loss of yang-qi, leading to the symptoms of profuse sweating, cold sensation in the skin, feet and hands, lying with the knees drawn up, spiritual lassitude and indistinct pulse, etc.

2. Loss of yin

Loss of yin is usually caused by exuberant pathogenic heat, violent vomiting, profuse sweating and diarrhea that result in loss of great quantity of body fluid with the symptoms of emaciation, curled skin, sunken ocular orbit, scanty and sticky sweating, irascibility and very weak pulse, etc.

Though loss of yin and loss of yang may appear solitarily, the loss of one side often leads to immediate exhaustion of the other because yin and yang depend on each other to exist. Thus untimely treatment of loss of yin or loss of yang may lead to death because "separation of yin and yang exhausts essence."

1. 亡阳

亡阳常见于邪盛而正不胜邪、素体阳虚而疲劳过度、误用汗法而汗出过多等原因,导致机体阳气突然脱失,症见大汗淋漓、肌肤手足厥冷、踡卧神疲、脉微欲绝等。

2. 亡阴

亡阴常见于热邪炽盛、大吐、大汗、大泄等原因,导致机体阴液大量丢失,症见身体干瘪、皮肤皱褶、眼眶凹陷、汗出少而粘、烦躁不安、脉细弱无力等。

亡阴和亡阳虽可单独出现,但由于阴阳必须相互维系才能内守而不失,任何一方亡失都会导致另一方也迅速消亡,所以亡阴以后阳气将无所依附而速亡,亡阳之后阴液也不能独存而速亡,最终导致阴阳俱亡。因此,出现亡阴或亡阳时,如不及时抢救,必然出现"阴阳离决,精气乃绝"的严重局面,导致死亡。

6.2.3　Disorder of qi, blood and body fluid

The disorder of qi, blood and body fluid includes two aspects respectively: insufficiency and disturbance. Insufficiency causes deficiency syndrome, such as qi deficiency

三、气血津液失常

气血津液失常,分为气失常、血失常和津液失常三个方面,每一方面又有不足和失调

syndrome, blood deficiency syndrome and body fluid deficiency syndrome. Disturbance of qi, blood and body fluid mainly refers to the abnormal flow of them.

6.2.3.1 Disorder of qi

1. Insufficiency of qi

Insufficiency of qi causes qi deficiency syndrome with the manifestations of sallow complexion, dispiritedness, lassitude and low and weak voice. On the other hand, qi deficiency may bring on hypofunction of the viscera, leading to deficiency of heart-qi, deficiency of spleen-qi, deficiency of lung-qi and deficiency of kidney-qi.

2. Disturbance of qi

The manifestations of qi disorder are various, such as qi exuberance, qi stagnation, adverse flow of qi, qi sinking, qi closure and qi leakage, etc.

Qi exuberance means that qi is excessive, usually leading to blockage of qi activity and transformation into fire. Take exuberance of lung-qi for example. If it accumulates in the chest and blocks the chest, it will cause oppression and distension of the chest and sonorous dyspnea; if it transforms into fire to scorch the lung, it will bring on fever, profuse sweating, thirst, cough with yellowish thick sputum.

Qi stagnation means unsmooth flow of qi and stagnation of qi in local areas, leading to distension, fullness and pain. Protracted stagnation of qi tends to transform into fire. For example, stagnation of liver-qi leads to hypochondriac distension and fullness or distending pain of lower abdomen and depression; transformation of stagnant qi into fire and upward surge of liver-fire may lead to reddish cheeks and eyes and irascibility.

Adverse flow of qi, sinking of qi, closure of qi and leakage of qi are caused by abnormal changes of ascent and descent. Excessive ascent of qi causes adverse flow of qi;

两类表现。其不足则形成虚证,如气虚、血虚、津液亏虚等;失调则主要表现为气血津液运行失常。

(一)气失常

1. 气不足

气不足则形成气虚证,主要表现为面色萎黄、精神不振、倦怠乏力、语声低弱等。气虚而导致脏腑功能减退,可出现心气虚、脾气虚、肺气虚、肾气虚等证。

2. 气失调

气失调的病机变化较多,有气盛、气滞、气逆、气陷、气闭、气泄等。

气盛即气有余,气有余则使气机壅塞,并可化热化火。如肺气有余,气满胸中,壅塞不通,则胸中闷胀、喘息声高;若气有余而化火灼肺,则出现发热、汗多、口渴、咳吐黄稠痰等症。

气滞即气机不畅,运行受阻,郁滞于局部,引起胀满、疼痛等症;气机郁滞日久,则易化火。如肝气郁滞,则胸胁胀满,或有少腹胀痛,心情抑郁;若气郁化火,肝火上冲,可出现面红目赤,急躁易怒等症。

气逆、气陷、气闭、气泄四证,是由气的升降出入失常所导致的病机变化。气升太过,

excessive descent of qi causes sinking of qi; failure of qi to disperse causes closure of qi; loss of qi fixation causes leakage of qi. Adverse flow of qi and stagnation of qi are excess syndromes while sinking of qi and leakage of qi are deficiency syndromes. For example, adverse flow of liver-qi causes dizziness, distension of head or syncope; adverse flow of lung-qi causes cough and asthma; adverse flow of stomach-qi causes nausea and vomiting. Sinking of gastrosplenic qi causes dizziness, diarrhea, visceroptosis and proctoptosis. Stagnation of lung-qi causes chest oppression, unsmooth breath, stuffy nose and anhidrosis. Loss of fixation of lung-qi causes spontaneous sweating; loss of fixation of kidney-qi causes incontinence of urine; excessive leakage of qi causes loss of qi.

6.2.3.2　Disorder of blood

1. Insufficiency of blood

Insufficiency of blood causes blood deficiency syndrome with the manifestations of pale complexion, dizziness, palpitation, insomnia, light-colored lips and nails, scanty and light-colored menses, etc. Blood deficiency causes malnutrition of the viscera with the manifestations of heart-blood deficiency syndrome and liver-blood deficiency syndrome.

2. Disturbance of blood

The manifestations of blood disturbance are blood stasis and hemorrhage. The former refers to unsmooth flow of blood and blockage of meridians and vessels, leading to various pathological changes, such as pain, swelling, distension and abdominal mass. The latter is caused by flow of blood outside the vessels due to impairment of the vessels, or by failure of the spleen to command blood, or by failure of the liver to store blood, leading to various kinds of hemorrhage, such as hematemesis, hemoptysis, epistaxis, hematochezia and hematuria.

则为气逆;气降太过,则为气陷;气失宣泄,不得外出,可形成气闭;气失固摄,不能内守,可导致气泄。气逆、气闭多为实证,气陷、气泄多为虚证。如肝气上逆则眩晕、头胀或昏厥;肺气上逆则咳嗽、气喘;胃气上逆则恶心、呕吐;中气下陷则头昏目眩、大便下利、内脏下垂、脱肛;肺气郁闭则胸闷、呼吸不畅、鼻塞、无汗;肺气不固而气泄则自汗;肾气不固而气泄则小便失禁;凡气泄过度,可致气脱。

(二) 血失常

1. 血不足

血不足则形成血虚证,主要表现为面色淡白无华、头晕眼花、心悸少寐、口唇爪甲色淡、妇女月经量少色淡等。血虚而脏腑失养,主要表现为心血虚和肝血虚证。

2. 血失调

血失调主要表现为血瘀和出血。血瘀是血行不畅,经脉瘀阻,可导致疼痛、肿胀、癥积等病理变化。出血是因血脉损伤,血液离经;或脾不统血,或肝不藏血,导致各种出血证,如吐血、咯血、衄血、便血、尿血等。

6.2.3.3　Disorder of body fluid

1. Insufficiency of body fluid

Insufficiency of body fluid usually causes dryness syndrome. If the body is attacked by pathogenic dryness and heat, external dryness syndrome will be caused. Internal dryness syndrome is usually caused by transformation of abnormal changes of emotions into fire, or by fever, profuse sweating, excessive vomiting and diarrhea and hemorrhage. Dryness syndrome is often marked by insufficiency of body fluid, insufficient moisture in the skin, the orifices and the viscera which lead to dryness of the skin, dry mouth and throat, dry eyes, scanty urine and dry feces. Severe deficiency of body fluid eventually leads to yin-deficiency syndrome.

2. Disturbance of body fluid

Disturbance of body fluid refers to internal retention of water and dampness due to disturbance of the metabolism of body fluid, leading to phlegm, rheum and edema, etc. The disturbance of body fluid results from dysfunction of the spleen, the lung and the kidney which leads to failure of the spleen to transport and transform water and dampness, or failure of the lung to regulate water passage, or failure of the kidney to control water metabolism.

Disorder of qi, disorder of blood and disorder of body fluid usually affect each other. For example, deficiency of qi causes deficiency of blood and vice versa; stagnation of qi causes blood stasis and vice versa; stagnation of qi causes metabolic disturbance of body fluid; insufficiency of blood causes insufficiency of body fluid, etc. Such pathological changes caused by abnormal changes of the relationships between qi, blood and body fluid are described in detail in the fourth section of the third chapter entitled "Relationships Between Qi, Blood and Body Fluid".

（三）津液失常

1. 津液不足

津液不足主要形成燥证。若感受燥热之邪气,则形成外燥证;若由五志化火,或发热、多汗、吐下过度、失血等原因使津液耗伤,则形成内燥证。燥证的特征是津液不足,皮肤、孔窍、脏腑皆失其滋润,从而出现皮肤干燥、口干咽燥、两目干涩、小便短少、大便干结等症。津液亏虚严重者,则演变为阴虚证。

2. 津液失调

津液失调即津液的运行代谢障碍,水湿内停,从而导致痰饮、水肿等病证。其形成原因,主要在于脾、肺、肾三脏功能失调,使脾不能运化水湿,或肺不能通调水道,或肾不能主水液代谢,都可使气化失司,水湿停聚。

气失常、血失常、津液失常三方面的病机也可相互影响。如气虚可导致血虚,血虚也可导致气虚;气滞可导致血瘀,血瘀也可导致气滞;气滞则津液代谢障碍;血不足也可导致津液不足等。此类由气血津液关系失常所导致的病机变化,可参阅本书第三章第四节"气血津液之间的关系"。

7 Prevention and therapeutic principles

第七章 预防与治则

In its long course of development, TCM has established a perfect theory of prevention based on the theories of yin-yang, five elements, qi-blood-body fluid, meridians, cause of disease and pathogenesis, still effectively guiding medical practice now. The core of this theory is prevention and therapeutic principles.

TCM pays great attention to prevention and takes prevention as the essential one of therapeutic principles, emphasizing the role of reinforcing healthy qi and eliminating pathogenic factors in restoring balance between yin and yang. With full consideration of individual, local and seasonal conditions, it has established an effective system of therapeutic methods.

中医学在长期的发展过程中,形成了一整套比较完善的防治学理论,至今仍然有效地指导着中医的医疗实践。预防原则和治疗原则是中医防治学理论体系的核心。

中医预防原则和治疗原则,都是在中医阴阳五行、藏象、气血津液、经络、病因、病机等理论基础上确立起来的。其中,中医学特别强调预防为主的原则,提出"治未病"的重要医学思想。在治疗原则中,中医学把"治病求本"作为根本原则,抓住扶正与祛邪这两个重要环节,以恢复人体的阴阳平衡为治疗的根本目的,并注意因人、因地、因时制宜,建立起一套科学有效的治疗方法体系。

7.1 Principles of prevention

第一节 预防原则

Prevention means to take measures to prevent the occurrence and development of disease. The principles of prevention in TCM cover two aspects: theory and methods.

预防,就是采取一定的措施,防止疾病的发生和发展。中医的预防原则,传统称为"治未病",包括中医预防思想和中医预防方法两方面内容。

7.1.1 Theory of prevention

7.1.1.1 Importance of prevention

TCM gives prevention the priority over treatment. Before the occurrence of a disease or at the primary stage of a disease, it is important to take measures in advance to avoid suffering or aggravation, which is helpful for protecting healthy qi and maintaining health. Though correct and timely treatment can eliminate pathogenic factors, restore healthy qi and cure disease, the attack of any disease inevitably damages healthy qi or causes sequelae. Up to now there are still some diseases incurable or irreversible. So no matter how excellent therapeutic methods are, they must be used as the last resort. That is why *Huangdi Neijing* says that "the best doctors are those who can prevent the occurrence of disease". It believes that resorting to treatment when disease has already occurred is just like drilling a well when one feels thirsty and manufacturing weapons when war has already broken out.

7.1.1.2 The theoretical basis of the principles of prevention

The principles of prevention are decided according to etiopathology and the transmission of pathogenesis in TCM. Etiopathology in TCM holds that the occurrence of disease results from insufficiency of healthy qi and attack of pathogenic factors, among which insufficiency of healthy qi is the key factor responsible for the onset of disease. That is why the principles of prevention in TCM

一、中医预防思想

(一) 预防的重要性

中医学认为,在预防和治疗的关系中,预防是首要的。在疾病尚未发生之时,或疾病尚处于萌芽时期,及早采取积极有效的预防措施,可以免受疾病痛苦的折磨,或防止疾病加深加重,这对于维护人体正气,保持健康状态具有重要意义。虽然正确而及时的治疗可以祛除邪气,恢复正气,使疾病痊愈,但每一次疾病都对人体正气造成某种程度的耗损,或留下后遗症;某些疾病甚至尚无有效的治疗手段,有些疾病可给人体带来不可逆的损害,所以再好的治疗手段都是不得已而为之的,人最好能避免疾病的伤害。因此,《黄帝内经》提出"上工治未病"的理论,认为有病而后治疗,犹如临渴掘井,上阵铸兵,已嫌太晚。

(二) 预防原则的理论基础

中医预防原则是建立在中医发病学和病机传变的理论基础上的。中医发病学认为,疾病的产生,是由于人体正气的不足和邪气的侵袭,其中正气不足是主导因素。因此,中医预防原则一方面强调

pays attention to both the protection and cultivation of healthy qi and avoidance of the invasion of pathogenic factors. According to transmission of pathogenesis, disease transmits among the viscera when it has emerged. The regions and organs that are weakened or insufficient of healthy qi tend to be affected. That is why the principles of prevention advocate early treatment and control of transmission.

7.1.1.3　The guiding ideology of the principles of prevention

1. Emphasis on holistic concept

The human body forms an integrated wholeness in itself and with the external environment. That is why TCM emphasizes both the harmonious relationship between the body and external environment and the interrelationships between the viscera and the meridians.

2. Emphasis on the protective effect of healthy qi

Among various preventive measures, the protection and cultivation of healthy qi is the most important one.

3. Emphasis on the integration of the body and the mind

The concept of health includes health of the body and health of the mind. Since psychological factors play a very important role in etiopathology, TCM gives psychological regulation and cultivation the priority over other preventive measures.

对人体正气的保护和培养,同时也重视避免邪气的侵袭。病机传变理论认为,疾病形成之后可以在脏腑经络之间传变,凡有虚弱不足之所,即是病邪最易传变之处,所以预防原则主张早期治疗和控制传变。

（三）预防原则的指导思想

中医预防原则的指导思想主要有以下三点。

1. 强调整体观念

人体与外界环境是一个息息相关的整体,人体自身也是一个有机的整体,所以在预防疾病过程中既要重视人体与环境的协调关系,又要重视人体脏腑经络形体之间的相互联系。

2. 强调正气的首要作用

在各种预防措施中,保护和培养正气是根本性的措施,所以在中医预防原则中特别重视养生。

3. 强调身心合一

健康不仅是身体的健康,也包括心理的健康。人的心理精神因素在疾病发生中具有不可低估的重要作用,因此中医预防原则把精神调养放在各种预防措施的首位。

7.1.2　The preventive methods

7.1.2.1　Giving prevention the priority

Giving prevention the priority means to take measures to prevent the occurrence of disease. Since the occurrence of disease is related to insufficiency of healthy qi and attack of pathogenic factors, the preventive measures taken should focus on reinforcing healthy qi and preventing the invasion of pathogenic factors by means of regulating psychological state, diet and living habit as well as doing physical exercise. Besides, cares should be taken to avoid attack of pathogenic factors.

1. Regulating psychological state

Regulating psychological state covers three aspects: avoiding direct damage of the viscera and disturbance of qi and blood; avoiding invasion of pathogenic factors due to deficiency of healthy qi caused by psychological factors; protecting and cultivating healthy qi to further strengthen constitution. There are various ways to regulate psychological state, the general principle is to be free from avarice. If one keeps the mind tranquil, qi and blood will flow normally, yin and yang in the body can communicate freely with that in the natural world, which can not only prevent the invasion of pathogenic factors but also strengthen constitution.

2. Proper diet

Diet provides necessary nutrients for the body, but unhealthy eating habits and improper food (such as intemperance or starvation, unhygienic food and food partiality) impair the viscera and damage harmonious state of qi and

二、中医预防方法

（一）未病先防

未病先防，就是在未病之前，先行预防，不使疾病发生。由于疾病的发生关系到正气不足和邪气侵袭两个方面的因素，所以只要从这两方面着手，使正气不虚，或不让邪气侵入，就可达到预防的目的。从保护和培养正气方面来说，可以采取精神调养、饮食养生、生活起居养生、锻炼身体等方法。此外，还要注意避免病邪的侵袭。

1. 精神调养

精神调养的目的有三：第一，避免七情直接损伤内脏，扰乱气血；第二，避免精神因素导致正气虚弱，邪气乘虚而入；第三，保护和培养正气，进一步增强体质。精神调养的方法很多，其总的原则是要求人们清心寡欲、恬淡虚无。人体在精神宁静的状态下，气血不乱，运行有序，天地阴阳之气能与人体相通相应，不但邪气不得侵入，而且体质也会越来越强。

2. 饮食养生

饮食养生的作用，主要是避免过饥过饱、饮食不洁、饮食偏嗜等因素损害和破坏人体脏腑、气血的平衡与协调，

blood. To cultivate health through regulating diet can supplement essence, adjust the state of yin and yang, improve constitution and strengthen body resistance. There are various ways to cultivate health through regulation of diet, these methods should be applied according to individual conditions. The general principle is to eat regularly at the right time in proper proportions with hygienic eating habits.

3. Proper living habits

Proper living habits include regular work and rest, temperance in sexual activity and proper clothing in different seasons. Proper living habits are effective in abiding by the variations of yin and yang in the natural world, protecting the viscera, qi, blood and body fluid, and preventing invasion of pathogenic factors.

4. Exercising the body

Exercising the body can promote the flow of qi and blood, reinforce the functions of the viscera and prevent retention of pathogenic factors. There are various ways to exercise the body. However traditional ways to exercise the body are more effective for strengthening constitution, eliminating disease and prolonging life, such as Wuqinxi (five-animals frolics), Baduanjin (eight-sections exercise), Yijinjing (tendon-relaxing exercise) and Taijiquan (taiji box), etc. These traditional exercises are slow in action and general in relaxation, very effective for directing the flow of qi and blood. They combine static actions with dynamic activities, effective for regulating both yin and yang without damaging tendons and exhausting qi and blood. People with different constitution should select

同时可从饮食获得人体所必需的营养物质。通过饮食养生,还可补益精气,调整阴阳,改善体质,进一步增强抗病能力。饮食养生的方法很多,应根据人的体质状况因人制宜地进行。其一般原则是,饮食应适时而有节,寒温适宜,精粗搭配,讲究卫生,无不良饮食习惯及嗜好等。

3. 生活起居养生

生活起居养生包括多方面内容,如作息应有规律,房事要有节制,衣着应适应时令气候变化,劳逸应当结合等。通过生活起居养生,可以顺应自然界阴阳变化,保护人体脏腑精气血津液而不使过分耗散,这样邪气就无侵入之机。

4. 锻炼身体

锻炼身体,可以促进人体气血流通,增进脏腑功能,防止邪气留着而致病。古今锻炼方法很多,但传统的锻炼方法更能增强体质,祛病延年,如五禽戏、八段锦、易筋经、太极拳等。传统锻炼方法的优点在于,其动作舒缓、全面,具有独到的导引气血的功效,而且动静结合,有双调阴阳的作用,而无伤损筋骨、耗散气血的不良作用。但对不同体质的人,应选择适宜的锻炼方法,量力而行。

different exercise.

5. Avoiding attack of pathogenic factors

Since pathogenic factors are the key elements in causing disease, measures have to be taken to avoid the attack of pathogenic factors in the cultivation of healthy qi. Some pathogenic factors are very toxic, even strong constitution cannot resist them. Thus the avoidance of these pathogenic factors is the only way to prevent the occurrence of disease.

7.1.2.2 Preventing transmission and change

When disease has occurred, it may transmit from a local area to the viscera and other regions. In this case, measures have to be taken to stop such transmission and change.

1. Early treatment

At the early stage, disease is easy to treat because it is still light and healthy qi has not declined yet. However, delayed treatment may worsen the disease and make it difficult to treat due to transmission of pathogenic factors from the external to the internal and damage of healthy qi. If healthy qi is seriously impaired and pathogenic factors become more and more predominant, the disease is hard to treat and tends to become aggravated. So early treatment is very important.

2. Controlling the transmission and change

Transmission and change refer to movement and change of disease in the external and the internal, the upper and the lower, the zang-organs and the fu-organs, the

5. 避免病邪侵袭

由于邪气是致病的重要条件,所以在培养正气的同时,也要注意避免被邪气所伤。有些病邪毒性很强,即使正气强盛,一般也难以抵御,只有不让邪气侵入,才能防止疾病的发生。

(二) 既病防变

疾病发生以后,开始可能只在人体的某个局部,以后会随其发展进程而向其他脏腑或部位传变。采取积极措施,阻断其传变途径,不使病邪传变,这就是既病防变的原则。既病防变也属于中医预防原则的范畴,它包括早期治疗和控制传变两方面。

1. 早期治疗

疾病初期,病情轻浅,正气未衰,比较易治。若治疗失时,病邪会由表入里,病情由轻变重,正气因此受到耗损,治疗就变得难了。若正气耗损严重,邪气日益亢盛,以致邪胜正衰,不但治疗棘手,而且有恶化死亡的危险。所以,早期治疗是中医学的一个重要原则。

2. 控制传变

传变,是指疾病在表里、上下、脏腑、经络、卫气营血等不同部位或层次之间的传移

meridians and the collaterals, wei, qi, ying and blood phases. The transmission and change of disease follow certain rules and routes. Measures can be taken according to these rules and routes to prevent the transmission and change of disease in advance.

The method for controlling the transmission and change of disease is to regulate and nourish the organs or areas that the disease is liable to transmit to by means of reinforcing healthy qi to prevent the transmission of the disease. For example, it is said in *Jingui Yaolüe* "measures must be taken to strengthen the spleen in the treatment of liver disease because liver disease tends to transmit to the spleen." That means to invigorate spleen-qi to prevent liver disease from transmitting to the spleen. Take febrile disease for another example. Since pathogenic heat damages yin, the impairment of stomach-yin can damage kidney-yin. Under such a condition, the prescription composed herbs sweet in taste and cold in nature for nourishing the stomach can be added with some herbs salty in taste and cold in nature for nourishing kidney-yin in order to prevent pathogenic heat from impairing the kidney.

7.2 Therapeutic principles

Therapeutic principles are decided according to the concept of holism and treatment based on syndrome differentiation, clinically guiding the composition of prescriptions and the selection of herbs.

Therapeutic principles and therapeutic methods are different. The former guides the latter and the latter specifies the former. Their difference is relative. In fact, some minor therapeutic principles are quite similar to certain major therapeutic methods and vice versa. The so-

变化,故也称"传化"。传变有一定的规律和途径,根据其传变的规律和途径,采取预防措施,不使疾病传变,是既病防变的又一重要内容。

控制传变的方法,是在疾病可能传变的下一个环节或层次的某一脏腑器官或部位,先进行调补,促使其正气转强而不受邪,就可以防止病邪的传变。如《金匮要略》提出"见肝之病,知肝传脾,当先实脾",就是指先充实其脾,令脾气得补而转旺盛,就可以切断其肝病传脾的病理进程,达到控制疾病传变的目的。又如温热病热邪伤阴,胃阴受损,进一步可耗伤肾阴,此时可在甘寒养胃之方中加入咸寒养肾阴的药物,防止热邪伤肾。

第二节　治疗原则

治疗原则,简称治则。治则是在整体观念和辨证论治精神指导下制定的,对临床治疗立法、处方、用药,具有普遍指导意义。

治则与治法不同,治则是用以指导治疗方法的总则,治疗方法是治则的具体化。因此,任何治疗方法总是从属于一定的治疗原则的。然而,治

called "major therapeutic method" in clinic can be taken both as a therapeutic method and a therapeutic principle.

7.2.1 Concentrating treatment on the root cause

7.2.1.1 Significance

"Ben" (root) and "biao" (branch) are two relatively opposite concepts with varied connotations in different cases. In exogenous diseases, the invasion of pathogenic factors is ben and the disorder of visceral qi and blood is biao. In endogenous diseases, the disorder of visceral qi and blood is ben and the clinical manifestations are biao. In terms of etiology and symptoms, the cause of disease is ben and the symptoms are biao. In terms of the sequence of diseases, old disease and primary disease are ben while new disease and secondary disease are biao. In the expression "concentrating treatment on the root cause", "ben" emphasizes the cause of disease while "biao" refers to the clinical manifestations.

Concentrating treatment on the root cause means to find the root cause of a disease and focus the treatment on it because the root cause is responsible for the emergence of syndrome. For this reason the process of searching root cause is the same as that of syndrome differentiation. That is why treatment based on syndrome differentiation

则与治法的区分只是相对的，某些较小的治则类似于较大的治法，某些较大的治法也可以归入治则的范畴。临床常说的"治疗大法"，就可以看作是界于治则和治法之间的概念。

本书介绍几个最基本的治则，包括治病求本、扶正祛邪、调整阴阳、因人因地因时制宜等。

一、治病求本

（一）治病求本的意义

"本"是和"标"相对而言的，两者是一组相对的概念。在不同的范围内使用，"本"与"标"具有不同的含义。在外感病中，外邪侵袭是本，脏腑气血失常是标；在内伤病中，脏腑气血失常是本，临床表现是标；从病因和症状来说，病因是本，症状是标；从疾病先后来说，旧病、原发病是本，新病、继发病是标。在治病求本的概念中，"本"着重于反映疾病的原因，"标"着重于说明疾病的临床表现。

治病求本，就是寻求疾病的根本原因，并针对根本原因进行治疗。从本质上讲，疾病的根本原因也是造成"证"的根据，求本的过程与辨证的过程是一致的，所

becomes a typical feature of TCM.

For each disease, there are various symptoms, but the root cause is just one. If you find the root cause, you can successfully treat any disease no matter how complicated it is. If you cannot find the root cause of a disease, it is very hard for you achieve successful treatment. Take headache for example. It may be caused by exogenous factors or endogenous factors. Only when the root cause is found can it be successfully treated. Exogenous headache can be treated by external relief therapy with acrid and warm herbs if it is caused by pathogenic wind-cold or by external relief therapy with acrid and cool herbs if it is caused by wind-heat. Endogenous headache may be caused by insufficiency of yin-blood, blockage of vessels, upward disturbance of phlegm-dampness and hyperactivity of liver-yang. So different therapeutic methods have to be used to deal with endogenous headache due to different causes, such as nourishing yin and invigorating blood, activating blood to resolve stasis, drying dampness and resolving phlegm, and soothing the liver and suppressing yang, etc.

7.2.1.2　Application

1. Treating biao in emergency

This means to treat the secondary symptoms first and then deal with the root cause in emergency. These symptoms are usually acute and bring on great suffering to the patients, or threaten life or tend to transmit and change. If they are overlooked, the pathological conditions may be

以治病求本实际上也就是辨证论治。辨证论治之所以能成为中医学一个基本特点，正是因为它符合了治病求本这一根本治则。

每一种疾病，其症状表现可以多种多样，但其根本原因（病机本质）只有一个。抓住了疾病的根本原因，也就是抓住了疾病的关键，针对疾病的关键进行治疗，无论多么复杂多样的症候表现都将随之而解。否则，抓不住疾病的本质，找不到正确的治疗方法，只能是头痛医头、脚痛医脚，也就达不到治疗的目的。如头痛一证，可由外感或内伤引起，必须找到其本质原因才能进行治疗。外感头痛，有属于风寒者，治宜用辛温解表法；有属于风热者，治宜用辛凉解表法。内伤头痛，又有阴血不足、血络瘀阻、痰湿上扰、肝阳上亢等不同病机，故其治疗应分别采用滋阴养血、活血化瘀、燥湿化痰、平肝潜阳等方法进行治疗。

（二）治病求本的运用

1. 急则治标

急则治标，是指当标症（病）紧急时，应当先治其标，然后再治其本。所谓标症紧急，是指所出现的标症比较急重，对病人造成很大痛苦时；

aggravated or make it difficult to treat "ben".

Clinically the following symptoms can be regarded as acute symptoms requiring immediate treatment: massive hemorrhage, extremely high temperature, sharp pain, violent vomiting or diarrhea, constipation and anuria, severe abdominal distension and fullness, serious ascites and edema, dyspnea and inhibited respiration, and mania, etc. In any case immediate measures should be taken to deal with these acute symptoms no matter what disease it is.

Treating biao in emergency does not contradict concentrating treatment on the root cause. The former paves the way for the latter. When acute symptoms are relieved, treatment can be concentrated on the root cause. In fact treating biao in emergency is an emergent treatment. For mild cases, the treatment should certainly focus on the root cause.

Clinically you may encounter disease marked by emergency or non-emergency of both the biao. In any case simple treatment of the biao or the ben is ineffective. The right way to deal with this case is to focus the treatment on both the ben and the biao. For example, impairment of yin by pathogenic heat and exhaustion of yin-fluid are the ben, while abdominal fullness, hardness and pain as well as retention of dry feces are the biao. This disease is obviously marked by emergency of both the biao and the ben. So the

或标症紧急可威胁生命时；或标症新起，有传变倾向时等。此时若不先治标，病情可能发生意外变化，或直接影响对"本"的治疗。

临床上见到如下情形时，可视为标症紧急：大出血、体温过高、剧烈疼痛、剧烈呕吐或泄泻、大小便不通、腹胀满甚剧、严重腹水及水肿、喘急而呼吸不畅、狂躁不宁等。此时不论病本如何，都应先治其标，立即采取止血、退热、止痛、止吐、止泻、通便、利尿、除胀、逐水、降气平喘、镇静安神等救急措施。

急则治标与治病求本并不矛盾，治标的目的正是为治本创造条件，待标症缓解以后，必须专一治本，所以与"急则治标"相对的一个概念就是"缓则治本"。所以，治标只是一种临时的应急措施，而以后的治本才是促使疾病痊愈的根本手段。

临床上还可出现标本俱急的情形，或标本虽皆不急，但单纯治标或治本都不易收效，此时可以把治标和治本结合起来，采取标本兼治的方法。如因邪热伤阴，阴液耗竭，此为本；同时腹满硬痛，大便燥结，此为标。显然此病标本俱急，必须泻下与滋阴同

treatment of purgation and nourishing yin has to be resorted to in order to relieve abdominal fullness, hardness and
pain, eliminate constipation and restore yin-fluid. If a
weak person is attacked by exogenous pathogenic factors,
simple treatment of supporting healthy qi to consolidate
constitution cannot remove exogenous pathogenic factors,
while simple treatment of eliminating pathogenic factors
and the biao will further exhaust healthy qi. The right
way to deal with this problem is to treat the ben and the
biao simultaneously by means of supporting healthy qi and
relieving the superficies.

2. Contrary treatment

Contrary treatment is just the opposite of routine
treatment. The latter refers to treatment opposite to the
nature of disease, suitable for the treatment of a majority
of diseases. For example, treating cold syndrome with
heat herbs, treating heat syndrome with cold herbs, treating deficiency syndrome with tonic herbs and treating excess syndrome with herbs for eliminating pathogenic factors are all routine therapeutic methods that are opposite
to the nature of disease and agree with the principle of
concentrating treating on the root cause.

Contrary treatment means treating disease according
to its false manifestations. The false manifestations of a
disease do not agree with the nature of the disease. Cares
should be taken to find the root cause and not be puzzled
by the false manifestations. Since contrary treatment just
agrees with the false manifestations, it is in fact opposite
to the nature of the disease. In this sense contrary treatment is also a kind of routine treatment.

用,既使腹满硬痛得解,大便
得通,又使耗竭之阴液得救,
起到一种双解危急、相辅相成
的作用。又如体虚之人,反复
外感,若单扶正治本,则其外
邪留连;若单祛邪治标,则更
耗伤正气。此时可以采用扶
正解表法,标本同治,就更切
合病情。

2. 反治

"反治"是与"正治"相对
而言的。所谓"正治",就是逆
其病证性质而治,故也称"逆
治"。对于大多数病证来说,
都适用正治法。如用寒药治
疗热证,用热药治疗寒证,用
补益药治疗虚证,用祛邪药治
疗实证等。逆治法是针对疾
病本质原因进行治疗的,它符
合治病求本的根本原则。

所谓"反治",就是顺从疾
病假象而治,故又称"从治"。
疾病的假象与疾病的本质不
符,治疗时不能被假象所迷
惑,而应透过假象看到疾病的
根本原因,然后针对其根本原
因进行治疗。由于治法与假
象的性质一致,所以就与其本
质相逆。也就是说,反治法表
面上与疾病的假象相顺从,实
质上仍与疾病的性质相逆,所
以归根结底仍属于正治。之

Routine treatment is an inhibiting therapy while contrary treatment is an inducing therapy. For example, emetic therapy, instead of the therapy for stopping vomiting, is used to treat nausea and vomiting caused by retention of phlegm in the upper energizer; purgation, instead of the therapy for stopping diarrhea, is used to treat diarrhea due to accumulation of dampness in the lower energizer. Contrary treatment also can be used to treat disease at the initial stage with predominant pathogenic factors which cannot be treated by inhibiting therapy.

The following are some of the commonly used contrary therapeutic methods.

(1) Treating false heat syndrome with hot-natured herbs: That means to use hot-natured herbs to treat disease with false heat symptoms. This therapy can be used to treat syndrome of real cold and false heat due to exuberant internal cold that drives yang outward. Take the case of extreme deficiency of kidney-yang and exuberance of internal cold for example. It is marked by cold feet and hands on the one hand, and no aversion to cold and reddish complexion on the other. These manifestations actually indicate predominance of cold drives yang floating outside. Since the root cause is internal exuberance of yin-

所以采取顺从疾病假象的治法，也是为了适应治病求本这一根本原则的需要。

反治的另一含义是"顺势"而治。一般治法是采取正面抑制的方法，"顺势"而治则采取因势利导的方法。如痰阻上焦，出现恶心呕吐，不用降逆止呕的方法，反用涌吐的方法，使痰吐出，其呕吐自止。湿聚下焦，出现便泄下利，不用收敛止泄的治法，反用通下利导的方法，使湿从下去，其下利自止。凡疾病初起，邪势正盛，不宜用抑遏之法，皆宜使邪有出路，所用治法往往与病势相顺从，所以也属于"从治"。这种从治，必须在认清疾病本质的基础上才能实施，因此也属于治病求本治则的一种运用。

常用的反治法如下。

（1）热因热用 热因热用就是以热治热，即用热性药物治疗具有假热症状的病证，适用于阴寒内盛，格阳于外，反见热象的真寒假热证。如肾阳虚衰至极，阴寒内盛，虽有手足厥逆，而身反不恶寒，面色红艳如妆，即是寒盛而浮阳外越之象。由于阴寒内盛是其本质，故仍用温热药治其真寒，其假热会自然消失。

cold, warm herbs should be used to treat real cold. When the real cold is eliminated, false heat disappears naturally.

(2) Treating false cold syndrome with cold-natured herbs: That means to treat disease with false cold symptoms with cold-natured herbs. This therapy can be used to treat syndrome of real heat and false cold due to exuberance of internal heat that drives yin outside. Take syncope in febrile disease for example. Though there are symptoms of high fever, dysphoria, thirst and preference for cold water, but the four limbs are cold and the pulse is deep. It is a syndrome caused by deep latent heat that prevents yang from extending to the external. Since exuberance of internal heat is the root cause, cold herbs must be used to treat real heat. When the real heat is eliminated, false cold disappears naturally.

(3) Treating blockage with tonic herbs: This therapy can be used to treat syndrome of real deficiency and false excess due to hypofunction of the viscera caused by decline of qi and blood. Take abdominal distension in patients with spleen deficiency, constipation in old people due to deficiency of qi and blood and amenorrhea due to exhaustion of blood for example. These syndromes are all marked by real deficiency and false excess and cannot be treated by purgation. Instead, nourishing therapy should be used to promote the flow of qi and blood, invigorate the functions of the viscera and dredge the meridians and collaterals.

(4) Treating outthrust with dredging therapy: This therapy can be used to treat outthrust syndrome due to internal accumulation of pathogenic factors. For example, sweating due to attack of pathogenic wind, diarrhea due to food retention, sudden uterine bleeding due to blood stasis

（2）寒因寒用　寒因寒用就是以寒治寒，即用寒性药物治疗具有假寒症状的病证，适用于里热盛极，阳盛格阴，反见寒象的真热假寒证。如温热病出现热厥，虽见壮热心烦，口渴而喜冷饮，但四肢厥冷，脉象反沉，即是热邪深伏而阳不外达之象。由于热盛于内是其本质，故须用寒凉药治其真热，其假寒方能消失。

（3）塞因塞用　塞因塞用就是以补开塞，即用补益药物治疗具有虚性闭塞不通症状的病证，适用于气血虚衰，脏腑功能减退，反见壅塞不通证候的真虚假实证。如脾虚病人出现腹胀，老年气血虚弱导致便秘，妇女血枯引起闭经等，都属于真虚假实的病证。此时不宜妄用攻伐，应用补益之法促进气血运行，增强脏腑功能，则经络气血得以疏通运行，其壅塞自然开通。

（4）通因通用　通因通用就是以通治通，即用通利的药物治疗具有实性通泄症状的病证，适用于邪气内聚，顺势外泄，而出现向外涌泄证候的

and urgent and frequent urination are all outthrust syndromes of excess in nature. However, they cannot be simply treated by astringing therapy, otherwise pathogenic factors will be retained inside. The right way to deal with them is to induce the pathogenic factors to leave the body with dredging therapy.

病证。如感受风邪而致出汗,食积而致泄泻,瘀血而致崩漏,湿热下注而致尿频尿急等,都属于实性通泄的病证。此时不宜误用收涩,以致闭门留邪,而应顺其势而仍用开通之法祛除邪气,疾病方能痊愈。

7. 2. 2 Strengthening healthy qi and eliminating pathogenic factors

The duration of a disease is a process of struggle between healthy qi and pathogenic factors, the result of which decides the development of the disease. If healthy qi succeeds, the disease gets improved and gradually heals; if pathogenic factors succeed, the disease becomes worsened or leads to death. In order to enable the disease to develop along a favourable route, it is necessary to support healthy qi and eliminate pathogenic factors. So supporting healthy qi and eliminating pathogenic factors is an important therapeutic principle in clinic treatment.

7.2.2.1 Significance
1. Strengthening healthy qi

Strengthening healthy qi usually refers to "nourishing therapy" which includes various methods, such as herbs, acupuncture and moxibustion, tuina therapy, diet regulation and exercise, etc. Nourishing therapy is usually used to treat deficiency syndromes such as qi deficiency, blood deficiency, yin deficiency, body fluid deficiency and kidney-essence deficiency. That is why it is said in TCM that "deficiency syndrome should be treated by nourishing therapy". Nourishing therapy can be further divided into different therapeutic methods to deal with different pathogenic factors, such as qi-nourishing therapy, blood-nourishing therapy, yin-

二、扶正祛邪

疾病的过程始终贯穿着邪正斗争,邪正斗争的盛衰与胜负,决定着疾病的发展演变与转归。若正胜邪退,则疾病好转并逐渐痊愈;若邪胜正衰,则疾病恶化或归于死亡。为了促使疾病向好转、痊愈方向转化,就必须扶助正气,祛除邪气,促使正气战胜邪气。因此,扶正祛邪是指导临床治疗的一个重要原则。

(一)扶正祛邪的意义
1. 扶正

所谓扶正,就是扶助正气,通常称为"补法"。补法有多种手段,如药物、针灸、推拿、饮食调理、气功锻炼等,都具有补益的功效。补法适用于虚证,故有"虚则补之"的理论。凡气虚、血虚、阴虚、阳虚、津液不足、肾精亏少等,都可用补法。针对不同的情况,补法可分为益气、养血、滋阴、温阳、生津、填精等多种具体

nourishing therapy, yang-warming therapy, fluid-genera-
ting therapy and essence-enriching therapy, etc. By
means of strengthening healthy qi, deficiency can be improved, body resistance can be reinforced and pathogenic
factors can be eliminated. In fact the purpose of strengthening healthy qi is to eliminate pathogenic factors. However, excess syndrome with predominance of pathogenic
factors cannot be treated by nourishing therapy because nourishing therapy may retain pathogenic factors in the body.

2. Eliminating pathogenic factors

Eliminating pathogenic factors refers to "purgation
therapy" (also known as "attack therapy") with herbs or
acupuncture and moxibustion. Purgation therapy is used to
treat excess syndromes such as attack of exogenous pathogenic factors, retention of food, internal accumulation of
phlegm-dampness, internal retention of water, internal
blockage of blood stasis, stagnancy of qi activity, exuberance of fire and stagnation of pathogenic cold, etc. That is
why it is said in TCM that "excess syndrome should be
treated by purgation therapy." Purgation therapy can be
further divided into different therapeutic methods to deal
with different pathogenic factors, such as diaphoresis
therapy, emetic therapy, defecation-promoting therapy,
water-draining therapy, blood-activating therapy, damp-
ness-resolving therapy, stasis-breaking therapy, heat-
clearing therapy and cold-dissipating therapy, etc. Eliminating pathogenic factors is helpful for restoring and
strengthening healthy qi. However, deficiency syndrome
due to insufficiency of healthy qi cannot be treated by purgation therapy because purgation therapy tends to impair
healthy qi.

7.2.2.2 Application of strengthening heal-
thy qi and eliminating pathogenic factors

In applying the principle of strengthening healthy qi

治法。通过扶正治法,可以纠
正虚损,增强正气,提高抗病
能力,从而有助于祛除邪气。
所以,扶正治法也起到了祛邪
的作用,扶正的目的也是为了
祛邪。但是,邪气亢盛的实证
不宜用补法,因为补法易使邪
气留恋于体内,不利于祛邪。

2. 祛邪

所谓祛邪,就是祛除邪
气,通常称为"泻法"(也称"攻
法")。泻法可以通过药物和
针灸来进行。泻法适用于实
证,故有"实则泻之"的理论。
凡有外邪侵袭、食积停滞、痰
湿内蕴、水气内停、瘀血内阻、
气机郁滞、热盛火旺、寒邪结
滞等,都可用泻法。针对不同
邪气,泻法可分别采用发汗、
涌吐、通下、利水、化湿、活血、
破瘀、消食、清热、散寒等多种
具体治法。通过祛邪治法,可
以祛除邪气,中止邪气对人体
正气进一步的损害,从而有利
于正气的恢复。所以,祛邪治
法也有扶助正气的作用,祛邪
的目的也是为了扶正。但是,
正气不足的虚证不能用泻法,
因为泻法易损伤正气,不利于
扶正。

(二) 扶正祛邪的运用

运用扶正祛邪的原则时,

and eliminating pathogenic factors, one must carefully analyze the state of pathogenic factors and the condition of healthy qi, differentiate the nature of the syndrome in question and distinguish the relationship between healthy qi and pathogenic factors in order to select the right therapy. Generally speaking, simple deficiency can be treated by strengthening healthy qi and simple excess syndrome can be treated by eliminating pathogenic factors. For the treatment of syndrome mixed with both deficiency and excess, the therapy for strengthening healthy qi and the therapy for eliminating pathogenic factors can be used simultaneously. Since the order and urgency of deficiency of healthy qi and excess of pathogenic factors are different, there are three methods for strengthening healthy qi and eliminating pathogenic factors, i.e. purgation prior to tonification, tonification prior to purgation and simultaneous application of purgation and tonification.

1. Purgation prior to tonification

Purgation prior to tonification means to eliminate pathogenic factors first and then strengthen healthy qi. If a syndrome mixed with deficiency of healthy qi and excess of pathogenic factors is marked by predomination of pathogenic factors that must be eliminated immediately and deficiency of healthy qi that still can bear attack, the therapy for strengthening healthy qi may reinforce pathogenic factors instead of strengthening healthy qi. In this case purgation should be used first. After pathogenic factors are reduced, nourishing therapy can be used to strengthen healthy qi. Take sudden uterine bleeding due to blood stasis for example. If blood stasis is not eliminated, hemorrhage cannot be stopped. Though hemorrhagia should be treated by nourishing therapy, tonic herbs may make it difficult to eliminate blood stasis. If hemorrhage continues, blood deficiency cannot be rectified. In this case

要仔细地分析邪正双方力量的对比情况,辨别证候的虚实性质,分清邪盛与正衰的主次关系,分别采用不同的治法。一般情况下,单纯虚证可以用扶正治法,单纯实证可以用祛邪治法,若属于正虚邪实相兼的虚实错杂证,则应扶正与祛邪并用。根据正虚与邪实的主次和缓急的不同,扶正与祛邪并用有三种不同的用法,即先攻后补、先补后攻和攻补兼施。

1. 先攻后补

即先祛邪后扶正。在正虚邪实的虚实错杂证中,若邪气盛,急待祛邪,而正气虽虚,尚可耐攻;若兼顾扶正反会助邪,此时应先攻邪,待邪气大势已去,然后再用补法。如瘀血所致崩漏证,因瘀血不去,出血不止,虽有失血当补,但恐滋腻之药不利于祛瘀,出血不止则血虚难复,此时可先行活血化瘀,以图血止,然后再用调经补血之法缓治其本。

measures should be taken to activate blood to resolve stasis in order to stop bleeding. Then nourishing therapy can be used to invigorate blood.

2. Tonification prior to purgation

Tonification prior to purgation means to strengthen healthy qi first and then eliminate pathogenic factors. This therapy can be used to treat syndrome mixed with deficiency of healthy qi'and excess of pathogenic factors. Though pathogenic factors should be eliminated，healthy qi is too deficient to bear attack. Early application of purgation may impair healthy qi. In this case tonifying therapy should be used first to strengthen healthy qi. Take ascites for example. Since healthy qi is deficient for a long time and cannot bear purgation，measures should be taken to strengthen healthy qi. After healthy qi is reinforced，purging therapy can be used to eliminate pathogenic factors and drain water.

3. Simultaneous application of purgation and tonification

This therapy means to strengthen healthy qi and to eliminate pathogenic factors simultaneously. It can be used to treat syndrome mixed with deficiency of healthy qi and excess of pathogenic factors. Because simple use of tonification may make pathogenic factors linger inside and simple use of purgation may impair healthy qi. Take common cold due to qi deficiency for example. It can be treated by supplementing qi and relieving superficies at the same time.

7.2.3　Regulation of yin and yang

TCM believes the root cause of disease is imbalance between yin and yang. So the sole purpose for treating disease is to readjust yin and yang and restore the normal balance between yin and yang. Since the main manifestations of imbalance between yin and yang are relative

2. 先补后攻

即先扶正后祛邪。适用于正虚邪实的虚实错杂证,此时虽有邪气当祛,但正气虚衰较甚,不耐攻伐,若过早地用攻法治疗,会更伤正气,恐有正气不支之虞,所以应先用补法扶正,使正气恢复到能承受攻伐时再攻其邪。如鼓胀病水邪盘踞腹中,而正气虚衰日久,正气不耐峻药攻逐,应先扶正,待时机成熟然后再用攻邪逐水之法,方为稳妥。

3. 攻补兼施

即扶正与祛邪兼用。适用于正虚邪实的虚实错杂证,若单用补则有恋邪之忧,单用攻又恐伤正,兼用则有相得益彰之利,此时应当攻补兼施。如气虚感冒,可用补气兼解表法治疗。

三、调整阴阳

中医学认为,疾病的根本原因是阴阳失调。因此,治疗疾病的关键在于调整阴阳,使之恢复阴阳平衡状态。由于阴阳失调主要表现为阴阳偏

predomination of yin and yang and relative decline of yin and yang, the purpose of regulating yin and yang is to reduce the excess and supplement deficiency.

7.2.3.1 Reducing excess

Relative predomination of yin or yang means excess. Relative predomination of yin means excess of yin and relative predomination of yang means excess of yang. Reduce excess means to reduce relative predomination and restore the normal state of yin or yang. Since the syndrome caused by excess of yin or yang is of excess in nature and the treatment of excess syndrome is purgation, the principle for "reducing excess" is also known as "excess should be treated by purgation" in TCM.

Relative predomination of yin causes excess-cold syndrome while relative predomination of yang causes excess-heat syndrome. The therapeutic principle for treating excess-cold syndrome is "to treat cold syndrome with heat therapy" while the therapeutic principle for treating excess-heat syndrome is "to treat heat syndrome with cold therapy."

Since yin and yang are opposite to each other, predomination of yin may damage yang and predomination of yang may impair yin. So in the treatment of syndromes due to predomination of yin or yang, cares should be taken to differentiate the state of the other side so as to take both sides into consideration if necessary, i. e. dispersing yin-cold in combination with strengthening yang and clearing yang-heat in combination with nourishing yin.

7.2.3.2 Supplementing insufficiency

Relative decline of yin or yang means insufficiency. Relative decline of yin means insufficiency of yin and

盛和阴阳偏衰,所以调整阴阳的意义就在于,通过损其有余和补其不足,纠正偏盛和偏衰的病理状态,达到恢复阴阳平衡的目的。

(一) 损其有余

阴阳偏盛都属于有余。阴偏盛为阴有余,阳偏盛为阳有余。损其有余,就是削弱其偏盛,使过于亢盛的阴或阳恢复到正常状态。由于阴阳偏盛所导致的证候性质为实证,治疗实证的大法为"泻",所以"损其有余"的原则在治疗学上也称"实则泻之"。

阴阳偏盛分为阴偏盛和阳偏盛,阴偏盛则形成实寒证,阳偏盛则形成实热证。针对实寒证,相应的治法是"寒者热之",即用温热药等以温散其阴寒;针对实热证,相应的治法是"热者寒之",即用寒凉药等以清泻其阳热。

由于阴阳是对立的,阴盛可以伤阳,阳盛可以伤阴,所以在治疗阴阳偏盛的病证时,应注意其相对一方受损伤的情况,必要时应当兼顾其不足,即在温散阴寒时兼顾扶阳,清泻阳热时兼顾滋阴。

(二) 补其不足

阴阳偏衰都属于不足。阴偏衰为阴不足,阳偏衰为阳

relative decline of yang means insufficiency of yang. Supplementing insufficiency means rectifying decline and restoring the normal state of yin or yang. Since the syndrome caused by relative decline of yin or yang is of deficiency in nature, the general principle for treating deficiency syndrome is "supplementation".

Relative decline of yin causes deficiency-heat syndrome while relative decline of yang causes deficiency-cold syndrome. For the treatment of deficiency-heat syndrome, yin-nourishing therapy can be used (to use tonic herbs to nourish yin and supplement blood); for the treatment of deficiency-cold syndrome, yang-supplementing therapy can be used (to use tonic herbs of warm nature to strengthen yang and supplement qi). However deficiency-cold syndrome due to relative decline of yang may result from retention of water in the body caused by failure of deficient yang to transform qi. In this case purging therapy cannot be used to eliminate retention of water. Instead, measures should be taken to warm and supplement yang-qi. When yang-qi is activated, qi will flow smoothly and retention of water will disperse naturally. That is why it was said in ancient times that "supplementing the source of fire can eliminate superabundance of yin." On the other hand deficiency-heat syndrome may result from endogenous fire due to failure of deficient yin to control yang. In this case purging and clearing therapy cannot be used to eliminate fire and heat. Instead, measures should be taken to enrich yin-essence. When yin-essence is enriched, the state of yin and yang will be normalized. When yang is able to maintain latent, fire will disappear naturally. That is why it was said in ancient times that "strengthening water source can control predominant yang."

不足。补其不足，就是补益其偏衰，使过于衰弱的阴或阳恢复到正常状态。由于阴阳偏衰所导致的证候性质为虚证，治疗虚证的大法为"补"，所以"补其不足"的原则在治疗学上也称"虚则补之"。

阴阳偏衰分为阴偏衰和阳偏衰，阴偏衰则形成虚热证，阳偏衰则形成虚寒证。针对虚热证，相应的治法是补阴（也称滋阴），即用滋补药等以滋阴补血；针对虚寒证，相应的治法是补阳（也称壮阳），即用温补药等以壮阳补气。特别需要注意的是，阳偏衰的虚寒证，可因阳虚气化无力而导致水饮等在体内滞留，此时不可妄用攻泻法以图祛除水饮，而应从根本上温补阳气，阳气一旦振兴，气化流通，其水饮自然消散，所以古人有"益火之源，以消阴翳"的说法；阴偏衰的虚热证，可因阴虚不能制阳而出现火热内生，此时不可妄用清泻法以图祛除火热，而应从根本上填补阴精，阴精一旦充满，阴阳调和，阳得以潜藏，其火热自然平息，所以古人有"壮水之主，以制阳光"的理论。

Since yin and yang depend on each other, relative decline of the one will certainly involve the other, eventually leading to decline of both yin and yang which will bring on deficiency of both yin and yang. For the treatment of such a morbid condition, both yin and yang should be supplemented. For this reason, simple yin deficiency syndrome can be treated by yin-nourishing therapy with the addition of herbs for strengthening yang for the purpose of promoting the transformation of yin with the qi-transforming function of yang, known as obtaining yin from yang; simple yang deficiency syndrome can be treated by yang-nourishing therapy with the addition of herbs for nourishing yin for the purpose of promoting the transformation of yang with the essence-nourishing function of yin, known as obtaining yang from yin.

Besides, the meridians, the viscera and the activities of ascent, descent, out-going and entering all pertain to yin and yang in nature respectively, the principles for regulating yin and yang can be used to generalize other related therapeutic methods. For example, the methods for regulating disorder of the meridians, qi and blood, zang-organs and fu-organs as well as ascent, descent, out-going and entering are all included in the concept of "regulating yin and yang."

7.2.4   Abidance by individuality, locality and seasons

The occurrence, development and change of disease involve a number of factors, including individual difference, geographical environment and seasonal variations which may affect the nature, duration and treatment of disease. So in treating disease, apart from following the principles of concentrating treatment on the root cause, strengthening healthy qi and eliminating pathogenic

由于阴阳是互根的,阴偏衰可以累及阳而导致阳衰,阳偏衰也可累及阴而导致阴衰,最终使阴阳俱衰。阴阳俱衰则形成阴阳两虚证,治疗时应阴阳并补。根据阴阳互根的理论,对于单纯的阴虚证,在滋阴方中可适当佐以补阳药,借阳的气化功能以帮助阴精的化生,这叫做"阳中求阴";对于单纯的阳虚证,在补阳方中可适当佐以滋阴药,借阴精的涵养功能以帮助阳的化生,这叫做"阴中求阳"。

此外,由于经络、气血、脏腑、升降出入等都具有各自的阴阳属性及其相互关系,所以"调整阴阳"的治疗原则也可以用来概括其他相关的治疗方法。如调理经络失常、调理气血失常、调理脏腑失常、调理升降出入失常等等,都可归属于"调整阴阳"的范畴。

四、因人、因地、因时制宜

疾病的发生、发展与转归,受多方面因素的影响,如个体差异、地理环境的不同及时令气候的变化等,都是影响疾病性质、程度及对治疗的反应性的重要因素。因此在治疗时,除了必须遵守治病求

factors as well as regulating yin and yang, one has to make corresponding changes according to individual condition, local environment and seasonal variations.

7.2.4.1 Abidance by individuality

Abidance by individuality means to decide treatment according to the age, sex, constitution and living habits of the patients.

1. Age

The physiological functions and the state of qi and blood vary with the age, so the use of herbs has to follow such variations. Generally speaking, infants are vigorous in physiological functions, but their qi and blood are not sufficient yet and their viscera are delicate. For this reason, infants are easy to be affected by cold and heat and tend to have deficiency or excess problems. Once they fall ill, their pathological conditions are prone to change. So in the treatment of infantile disease, drastic herbs are forbidden to use and tonic herbs should be used infrequently with small dosage. In selecting prescription form and taking method, the characteristics of infants have to be taken into consideration. As to the old people, their physiological functions, qi and blood have all declined, so they are easy to have deficiency problems. For the treatment of old people, purgation should be used with great care even for treating excess syndrome because their constitution is weak. Since qi and blood in the aged have declined, their reaction to herbs is slow. So the treatment of deficiency syndrome for the aged with nourishing therapy needs large dosage of herbs and longer course of treatment.

本、扶正祛邪、调整阴阳的基本原则外,还应根据不同情况进行灵活变通,采取适宜的治疗方法。因人、因地、因时制宜,就是这样一种灵活变通的原则。

(一)因人制宜

因人制宜,是根据病人的年龄、性别、体质和生活习惯的不同特点,来考虑治疗用药的原则。

1. 年龄

人体的生理功能和气血的盛衰,随着年龄的变化而有不同,治疗用药也应有区别。一般地说,小儿生机旺盛,但气血未充,脏腑娇嫩,易寒易热,易虚易实,病情变化较快,故治小儿病,忌用峻攻,少用补益,用药量宜轻,剂型及服药方法也应考虑小儿的特点;老年人生机减退,气血渐衰,患病多虚,即使是实证也应考虑其体质偏虚的一面,用攻邪法要慎重,但老年人气血虚衰后对药物的反应性也降低,因此老年虚证用补益法往往需要更大的剂量和较长的疗程。

2. Sex

Different sex has different physiological characteristics. TCM emphasizes that women are different from men because they have menstruation, leukorrhage, pregnancy and labor which have to be taken into consideration in treating women diseases. For example, herbs used during menstruation should not hinder menses, avoiding the use of herbs of cold and astringent nature; herbs used after menstruation mainly concentrate on supplementation because the vessels are deficient because of menses; during pregnancy, cares should be taken to protect fetus and herbs for drastic purgation, breaking blood and lubrication or herbs tending to migrate or poisonous herbs should not be used or used with great care; after labor, qi and blood are seriously deficient, cares should be taken to supplement more and purge less. If there is lochiorrhea, warming and supplementing therapy can be used to dredge and disperse, cold tonifying and astringing therapy should not be used lest lochia be retained. Since the liver is regarded as the congenital base of life for women and liver-qi is easy to stagnate, the treatment of women diseases often needs to soothe and regulate liver-qi.

3. Constitution

There are different types of constitution which should be treated by different herbs. Generally speaking, strong constitution bears more purgation but less tonification, so it can be treated with large dosage of herbs for purgation but small dosage of herbs for tonification; weak constitution bears more tonification but less purgation, so it can be treated with small dosage of herbs for purgation but large dosage of herbs for tonification. For the treatment of people with frequent predominance of yang or frequent deficiency of yin, warm-natured herbs should be used with great care lest fire be strengthened or yin be impaired.

2. 性别

男女性别不同,各有其生理特点。中医学主要强调女子有经、带、胎、产等情况,有别于男子,治疗时应加以考虑。如在月经期,用药不应有碍经血运行,一般忌过用寒凉收涩药;经期后血去脉虚,宜多补少泻。妊娠期需注意护胎,凡峻下、破血、滑利、走窜伤胎或有毒药物,当禁用或慎用。产后大多气血亏虚,应多补少泻,但同时应兼顾恶露的排出情形,若恶露未净,一般宜用温补疏通之剂,不宜用凉补敛涩之剂,以免留瘀不去。由于女子以肝为先天,肝气易郁,故治疗妇科病常需疏理肝气。

3. 体质

人的体质有不同的类型,对于不同类型的体质,治疗用药应有不同。一般来说,体质强者耐攻伐而不耐补益,故用攻邪法药量可大,而用补益法不宜过量;体质弱者耐补益而不耐攻伐,故用攻邪法药量宜小,而用补益法药量可大。素体阳盛或阴虚之人,慎用温热之剂,若过量则有助火或伤阴之虞;素体阳虚或阴盛之人,

For the treatment of people with frequent deficiency of yang or frequent predominance of yin, cold-natured herbs should be used with great care lest yang-qi be impaired or phlegm be caused.

4. Living habits

Different living habits may exert different effect on constitution. For example, frequent indulgence in drinking of wine may cause insufficiency of liver-yin complicated by phlegm-dampness encumbering the spleen; frequent food partiality tends to cause decline of qi and blood or disharmony between yin and yang; lack of physical exercise often leads to hypofunction of the viscera and slow flow of qi and blood. People in different regions, countries and nations differ greatly in living habits. Such a difference in living habits can be used as evidence to analyze their types of constitution.

7.2.4.2 Abidance by locality

Locality means to decide treatment according to geographical difference.

People in different regions differ in physiological functions and pathological changes because of geographical location, weather condition and living habits. Take China for example. The plateaus in the west regions are cold and dry with insufficient rain. People live in the mountains, mainly taking milk and meat. So their constitution is strong and their muscular interstices are dense, making it difficult for pathogenic factors to invade them. When attacked by exogenous pathogenic factors, they can be treated by dispersing therapy with large dosage of herbs for relieving the superficies. The regions in the east and south and along the seas are low and warm with sufficient rain. People live beside water and mainly eat fish and

慎用寒凉之剂,以防损伤阳气或助湿生痰。

4. 生活习惯

生活习惯不同,对体质的影响也不同,治疗时必须加以注意。如一贯嗜酒,往往肝阴不足与痰湿困脾夹杂;长期偏食,易致气血偏衰或阴阳不和;运动不足,缺少锻炼,往往脏腑功能减退,气血运行迟缓等。不同地区、不同国家、不同民族的人,其生活习惯上的差异更大,从这些生活习惯的差异可以推断其体质的倾向,作为治疗时的重要参考。

(二) 因地制宜

因地制宜,是根据不同地区的地理特点,来考虑治疗用药的原则。

不同地区,由于地势的高低,以及气候条件与生活习惯的不尽相同,人体生理功能特点和病变特点也有相应的差异,所以治疗用药应根据当地环境和生活习惯而有所变化。如中国西北高原地区,气候寒冷,干燥少雨,人们依山陵而居,多食乳酪及肉类,故体质壮实,腠理致密,外邪不易侵犯,若感受外邪需用发散法治疗,当用解表重剂;东南沿海地区,地势低洼,温热多雨,人

rice. Their constitution is weak and their muscular interstices are loose. So they are easily to be invaded by exogenous pathogenic factors. When attacked by exogenous
pathogenic factors, they can be treated by dispersing therapy
with small dosage of herbs for relieving superficies.

7.2.4.3 Abidance by seasonal variation

Seasonal variation means deciding treatment according to seasonal changes of weather.

Seasonal variations of weather exert certain effect on
the physiological functions and pathological changes of the
body. Generally speaking, the muscular interstices are
loose in spring and summer because the weather becomes
warmer and warmer and yang-qi gradually elevates. So
herbs acrid in taste and warm in nature cannot be used in
large dosage even for wind-cold attack, avoiding excessive
purgation and damaging qi and yin. In autumn and winter,
the muscular interstices are dense because the weather
becomes colder and colder, yin becomes predominant and
yang deficient. In these two seasons cold-natured herbs
should be used with great care except great heat syndrome. In *Huangdi Neijing* such a use of herbs according
to seasonal variation is summarized as "avoiding using
cold-natured herbs in winter, cool-natured herbs in autumn, warm-natured herbs in spring and hot-natured
herbs in summer."

TCM analyzes the five zang-organs according to the
four seasons, believing that liver-qi is predominant in
spring, heart-qi is predominant in summer, spleen-qi is
predominant in late summer, lung-qi is predominant in autumn and kidney-qi is predominant in winter. In each season one zang-organ is in predomination, the zang-organ
that it generates is promoted while the zang-organ that it

们傍水而居,多食鱼米,故体
质较弱,腠理疏松,易受外邪
侵袭,若感受外邪需用发散法
治疗,当用解表轻剂。

(三) 因时制宜

因时制宜,是根据时令气
候的不同特点,来考虑治疗用
药的原则。

四时气候的变化,对人体
的生理功能、病理变化均能产
生一定的影响,因此在治疗上
应根据这种气候变化的特点
来考虑用药。一般来说,春夏
季节,气候由温渐热,阳气升
发,人体腠理疏松开泄,即使
患外感风寒,也不宜过用辛温
发散药物,以免开泄太过,耗
伤气阴;而秋冬季节,气候由
凉变寒,阴盛阳衰,人体腠理
致密,阳气内敛,此时若非大
热之证,当慎用寒凉药物,以
防伤阳。《黄帝内经》把这种
春夏慎用温热、秋冬慎用寒凉
的治疗思想归纳为"用寒远
寒,用凉远凉,用温远温,用热
远热"。

中医学根据"五脏法四
时"的理论,认为春天肝气旺,
夏天心气旺,长夏脾气旺,秋
天肺气旺,冬天肾气旺。每一
季节有一脏气旺,则其所生之
脏受气,所胜之脏受制。因此
在治疗时,必须考虑五脏之气

dominates is restricted. Only when such a corresponding change of the five zang-organs in the four seasons and their interrelationships have been taken into consideration in treating disease can damage of healthy qi and promotion of pathogenic factors be avoided. Besides, interrelationships among the five zang-organs in the four seasons also can be used to decide therapeutic principle and select herbs. Take spring for example. In spring, liver-qi is predominant, but spleen-qi must be restricted. So patients with frequent deficiency of the spleen has to be treated by strengthening spleen-qi in spring. Since predomination of liver-qi can reinforce heart-qi, the syndrome of heart-qi deficiency can be more effectively treated in spring. If it is treated in winter, the therapeutic effect is not so easy to obtain because heart-fire is restricted by kidney-water.

的旺衰和相生相克情形,才不至于助邪伤正,并且还可以利用这种五脏之气相互作用的原理设计治疗方案和选择用药,这也符合因时制宜的原则。如春天肝气旺则脾气受制,若脾虚体质者患病,到春天应注意扶助脾气。肝气旺则能资生心气,所以心气虚证在春天治疗较易收效。若在冬季治疗心气虚之证,则因心火受肾水的制约而不易收效。

Postscript

The compilation of *A Newly Compiled Practical English-Chinese Library of TCM* was started in 2000 and published in 2002. In order to demonstrate the academic theory and clinical practice of TCM and to meet the requirements of compilation, the compilers and translators have made great efforts to revise and polish the Chinese manuscript and English translation so as to make it systematic, accurate, scientific, standard and easy to understand. Shanghai University of TCM is in charge of the translation. Many scholars and universities have participated in the compilation and translation of the Library, i.e. Professor Shao Xundao from Xi'an Medical University (former Dean of English Department and Training Center of the Health Ministry), Professor Ou Ming from Guangzhou University of TCM (celebrated translator and chief professor), Henan College of TCM, Guangzhou University of TCM, Nanjing University of TCM, Shaanxi College of TCM, Liaoning College of TCM and Shandong University of TCM.

The compilation of this Library is also supported by the State Administrative Bureau and experts from other universities and colleges of TCM. The experts on the Compilation Committee and Approval Committee have directed the compilation and translation. Professor She

后　记

《(英汉对照)新编实用中医文库》(以下简称《文库》)从2000年中文稿的动笔，到2002年全书的付梓，完成了世纪的跨越。为了使本套《文库》尽可能展示传统中医学术理论和临床实践的精华，达到全面、系统、准确、科学、规范、通俗的编写要求，全体编译人员耗费了大量的心血，付出了艰辛的劳动。特别是上海中医药大学承担了英语翻译的主持工作，得到了著名医学英语翻译家、原西安医科大学英语系主任和卫生部外语培训中心主任邵循道教授，著名中医英语翻译家、广州中医药大学欧明首席教授的热心指导，河南中医学院、广州中医药大学、南京中医药大学、陕西中医学院、辽宁中医学院、山东中医药大学等中医院校英语专家的全力参与，确保了本套《文库》具有较高的英译水平。

在《文库》的编撰过程中，我们始终得到国家主管部门领导和各中医院校专家们的关心和帮助。编纂委员会的国内外学者及审定委员会的

Jing, Head of the State Administrative Bureau and Vice-Minister of the Health Ministry, has showed much concern for the Library. Professor Zhu Bangxian, head of the Publishing House of Shanghai University of TCM, Zhou Dunhua, former head of the Publishing House of Shanghai University of TCM, and Pan Zhaoxi, former editor-in-chief of the Publishing House of Shanghai University of TCM, have given full support to the compilation and translation of the Library.

With the coming of the new century, we have presented this Library to the readers all over the world, sincerely hoping to receive suggestions and criticism from the readers so as to make it perfect in the following revision.

Zuo Yanfu
Pingju Village, Nanjing
Spring 2002

专家对编写工作提出了指导性的意见和建议。尤其是卫生部副部长、国家中医药管理局局长佘靖教授对本书的编写给予了极大的关注,多次垂询编撰过程,并及时进行指导。上海中医药大学出版社社长兼总编辑朱邦贤教授,以及原社长周敦华先生、原总编辑潘朝曦先生及全体编辑对本书的编辑出版工作给予了全面的支持,使《文库》得以顺利面世。在此,一并致以诚挚的谢意。

在新世纪之初,我们将这套《文库》奉献给国内外中医界及广大中医爱好者,恳切希望有识之士对《文库》存在的不足之处给予批评、指教,以便在修订时更臻完善。

左言富
于金陵萍聚村
2002年初春